Indian Medicine in Highland Guatemala

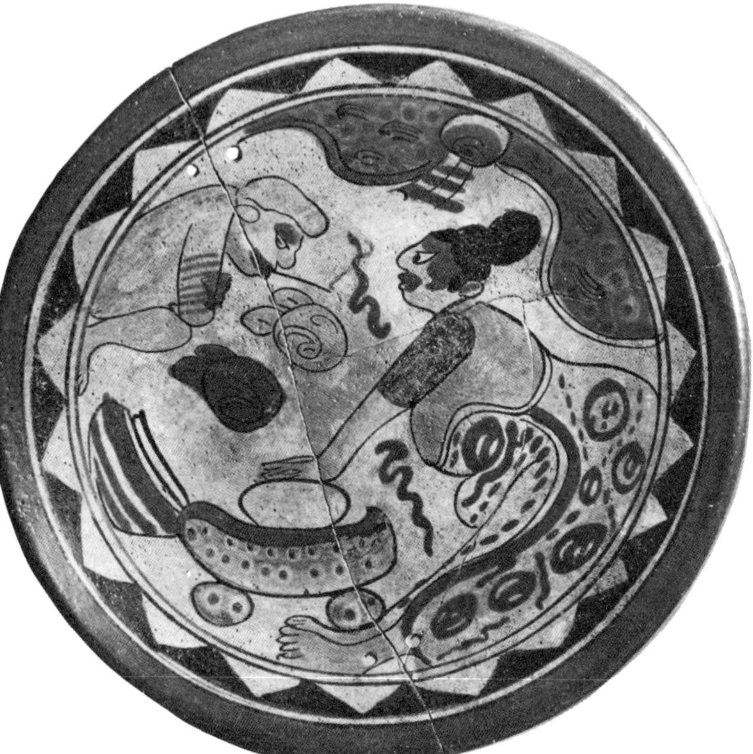

Indian Medicine in Highland Guatemala

The Pre-Hispanic and Colonial Periods

by Sandra L. Orellana

Pen-and-ink drawings by Fred Folger

University of New Mexico Press : *Albuquerque*

Library of Congress Cataloging-in-Publication Data

Orellana, Sandra L. (Sandra Lee), 1941–
Indian medicine in highland Guatemala.

Bibliography: p.
Includes index.
1. Mayas—Medicine. 2. Indians of Central America—Guatemala—Medicine. I. Title. [DNLM: 1. Medicine, Traditional—history—Guatemala. WZ 309 066i]
F1435.3.M4074 1987 615.8'82'097281 86-24943
ISBN 0-8263-0931-3

Contents

Illustrations and Maps

Preface

There is no comprehensive study of the native Guatemala highland Maya medical system of late pre-Hispanic and early colonial times. Most studies of Indian medicine in that area concentrate on the contemporary period and deal with the impact of modernization upon traditional healing practices. In this work the focus will be on the immediate pre-Conquest period through the beginning of the eighteenth century.

The primary data have survived mainly in the writings of colonial Guatemalan historians, and it is regrettable that there are no works on aboriginal or colonial native medicine written by the highland Indians themselves. The Indian medical system is therefore presented mainly as it was observed by non-natives in post-Conquest times, and it had already changed due to introductions of European beliefs and practices. Ethnographic and botanical studies have also been used to compare and augment the material contained in colonial sources. The variety of practices still in existence today indicates how extensive ancient medical lore may have been.

Part I begins with a discussion of pre-Hispanic medicine in the Guatemala highlands and establishes the context within which treatment of illness occurred in those times. The important relationship between medicine and religion is discussed and the types of medical practitioners defined. Herbal medicines used by the Indians in colonial times are mentioned under the endemic illnesses they were believed to cure or alleviate. Although this information was written in post-Conquest times, it is primarily a description of aboriginal herbal remedies. Western categories of illness are used in Part I because these were the ones ordinarily given by the colonial authors who provided the data. Many of the same illness categories given by Guatemalan historians were also listed by Fray Pedro Beltrán who in 1746 published a lexicon of anatomical terms and illness syndromes present in Yucatán around the time of the Conquest (Guerra 1964:38–39).

Part II deals with the post-Conquest period when European medical concepts were introduced into Guatemala and began to restructure and merge with native medical beliefs and practices. The arrival of the Spanish also signaled the beginning of new and terrible epidemics.

Both groups exchanged illnesses, but the Indians fared worse than the Spaniards due to the severity of effect of the Old World epidemics on a host population which had no immunities against them. Native New World epidemic diseases seem to have been fewer in number and less sweeping in effect on the Spanish population. Neither Indian nor European medicine had much curative value when it came to epidemic diseases. Introduced non-epidemic diseases are included in Part II as well as discussion of European medicine in early colonial times, the influence of Catholicism on native medicine, and humoral theory.

Part III contains a discussion of constituents and an evaluation of their clinical effectiveness for many of the medicinal plants included in the text. A search of the medical and botanical literature revealed that some plants have been well studied while others have been neglected or totally ignored. Coverage is therefore uneven, and it is clear that many plants used as medicines have not yet been studied to see if they have any therapeutic value.

I wish to thank several of my colleagues who were particularly helpful in aiding me in completing this manuscript: Dr. Frank Almeda, Associate Curator of the Department of Botany, California Academy of Sciences, who checked the plant identifications; Dr. Benjamin Paul, Department of Anthropology, Stanford University, who made many useful comments on the ethnographic portions of this manuscript; and Dr. Henry B. Nicholson of the Department of Anthropology, University of California, Los Angeles, who has a wide knowledge of ancient and colonial Mesoamerica, and made many useful suggestions.

I would also like to thank other colleagues and friends who discussed various aspects of this work with me and who provided me with constant support: Patricia Rieff Anawalt, Robert M. Carmack, Juan Ajtzip Alvarado of Santiago Atitlán, Guatemala, and Barbara Goldfus who typed the final draft of the manuscript. My special thanks goes to Fred Folger who made the pen and ink drawings used in the text. Special Collections of the University Research Library and the Rare Books Section of the Biomedical Library of the University of California, Los Angeles generously allowed me to photograph several books and manuscripts. The British Library of London supplied the photograph from the Luttrell Psalter, Ms. Add. 42130, *F.* 61.

My research in Guatemala was made possible by a grant from the American Philosophical Society. I was able to do research in the Archivo General de Centroámerica in Guatemala City and to visit several Indian towns in the highlands in 1973, 1975, and 1979.

Los Angeles 1987

CHAPTER ONE

Sources

Modern medical anthropology includes two distinct trends. In one, the concepts, classifications, and causative chains of Western medicine are used to investigate native medical systems. Disease etiology, symptomatology, prevention, and cure are defined within a Western framework. The second, ethnomedicine, is based on the premise that not only states of health and illness, but also specific illnesses recognized in a particular society are culturally defined (Méndez Domínguez 1983:267–68).

The emphasis of the present study is the former. The data used are ethnohistoric and ethnographic and were given by chroniclers and researchers who used mainly Western disease categories. The approach involves primarily etic analytic categories, or those derived from Western culture, as opposed to emic, where the ethnographic categories are those derived from the culture being studied (Cosminsky 1972:7).

Although this is primarily an etic study, some contemporary native-defined illnesses which are common today throughout Mesoamerica and have a large body of data which refers to them are included. Such illnesses as fright (*susto,* Spanish), evil eye (*ojo, mal de ojo,* Spanish), fallen fontanel (*caída de la mollera,* Spanish), and others are discussed because they are so prominent in today's native medical system and appear to have pre-Columbian antecedents. Others, such as the snake illness (*cumatz* in Quiché) and *pasmo* (from *pasmada* in Spanish meaning chilled), are of interest because they were common during the colonial period.

Guatemalan Colonial Sources

Recordación Florida

The most comprehensive treatment of native Guatemalan plants and their medicinal applications during colonial times is contained in *Recordación Florida* written by the chronicler Francisco Antonio de Fuentes y Guzmán in the late seventeenth century. He served as a government official in Totonicapán and Sonsonate and observed many local customs in those and other Guatemalan areas.

The complete text of the original manuscript is in the Archivo General de Centroámerica in Guatemala City. It was first published in its entirety in the Biblioteca "Goathemala" series of the Sociedad de Geografía e Historia de Guatemala in 1932–33 under the title *Recordación Florida: Discurso historical y demostración natural, material, militar y política del Reyno de Guatemala* (Carmack 1973:184). Another edition was published in 1969–72 in Madrid under the title *Obras Históricas de Don Francisco Antonio de Fuentes y Guzmán.*

Fuentes y Guzmán was interested in Indian medicine and included quite a bit of material on the subject in *Recordación Florida.* Although not a doctor, Fuentes y Guzmán did try many of the remedies he observed and noted that some were useful. He also obtained opinions from others, such as doctors and writers, who had knowledge of medicinal plants.

Fifty-nine plants included in *Recordación Florida* were identified by Horacio Figueroa Marroquín (1957) who provided both Latin binomial and common names—the latter in Spanish, Nahua, and Maya. The drawings of forty-nine medicinal plants made by Fuentes y Guzmán aided in plant identification, but the chronicler referred to the plants in his work only by common names. Some could be easily identified because they were commonly known or because a drawing was provided. In other cases it was more difficult because many similar plants with the same name existed or because only Nahua names were given (Figueroa Marroquín 1957:87).

Some plants were described by Fuentes y Guzmán in lengthy paragraphs but others in only a few lines. Twenty-six plants were merely mentioned as having medicinal value but no physical description or uses were given. Most of these plants have been discussed in the present study. It is possible that some of the plants have not been correctly identified by Figueroa Marroquín. Therefore, in this work every effort has been made to check uses given by Guatemalan colonial authors with those given in Mexican and contemporary Guatemalan ethnographic accounts.

Fuentes y Guzmán knew of the work on Mexican medicinal plants written by the Spanish physician Francisco Hernández (see pp. 9–11). He made some annotations from this work or from another author who had taken material from it. By comparing the plants described by Fuentes y Guzmán with their counterparts described by Hernández, it can be seen that some uses do appear to be similar if not identical. This does not necessarily mean that Fuentes y Guzmán copied Hernández—he also cited José de Acosta (1969:1:239), and Nicolas Monardes (1969:1:243).

However, in some instances the passages in both works were very close which would indicate that Fuentes y Guzmán did copy from Hernández (e.g., passages dealing with maize, the century plant, and the Aztec marigold). In most instances, this does not appear to have been the case, and perhaps Fuentes y Guzmán only took material from Hernández when he felt that it also described the Guatemalan situation. And, though Fuentes y Guzmán used a Nahua term for a plant, this did not mean that he borrowed from Hernández since a form of Nahua was spoken in some areas of Guatemala in pre-Columbian times. Also, the Nahua language tended to increase in importance after the Conquest because it was more familiar to the conquerors and their native allies. Most of the herbal treatments included in *Recordación Florida* were probably observed by Fuentes y Guzmán himself in Guatemala.

Historia Natural del Reino de Guatemala

Another important colonial source on Guatemalan native medicinal plants is the *Historia natural del Reino de Guatemala* written in 1772 by Fray Francisco Ximénez. Fray Ximénez lived for many years among the Quichés and Cakchiquels, spoke Quiché, and included much information relating to native peoples in his work (Carmack 1973:189–92). He is, however, less comprehensive on the subject of native medicine than Fuentes y Guzmán.

The *Historia natural* was preserved for posterity by don Ignacio Solís who had it in his library until it was deposited in the Sociedad de Geografía e Historia in 1932 (Chinchilla Aguilar 1967:5–6). It was not published until 1967 when the Sociedad de Geografía e Historia de Guatemala put out the first edition.

Two chapters of the work, 10 and 11, were devoted to plants. The former dealt with trees and the latter with flowers. Around twenty-five medicinal plants were included in the *Historia natural,* some being discussed at length and others briefly. Latin binomials were given by Francis Gall in footnotes below the text. The identifications are not always accurate and there are no illustrations provided by Ximénez to facilitate identification. The illustrations in the 1967 edition were taken from Fuentes y Guzmán.

Ximénez does not appear to have copied from any other works on medicinal plants. He described what he observed himself and tried some of the remedies. However, Ximénez did not know a great deal about native medicine. There are other plants in his work that were known to have had medicinal properties and Ximénez made no reference to them. For example, he discussed balsam (1967:244), American storax (1967:244–45), and the goldenshower senna (1967:249)—three commonly known medicinal plants in colonial times—but said nothing regarding their curative properties.

A few remedies given by Ximénez are similar to those in the *Recordación Florida,* but this is probably due to the fact that both authors were talking about similar geographical and cultural areas. Although Ximénez made little, if any, use of Fuentes y Guzmán's work, he did know about Hernández's and may have drawn some material from that source.

The Popol Vuh

The Popol Vuh, the legendary book of the Quiché Mayas, is one of the most important native written documents of the Guatemala highlands. It describes the early history of the Quichés. Unfortunately, it does not contain a great deal of information on native medicine, but the material given is invaluable in that it presents the native view of curing and illness. It is particularly useful in reconstructing pre-Hispanic illness etiology.

The Popol Vuh was written sometime around the mid-sixteenth century by descendants of the royal lines at K'umarcaaj, the ancient Quiché capital. It was discovered in Chichicastenango by Fray Ximénez around 1701. He translated it into Spanish and that version was published by the Sociedad de Geografía e Historia de Guatemala as part of the "Biblioteca Goathemala" series in 1929. There have been many translation of the *Popol Vuh* into Spanish, some including the Quiché text as well, and two into English. (See Carmack 1973:24–28 for a review of these translations.) The English translation of Munro Edmonson (1971) was used in the preparation of this work.

The Annals of the Cakchiquels

The Annals of the Cakchiquels was written at Sololá in Cakchiquel mainly by two members of the Xajil line which ruled in aboriginal times. A copy was made of the original Cakchiquel text, probably in the seventeenth century, and most translations are based on that copy. Several translations have been made into French, Spanish, and English (Carmack 1973:47–48). The English version of Adrián Recinos and Delia Goetz (1967) was used in this work.

Like the *Popol Vuh,* the *Annals* provide information on early history, but from the Cakchiquel viewpoint, and it continues until the year 1601. For the study of medicine, the post-Conquest material is more useful because it presents the native view of the devastation caused by early epidemic diseases.

Apologética Historia de las Indias

In his *Apologética historia* Bartolomé de Las Casas included thirteen chapters on the Indians of Guatemala. This information is the best early account of the Indians of the Verapaz and K'umarcaaj areas, though it is far less complete than the works of Fray Bernardino de Sahagún on Mexico. The Las Casas manuscript was finished in 1550, but most of the observations were made between 1536 and 1544 when he was in Guatemala. Las Casas finished the manuscript after returning to Spain, where it was subsequently placed in the library of the Academy of History in Madrid (Carmack 1973:101). It was first published in 1909, and there have been several modern editions. The critical edition edited by Edmundo O'Gorman published in Mexico in 1967 was used in preparing the present work (Warren 1973:52).

Las Casas drew his information from various sources: Spaniards, Indian lords and commoners, other priests, and written accounts. He had some knowledge of the Quiché and Cakchiquel languages, and his account is generally accurate as is demonstrated by the correlations between it and other native sources (Carmack 1973:101–102, 105).

Las Casas did not say a great deal about medicine, but his account is the only one which described the role of the physician in the pre-Hispanic highland area. He also provided important information on ceremonies, sacrifice, birth rituals, temple rituals, diviners, and illness etiology. It is difficult to know at times to which group he is referring, but he focused on K'umarcaaj and Verapaz. Unfortunately, Las Casas did not say anything about herbal medicine; therefore, it is necessary to rely on Fuentes y Guzmán and Ximénez even though their accounts were written at a much later time.

Parts of Las Casas's work have been incorporated into S. W. Miles's study on "The Sixteenth-Century Pokom-Maya: A Documentary Analysis of Social Structure and Archaeological Setting" (1957). She focused on the Pokomans who lived east of the Quichés and also used information drawn from dictionaries written by the Dominican Dionysius Zuñiga, who arrived in Verapaz in 1597, and Pedro Morán (also a

Dominican) who copied the work of Zuñiga in 1720 (Carmack 1973:120–21).

The following colonial sources provided some information on native medicine in Guatemala, but to a lesser extent than those discussed already; thus, they will only be briefly mentioned here.

Historia General de las Indias Occidentales y Particular de la Gobernación de Chiapa y Guatemala

The *Historia general* of the Dominican Antonio de Remesal was written between 1615 and 1617 and was first published in 1620. In 1932, it was published in two volumes by the Sociedad de Historia e Geografía de Guatemala as part of the "Biblioteca Goathemala" series. In 1964, it was published as part of the *Biblioteca de Autores Españoles* in Madrid.

Remesal had only been in Guatemala for two years when he began his manuscript, and it is primarily of interest here for the accounts of hospital building in the first and second post-Conquest capitals, epidemics, and the notorious Dr. N. who resided in the Guatemalan capital. He relied on documentary sources, many of which contained references to the Indians (Carmack 1973:178).

Crónica de la Provincia del Santísimo Nombre de Jesús de Guatemala

The *Crónica* was written by the Franciscan Francisco de Asís Vázquez de Herrera between 1683 and 1713 or 1714 and contains a number of passages referring to native medicine and early Spanish hospitals in Guatemala. Vázquez de Herrera also provided information on diviners, epidemics, and the role of the lay brotherhoods (*cofradías,* Spanish) in treating the sick.

The *Crónica* was first published in Guatemala in 1716 and more recently in 1937–44 as four volumes of the "Biblioteca Goathemala" series. Although Vázquez de Herrera apparently used a few native documents, most of his information was based on his own observations or those of other Franciscans. His account is somewhat marred by his view of the Indians as a people who were rebellious against Christianity and who were deceived by the devil (Carmack 1973:187–89).

The Relaciones Geográficas

The *Relaciones Geográficas* were compiled in many areas of the New World by order of Philip II of Spain. They were mainly written up by local Spanish officials who obtained answers to a standard questionnaire of fifty questions which had been developed in Spain (Cline 1972:183). Only two *Relaciones Geográficas* are extant for Guatemala, those of Atitlán and its dependencies (1585) and that of Zapotitlán and Suchitepéquez (1579) (Cline 1972:225,227).

The *Relación Geográfica* from Atitlán contains responses from elderly Indian leaders of both the capital and dependencies who were questioned about pre-Hispanic times. The originals of both of the *Relaciones Geográficas* are now in the University of Texas collection (Carmack 1973:131, 133–34). The *Relaciones Geográficas Atitlán, Aguacatepec,* and *Zapotitlán and Suchitepéquez* have been published by the Sociedad de Geografía y Historia de Guatemala (see bibliography). Those of San Andrés and San Francisco are given in Broussard (1952). In the *Relaciones Geográficas* of Atitlán and its dependencies the answer to question 5 contains information on epidemic diseases, question 14 yields a description of sacrifice, the role of the idols in divination of epidemics, and casting of lots, and questions 17, 22, and 26 contain information on the illnesses which affected the towns and the herbs used to treat them.

The questionnaire sent to Zapotitlán and Suchitepéquez was answered by the resident local Spanish official, Capitán Juan de Estrada. He asked the priests in his jurisdiction for help and got information from Indian leaders and documents. Since he did not speak any native language, he received his data second-hand or from Indians who spoke Spanish (Carmack 1973:131–32). He discussed the effects of epidemic diseases in response to question 5, sacrifice, divination, nagualism, and beliefs concerning illness in question 14, illnesses and remedies in question 17, and medicinal herbs in question 26.

Relación García de Palacio

Licenciado Diego García de Palacio was an official of the *audiencia* (Spanish) of Guatemala. His *relación* of 1574 was a report concerning the eastern area of Guatemala, and it was sent to Philip II as a response to one of the questionnaires about native life which had been sent to colonial officials prior to that of the *Relaciones Geográficas*. The complete Spanish text of García de Palacio's report was first published in 1860, and it appeared in the *Colección de documentos inéditos . . . de Indias* in 1866. It was also published in the *Anales* of the Sociedad de Geografía e Historia de Guatemala in 1927.

García de Palacio asked questions of elderly Indians and possibly priests concerning aboriginal history and customs and made geographical observations of the areas he visited (Carmack 1973:127–28; Warren

1973:103). He gave information on poisonous animals and birth rituals of the Pipil of the Asunción Mita area, which is of particular interest to this study.

Compendio y Descripción de Las Indias Occidentales

Between 1612 and 1621 Antonio Vázquez de Espinosa, a Carmelite friar, traveled throughout Latin America studying geography, society, and economic conditions. He returned to Spain and prepared his account. This manuscript was eventually discovered in the Vatican Library by Charles Upson Clark of the Smithsonian Institution. Clark translated it into English, and it was published in 1942 and in 1968 under the titles *Compendium and Description of the West Indies* and *Description of the Indies* respectively. In the eleven chapters devoted to Guatemala there are a few references relevant to a study of native medicine—mainly pertaining to the sweatbath, sulphur baths, and herbal medicines (Carmack 1973:192; Warren 1973:53–54, 136).

Thomas Gage's Travels in the New World

The English Dominican friar, Thomas Gage, lived in Chiapas and Guatemala from 1625 to 1637, and wrote his account after he returned to England and denounced the Catholic church. Most of the information he included concerning native life was based on his own observations of Pokoman Indians while he was living in Mixco, Pinula, Petapa, and Amatitlán. He understood and spoke Pokoman, and his book was based on a journal he kept while in the New World (Carmack 1973:180–82).

His book was first published in 1648, under the title *The English-American, his travail by sea and land:* Or, *A new survey of the West-India's.* Several editions have been published since that time—two being edited by J. Eric S. Thompson in 1958 and 1969. Gage's account provides some information of illnesses, medicinal remedies, and the sweatbath.

Compendio de Nombres en Lengua Cakchiquel

Fray Pantaleón de Guzmán wrote a dictionary (dated to 1704) in which Cakchiquel-to-Spanish entries were listed according to topical subjects. Those particularly relevant to this study are medicinal herbs and trees. On the few topics he covered, Pantaleón de Guzmán defined the meanings of more words on the topics covered than any other dictionary source. Some entries may have come from earlier sources, but many came from his own studies of the Cakchiquel language (Carmack 1973:161). Copies of this work may be found in the Library of Congress and the Newberry Library.

Calepino en Lengua Cakchiquel

This dictionary, published in 1940 by Carmelo Sáenz de Santa María under the title *Diccionario Cakchiquel-Español,* was the work of Francisco Varela who composed it around 1600. There are two copies of the Varela dictionary extant today. One copy with the title of *Calepino en Lengua Cakchiquel* is in the American Philosophical Society in Philadelphia. A second copy was obtained from the Maya Society shortly before 1940 by Father Rossbach of Chichicastenango. He provided Sáenz de Santa María with a copy, and most of its contents are found in his published version (Carmack 1973:116–17). This work provided entries which were useful in reconstructing the Cakchiquel medical hierarchy and gave some names of illnesses.

Mexican Colonial Sources

Historia General de Las Cosas de Nueva España

Although this work by Francisco Hernández deals only with Mexican medicinal plants, it is useful as a source of comparison with those of Guatemalan origin. Plants from Mexican sources are included in the present text only when they were also mentioned by Guatemalan writers.

Hernández, a Spanish physician, was named *Protomédico general* of the New World by King Philip II of Spain and was charged with the task of finding out about native medical knowledge in the new land. He left for Mexico in 1571 and stayed there until 1577.

All of the information collected by Hernández came from native informants who understood Aztec herbal medicine. He traveled throughout a large part of the country collecting medicinal plants, studying, and describing natural history and antiquities (Warren 1973:74). Much of his material was collected while visiting the gardens of Atzcapotzalco, Texcoco, Huaxtepec, and many of the hospital and convent gardens of Mexico (Emmart 1940:xiv).

Hernández worked directly with his informants and took data down orally. From time to time he checked out the veracity of the data on himself. He did not always approve of native medical practices, as he occasionally mentioned in the *Historia*. Before saying that he did not believe a remedy would work, however, he accurately recorded it. In some instances, he used native medicine to cure himself, as when he suffered from a urinary infection (Hernández 1960:1:175–76, 185).

After Hernández had gathered many plants, he returned to Mexico City and began to systematically experiment with the flora at the Hospital Real de Naturales. There was adequate land there where he could grow plants, and there were other doctors to help him (Hernández 1960:1:228–29). Neither Fuentes y Guzmán nor Fray Ximénez, who were not doctors, performed this type of experimentation.

When Hernández's work was completed, it was sent to Spain and included magnificent color illustrations drawn by native artists. The *Historia* was eventually placed in the library of the Escorial. Unfortunately, the original manuscript and illustrations were almost certinaly lost in the Escorial library fire of 1671 (1960:1:309–10). The work of Hernández is known to us today through various publications based on extracts, a severely edited summary, and a contemporary copy (Glass and Robinson 1975:131–32).

In 1580 the King named Dr. Nardo Antonio Recchi as chamber physician and charged him with the task of revising and ordering the work of the ailing Hernández who had by then returned to Spain. Recchi eliminated things which did not deal directly with medicine (1960:1:278–79, 281). This manuscript was published in Europe by the Accademia dei Lincei in 1651 (some copies bear dates of 1630, 1648, or 1649) under a Latin title, *Rerum medicarum Novae Hispaniae thesaurus, seu plantarum, animalium, mineralium mexicanorum historia* (Emmart 1940:xiv), and it contained references to some 1,200 medicinal plants.

In making cuts for the first illustrated European edition, the original native illustrations were redrawn following the European style (Emmart 1940:37). A copy of the rough drafts of Hernández in his own hand, but without illustrations, also survived in the library of the Jesuit Colegio Imperial of Madrid (Hernández 1960:1:330). This was partially published in Madrid in 1790 (Glass and Robertson 1975:132). Other editions, such as the *Quatro libros de la naturaleza y virtudes medicinales de las plantas y animales de Nueva España* (1615), published in Mexico by Francisco Ximénez (not related to the Guatemalan writer of the same name) were based on copies of the Recchi Manuscript (Hernández 1960:1:282). In his *Historia naturae maximae peregrinae* (1635), Juan Eusebio Nieremberg drew heavily upon the original Hernández manuscript contained in the Escorial (Emmart 1940:38). The modern critical edition of the *Historia* is entitled *Obras Completas* and was published in Spanish in three volumes based upon the texts from the 1651 and 1790 editions. It contains illustrations from the 1651 edition and from Nieremberg's work (Glass and Robertson 1975:132).

It is difficult to correctly identify the plants mentioned by Hernández because he only provided Nahua names, and the same name was used at times for different plants. Drawings in Hernández were matched with those provided by Fuentes y Guzmán to see if they were the same or similar. If two plants had the same use, they were considered to be the same plant.

The Florentine Codex

Another Mexican source that has comparative value is the *Florentine Codex* written by the Franciscan Bernardino de Sahagún. Fray Sahagún, now considered to be the most prominent ethnographer of sixteenth century Mexico, arrived in Mexico in 1529 and devoted much of this life to studying the Aztecs (Guerra 1966a:317).

Sahagún began his systematic collection of information on Aztec culture in the 1540s. He used a questionnaire to gather data from the elderly Indians who remembered pre-Hispanic days. These informants used oral explanations and native pictorials to respond to Sahagún's questions. Students from the Colegio Santa Cruz de Tlatelolco, who were trilingual, wrote down what the old Indians said (Robertson 1959:46–47).

Sahagún completed the final version of his work today known as the *Florentine Codex* around 1575 to 1577 or 1578 to 1580 in the Convento de San Francisco in Mexico City. This codex is now located in the Laurentian Library in Florence. It is a final and complete version which contains twelve books and a Nahua text (Glass and Robertson 1975:190). The *Florentine Codex* is beautifully illustrated and includes information on 360 illnesses (López Austin 1974b:215–16). Volume 10 contains the discussion of ailments and cures and Volume 11 (containing over half of the 1,846 drawings), is a natural history. Chapter 7 of the latter volume discusses medicinal plants (Guerra 1966a:332). Sahagún mentioned 225 medicinal plants (Andrews and Hassig 1984:29).

The *Florentine Codex* was compiled to be sent to King Philip II of Spain and his Council of the Indies, but the church had banned all books relating to pagan customs. It is possible that the codex was sent to Rome to be judged (Cline and Nicolau d'Olwer 1973:194, 196, 198). It appears to have then been forgotten and remained generally unknown until 1883.

There have been six editions of the Spanish text entitled *Historia general de las cosas de Nueva España,* one French translation, and one incomplete English translation (Glass and Robertson 1975:191). The only complete translation of the Nahua text is that of Anderson and Dibble (1950–69). In this work, plants were identified with Latin binomials in footnotes below the text. Irene Rivera identified those in Book 10, Chapter 28, and Emily Walcott Emmart those in Book 11. Several valuable modern studies analyzing the Sahagún corpus and other works relevant to early medicine have been published by Alfredo López Austin. (See bibliography.)

The Cruz-Badianus Herbal

Although used to a lesser extent in the present work, the *Cruz-Badianus Herbal* (1552) also contains valuable comparative information on illnesses and native herbal treatments. There are 251 plants mentioned (Guerra 1966a:332) and 184 are drawn in color. The herbal was written by Martín de la Cruz, a physician, who was a student at the Colegio Santa Cruz de Tlatelolco. He obtained his information from elderly Indians who remembered pre-Hispanic times. Juan Badiano, a teacher of Latin at the Colegio, prepared the Latin version of the medical information given in Nahua by De la Cruz. The work was titled *Libellus de medicinalibus Indorum herbis* (Guerra 1966a:317–18). The original, called the *Codex Barberini* (Latin 214), is presently located in the Vatican Library (Gates 1939:iii). A later copy of the late sixteenth or seventeenth century, probably by Cassiano dal Pozzo, exists at the Royal Library, Windsor (Guerra 1966a:317).

There are several modern editions of the *Cruz-Badianus Herbal.* The earliest, an English translation, was published by William Gates of the Maya Society in 1939. Emily Walcott Emmart published a beautiful color facsimile in 1940. Two Spanish versions, the latter in color, were published in 1952 and 1964. The *Cruz-Badianus Herbal* contains the earliest illustrations of many of the native flora of Mexico (Emmart 1940:xiii). Plant names were given in Nahua, but there is no Nahua text.

The herbal is divided into 13 chapters of groups of illnesses of either similar type or which attacked similar locations of the body. Plants were only used in the present study if the use given was the same as that mentioned by Fuentes y Guzmán or Ximénez. The *Cruz-Badianus Herbal* is particularly important to the study of native medicine because it is the only one extant that may be totally native in design and execution. However, the description of illnesses in this herbal and in the work of Sahagún follows the medieval schema of order which groups under the same heading pathological entities of the most opposite etiology. This had led some writers to believe that both works show some traces of European influence (Andrews and Hassig 1984:29; Guerra 1966a:324).

Tractado Brebe de Chirurgia y del Concocimiento y Cura de Algunas Enfermedades que en Esta Tierra mas Comunmente Suelen Haber

The *Tractado brebe* was published in Mexico in 1579 and was the work of Fray Agustín Farfán of the religious order of San Agustín. Fray Farfán was a doctor and supposedly was the first to graduate from the University in Mexico in medicine and surgery in the year 1567. There is some doubt as to whether he could have graduated in those fields in 1567 as medicine and surgery were not taught there at that time, and there were no professors available to teach those subjects.

A second edition of Farfán's work entitled *Tractado brebe de medicina, y de todas las enfermedades,* appeared in 1592 and was a modification of the 1579 work (Comas 1954:344). This work was also published in Madrid in 1944 under the title *Tractado breve de medicina.* Farfán discussed medicinal remedies mainly within illness categories although some chapters focused on a particular plant and gave several ways in which it was used. He included information on anatomy, medicine, pharmacology, and surgery.

Historia Medicinal de Todas Las Cosas que Se Traen de Nuestras Indias Occidentales, que Sirven al Uso de la Medicina

Although Nicolas Bautista Monardes, the author of the *Historia medicinal* was actually a Spaniard, his work will be considered here with Mexican sources. The *Historia medicinal* was published in 1565. Monardes was a well-known physician in the sixteenth century who was one of the most learned in Europe. The work was translated into several languages, and even though Monardes was never in the New World, his book was instrumental in informing Europeans about

New World medicine (Guerra 1961:1). Monardes obtained the data for his book by collecting information from conquistadors and travelers who returned from the Americas (Comas 1954:331).

Several medicinal plants were described for the first time in Monardes's text. He included information on two types of plants: food plants and medicinal plants. Monardes, being a good physician, attempted to verify the action of some of the medicines by experiment. However, though he represents the level of thought attained in medicine in the mid-sixteenth century in Europe, we should note that as a product of his times, he also believed in such things as the usefulness of bezoar stones in cases of poison (Guerra 1961:74–75).

Monardes's work was published in Spanish in 1565, in Seville. The book was translated into English by John Frampton who was in Spain when the book first appeared. Frampton's first edition was published in 1577, and the most well known variant, *Joyfull Newes Out of the Newe Founde Worlde,* did not contain the complete work of Monardes but only a translation of the first three parts. The complete work was contained in the later 1580 and 1596 editions of Frampton's translation (Guerra 1961:97–99). The version published in London in 1925 was used in the preparation of the present study.

Descripción de los Nombres y Virtudes de Las Yerbas de Yucatán y Las Enfermedades a que se Aplican

Ricardo Ossado (el Judío) was a physician who wrote the *Descripción de los nombres* which was published in Mérida in 1834 but was written in the late eighteenth century. The real name of the author was Juan Francisco Mayoli who lived in Valladolid de Yucatán and died in May of 1770. He was born in Rome and was called el Judío, not because he was Jewish, but because the common people called all foreigners Jews, seeing as there were so few of them in those times.

The work of el Judío is contained in Maximino Martínez (1944:527–78). Around 250 plants were listed, mainly in Yucatec Maya but some in Spanish, and a few have been identified by Latin binomials. Cures were given for each. In some instances, especially if the Spanish name was used, a plant can be recognized, but ordinarily only those which were identified in Latin terms were used in this work. In a second section illnesses were given and cures were provided for them. Some plants were also given with illnesses they were said to cure. Names of illnesses were given in Yucatec or Spanish.

Botanical, Ethnobotanical, and Ethnographic Sources

Atlas of Medicinal Plants of Middle America: *Bahamas to Yucatán*

Julia F. Morton is the Director, Morton Collectanea, of the University of Miami in Coral Gables, Florida. She has collected many medicinal plants in Middle America from northern Venezuela through the West Indies and the Bahamas, and in Central America and Yucatán. In her monumental work *Atlas of Medicinal Plants of Middle America,* Dr. Morton assembled data in a tabular format. She included information on the medicinal uses, properties and effects, including toxicity, of each plant specimen listed, numbering more than one thousand. Her descriptions were based on contemporary sources and herbs collected from local vendors (1981:xi). She also included information on food and other uses of the plants.

The book is a comprehensive guide to medicinal plants known or reasonably assumed to be in current use in Middle America. Plants are grouped according to families which brings together those most likely to have similar properties or physiological effects. Within each family the genera appear in alphabetical order, and the species are alphabetically arranged under each genera. Dr. Morton has also assembled all possible common names recorded throughout Middle America. She notes that even locally, different vendors may use different names for the same plant, or the same name may be applied to two or more species; therefore, the only safe course is to see or collect a specimen of each plant (1981:xix). A classified list of medicinal plants, according to principal uses, a vernacular index, and many illustrations help to make this work the best contemporary source on medicinal plants for the area. It is particularly useful in determining the effectiveness of plant medicines.

Practicas Medicas Tradicionales de Los Indígenas de Guatemala

Francisco Rodríguez Rouanet coordinated an extensive study of contemporary Indian medical practices under the auspices of the Instituto Indígenista Nacional of Guatemala. *Practicas medicas* (1969) presents a list of plants used by sixty-two native curers from a variety of native towns. In the later survey entitled *Aspectos de la medicina popular en el area rural de Guatemala* (1971), Indians and non-Indians were observed using medicinal plants in thirty-eight communities with a minimum of five informants in each community.

The major difficulty in using these two studies is that only the native names for the plants were given. In some cases, one name was used for several different plants. If the use given for a particular plant matched that given in another source, it was assumed that the same plant was discussed by both authors. A particularly useful source in identifying plants included in these studies was the work of Martínez (1944). Plants contained in Rodríguez Rouanet which could not be identified according to Latin binomials were not included in the present study.

Rodríguez Rouanet grouped plants under the illnesses they were reputed to help, stated how they were used, and gave the location where the cure was observed. It is evident from his works that treatment varied from locality to locality, and this is probably true of much of the material collected by colonial and contemporary authors. Some cures had a more restricted use than others. When specific localities were not given for the use of medicinal plants, as is true for many of the sources, it cannot automatically be assumed that such uses were widespread.

Recordación de Unos Aspectos de la Flora Util de Guatemala

This work, written by the Guatemalan botanist, José Ignacio Aguilar Girón, was published in Guatemala in 1966. It is one of the best sources on Guatemalan flora other than the Fieldiana series, *Flora of Guatemala* (1946-77). The latter, however, did not focus on medicinal properties of plants and included only occasional references to their curative uses.

Aguilar Girón became the administrator of the zoological and experimental station of Aurora Park in Guatemala City. He also worked for the Ministry of Agriculture and taught at the National School of Agriculture (1966:11, 13–14). He identified many plants according to their genus names, Latin binomials (sometimes spelled incorrectly), and common names, usually in Spanish. The sources of his information on medicinal plants were not identified nor were the specific localities where cures were used. Much of his information was probably based upon his extensive notes on all matters pertaining to Guatemalan flora.

Some illustrations were provided. Aguilar Girón supplied a fairly lengthy list of medicinal plants, but there were other references to them scattered throughout the text.

El Uso de Las Plantas Medicinales en Guatemala

George-Ann Mellen (1974) gave an extensive list of medicinal plants which were grouped under illnesses they were said to cure. Latin binomials, native names, parts of the plant used, the manner of preparation, and the habitat range of each plant were included in her discussion. Some illustrations were provided at the end of the text.

Mellen obtained her information from the Botanical Garden of Guatemala, and she stated that her article contained only a small sample of the many medical plants located there. This garden may give some idea of how extensive the pre-Columbian Guatemalan knowledge of medicinal plants may have been. Mellen did not say which Indian groups used the remedies given, but the general geographical distribution of each plant was included. Latin binomials were sometimes incorrectly spelled, but they are generally recognizable.

Las Plantas Medicinales del Departamento de Alta Verapaz

In 1940, Erwin Dieseldorff discussed around sixty medicinal plants in use among the Indians of Alta Verapaz. He supplied Latin binomials for most of the plants, but in some instances only the common name was given. Dieseldorff gave a brief description of each plant, some illustrations, native names, and medicinal uses. Sometimes the Latin binomials were incorrectly spelled, and some of the plants identified only by native names could not be correlated with Latin terminology. They were not included in the present study.

Monografía del Departamento de Guatemala

The Guatemalan anthropologist and historian José Antonio Villacorta Calderón published his study of the Department of Guatemala in 1926. As part of this regional study, he included a chapter on plants which included a list of medicinal plants used in various towns located in the area. Common plant names were given for 140 plants along with their medical uses and the towns in which they were used. Villacorta Calderón drew his information from a work entitled *Catalogo de Plantas reputadas medicinales en la República de Guatemala* published in 1923. The uses mentioned are quite brief but do supplement information already given in greater detail in other sources.

There are many other modern studies which are useful in elucidating current native medical beliefs and practices, and many other have been utilized in this work. The studies of Sheila Cosminsky, especially those relating to the Quiché hamlet of Chuchexic (1972); Barbara Tedlock on the Quichés of Momostenango (1982); William Douglas on the Tzutujil of Santiago Atitlán (1969); Benjamin and Lois Paul (1975) and Lois Paul (1974) on the Tzutujil of San Pedro la Laguna have been particularly helpful. These are in-depth studies of native medical systems carried out by anthropologists. There are also helpful general surveys of native medical beliefs and practices by Richard N. Adams (1952), Adams and Arthur J. Rubel (1967); and, more recently, by Alfredo Méndez Domínguez (1983). The study by Jorge Luís Villacorta Cifuentes (1976) on pre-Hispanic medicine in Guatemala and the comprehensive study by Alfredo López Austin (1980) on Aztec medicine were invaluable in reconstructing aboriginal illness etiology, treatment, and endemic ailments.

The contemporary sources often give a more complete picture of the uses of a medicinal plant by providing data on uses not discussed in the colonial sources. These additional uses have been included to give some idea of the complexity of native herbology. Some plants mentioned in the modern sources but not in those of colonial times are also incorporated here to supplement early data and give a broader view of the different plants used in treating a particular illness.

Contemporary sources also provide information on illness etiology, curing rituals, and non-herbal therapies that is essential in fleshing out the scant data present in the Guatemalan colonial sources. Modern studies of highland Guatemalan medical systems contain valuable data that can also be compared with the more comprehensive corpus of material relating to early medicine in Mexico. This must be done with care as the two areas were not the same in pre-Hispanic times; however, many parallels do seem to have existed between the Aztecs and Mayas.

Nomenclature Sources

In the text plants are usually identified according to the Latin binomial and English names. In some cases there is no English name so the Latin name is given along with the Spanish or Nahua common name. In other instances only the native name is given. Sometimes it was not possible to identify a plant given by the colonial authors. In Chapter 7 and Appendix I, Latin binomials, English, Spanish, and some Nahua and Maya (primarily Quiché and Cakchiquel) names are given for plants included in the text.

Latin binomials given by the various authors were checked with *Standardized Plant Names* (1942) by Harlan P. Kelsey and William A. Dayton, *Hortus third* (1976) by Liberty Hyde Bailey and Ethel Zoe Bailey, *Flora of Guatemala* (1946–77) by Paul C. Standley and Julian A. Steyermark, and *Atlas of Medicinal Plants of Middle America: Bahamas to Yucatán* (1981) by Julia F. Morton.

When only common names were given by an author, it was necessary to compare those with common names given by other authors who also supplied Latin binomials. Then the medicinal uses given by each author were checked to see if they were similar. If so, the plant was considered to be identified.

PART I

Indian Medicine in Aboriginal and Colonial Times

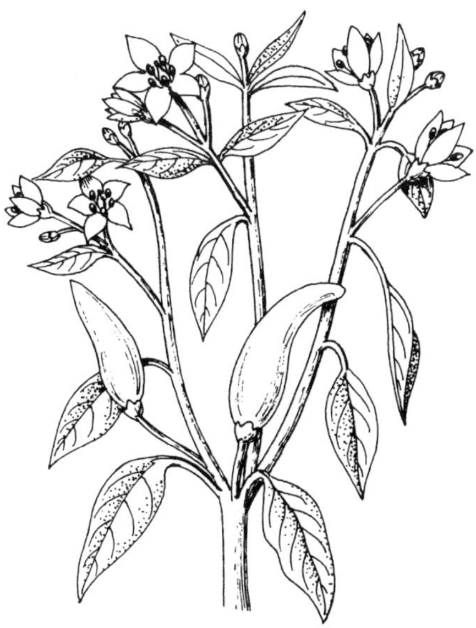

CHAPTER TWO

The Causes of Illness

The first part of this work presents a reconstruction of the native medical system which existed in the Guatemala highlands before the Conquest and during the early colonial period. Although the sources are primarily colonial or contemporary, it is possible to derive a picture of the pre-Hispanic situation by comparing the information contained in the Guatemalan colonial sources with that found in central Mexican documents written shortly after the Conquest. Even ethnographic sources are useful since highland Guatemala is culturally conservative and has retained much of the native way of life until present time.

During the colonial period, few Spaniards lived in remote Indian towns and not much European influence was evident. The Spaniards tended to respect native herbology, and that explains why so much of it has survived into our own time. There was also a shortage of European-trained doctors in the Guatemalan countryside until recent times. Religious beliefs, which were closely related to medicine in pre-Hispanic times, proved to be very difficult to eradicate, and much of the ancient illness etiology and curing practices apparently continues to exist among today's Indian groups. Change did occur during the colonial period, however, and much of the aboriginal medical system was lost.

HIGHLAND GEOGRAPHY AND HISTORY

The Guatemala highlands run the length of Guatemala from the northeast to the southwest and form a mountain plateau which is an extension of the Andean cordillera. West of Guatemala City, which lies almost in the center of the highlands, are the western highlands. East of the capital are lower hills called the eastern highlands. The

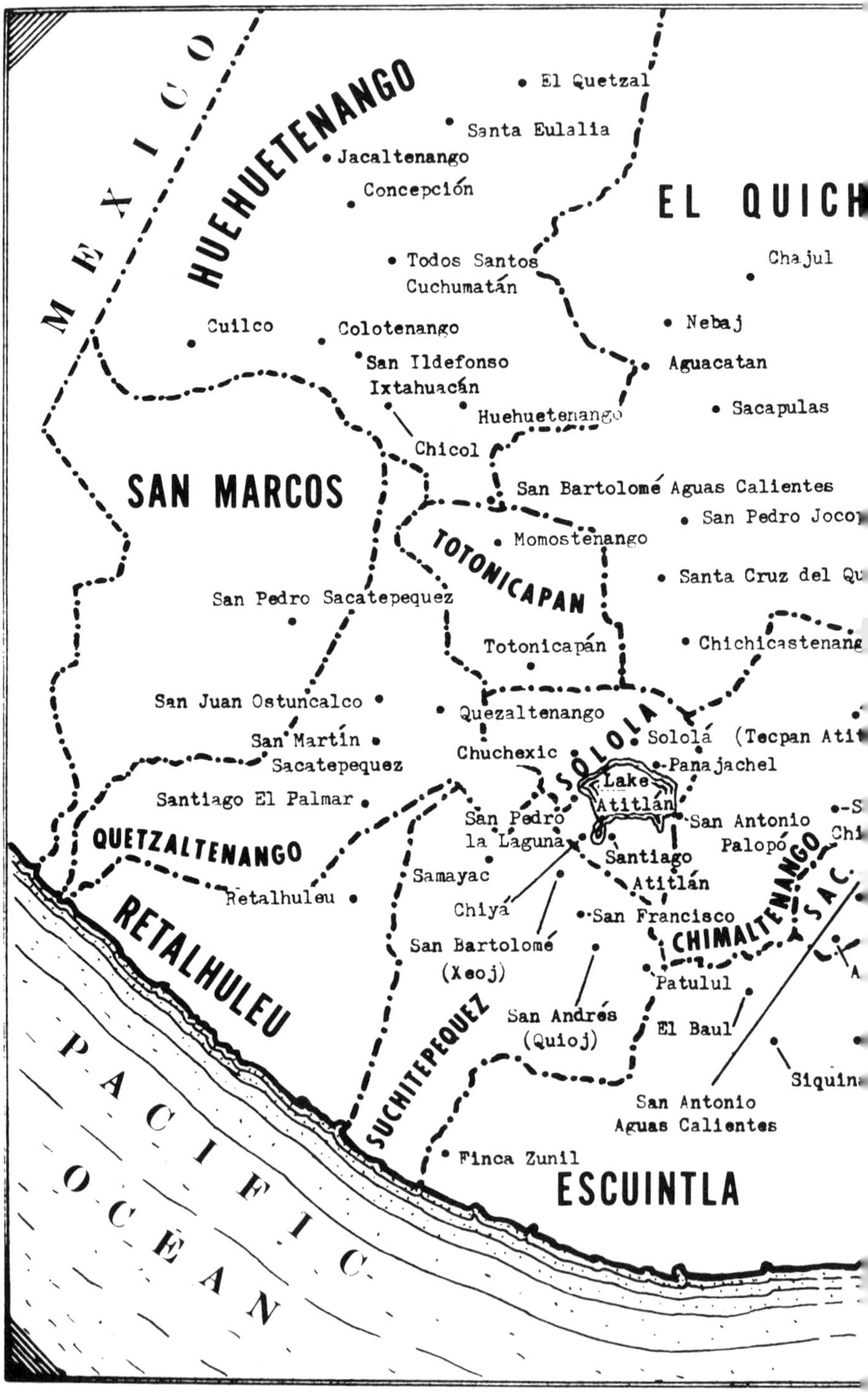

Figure 1
Map of Guatemala.

region around the Cuchumatanes is the northwest highlands. The majority of the Indian population can now be found in the western and northwestern highland areas (Nash 1969:30,35).

During the Late Postclassic (A.D. 1400–1542), the highland Maya area was divided into several political entities which had achieved a fairly advanced level of civilization. The people were stratified into hierarchically organized descent groups which monopolized specific offices. The ruling dynasties inhabited fortified hilltop centers (*tinamit,* from Nahua), and the commoners lived scattered over the land in small hamlets (*amak,* Quiché). The tinamit were administrative and religious centers with the main temples and idols being located there. The commoners paid tribute to their lords and made their living by farming the land.

Around the beginning of the fifteenth century, the Quichés conquered an extensive portion of the highland and nearby lowland area and forced neighboring groups to pay them tribute. By the late fifteenth century, their hold had begun to weaken, and the Quiché empire fragmented into several independent kingdoms. Although these groups fought against each other right up until the Spanish entered Guatemala, each maintained political, social, economic, and cultural ties with the others. They also shared a common body of ritual, mythological, and political knowledge. The medical system was part of this shared cultural tradition which existed among the highland peoples of Late Postclassic times.

General Beliefs Regarding Illness Causation

In this work *disease* is considered to be a pathological state of an individual whether or not it is socially or culturally recognized and whether or not the patient and his or her treatment specialist are aware of its existence. Illness takes into consideration the patient's conscious awareness that there is something wrong and the societal reaction to the disease (Frankenberg 1980:199). Disease, therefore, is defined from the perspective of biomedical science. Illness is a cultural category applied to individual experience. Sickness is a category of social behavior (McElroy and Townsend 1979:49).

There are two broad categories of illness etiology that were recognized in pre-Columbian Mesoamerica. Illness was thought to be caused by nonhuman beings or by human beings who possessed supernatural powers. It was also thought to be the result of natural causes such as accidents, deficiencies, or excesses (López Austin 1974b:216). A study of the existing documentary sources does not reveal any all-embracing theory or mechanism of illness such as the humoral pathology which existed in sixteenth century Europe (Guerra 1966a:324).

Once the cause of an illness was discovered, it was possible to treat it. For example, illnesses believed to come from offenses against the gods required confession of sin and performance of penance. Those resulting from witchcraft required measures against the witchcraft, divination, and magic. Those resulting from natural causes required the use of medicines discovered empirically. All three remedies could be used (Ortíz de Montellano 1980:295). Incantations may have accompanied all types of curing.

If an illness were judged to be a common one which was not considered serious, then it was probably treated at home by the sufferer or by a non specialist known to be good with simple remedies as is done in modern times (Adams and Rubel 1967:347). If a person became seriously or chronically ill, then the possibility that the illness was sent by the gods as a punishment for an unconfessed sin would be considered (Las Casas 1967:2:226). Today individuals do not usually classify illnesses according to whether they are of supernatural or natural origin since all illnesses are believed to be caused ultimately by the supernatural. This belief may have been true in ancient times as well (Cosminsky 1977c:328). For example, in Chichicastenango if the symptoms of an illness are obscure, or if it fails to respond to treatment, then it is said to have meaning. A diviner will then be called in to find out if the illness has been caused by some fault of the patient or if it is the work of an enemy (Bunzel 1967:146).

Illness and the Animate Entities

The Teyolía

In ancient Mexico the main organ of the body was believed to be the heart, and it was there that the seat of illnesses was found. The heart was also considered to be the source of feeling and thought (Viesca Treviño and De la Peña Páez 1976:80). Similar concepts were also present among the Quichés. The Quichés believed that all of the psychic powers, memory, will, faculties of reasoning, life, spirit, and soul were found in the heart (López Austin 1980:1:255). Today among the Tzutujil Maya of Santiago Atitlán, the heart is still considered to be the major organ of the body and the seat of the soul (Douglas 1969:264).

In Mexico the soul associated with the heart was called the *teyolía* (Nahua), and it was that entity that went to the underworld after an individual's death. (It is this type of soul that is associated with the Spanish terms *ánima* and *alma*.) It was thought never to leave the living body until the death of an individual (López Austin 1980:1:253).

Among the Aztecs harm to the teyolía and to the heart was attributed to several causes—among them immoral sexual conduct. The cure involved confession, sacrifice, and penance (1980:1:256). This sounds similar to what Las Casas said about grave illnesses and their particular relationship to sexual conduct (1967:2:522–23). The teyolía was also thought to be harmed by certain illnesses that covered the heart with phlegm and by sorcery (López Austin 1980:1:256).

The Tonalli

Another conception of the soul that is relevant to pre-Columbian illness etiology is the *tonalli* (Nahua). The modern belief in the *tona* (Spanish) has been intertwined with that of a second aboriginal concept, the *nagual* (Spanish, *nahualli* in Nahua). (See pp. 32–33 for a discussion of nagualism.) The tonalli was a life force received by each individual depending upon the day of his or her birth (López Austin 1980:1:223) and was essential to an individual's vigor, heat, valor, and growth (1980:1:225). In ancient Mexico it was associated with the head, and cures of illnesses related to the tonalli were directed principally at the head (1980:1:234). It was a very important element in the functioning of the organism, a regulator of body temperature, a conditioner of health, and a generator of pathological processes (1980:1:401). The primary way the tonalli could cause illness was to leave the body for too long a time, e.g. when hair which protected the head (*mollera*) was cut, sexual transgression occurred, or a person was badly frightened (1980:1:245, 246). In adults there was also the possibility of loss of the tonalli due to divine wrath. The tonalli had to be restored to the body or the individual would die (López Austin 1980:1:224, 235).

Today in highland Guatemala fright is one of the most important causes of soul loss, and this contemporary illness is similar in conception to the ancient beliefs regarding the tonalli. Fright refers to being shocked or frightened by something. This is believed to result from a bad experience or suddenly seeing an animal, spirit, or ghost. It is also thought to result from falling into the water or from fear of drowning. The person may become ill, or the soul may be said to be jarred loose, remaining at the place where the incident occurred. Prolonged absence of the soul will bring death according to common belief (Adams 1957:366; Adams and Rubel 1967:346–47).

The simplest and most common form of fright is said to be caused by a fall and is frequently seen in children (Tenzel 1970:374). To bring about a cure, the curer will usually go with the patient to the place where the soul was lost and attempt to restore it to the victim's body (Adams 1957:366). In eastern Guatemala the image of the person, animal, or event which occurred and caused the fright is thought to impress the victim. The image must be expelled or the soul (called heart, or spirit) rescued to bring about a cure (Méndez Domínguez 1983:280–82).

A more severe form of fright (*espanto,* Spanish) can also occur. Espanto is used to stand for the agent of illness as well as the illness itself. In San Antonio Palopó it is thought to be caused by a "being" such as a witch who has transformed into an unusual beast. When seen, it causes great fright, and the soul leaves the body (Tenzel 1970:374–75). Espanto is used as the equivalent of susto (Spanish) in some areas (Adams 1957:366).

Fright may also result without the loss of the soul. In this instance the person is said to be made ill from a sudden emotional experience (Adams and Rubel 1967:346–47). This form of fright seems to appear when a person is in a stressful social situation. The syndrome is a vehicle by which people of Hispanic-American peasant and urban societies manifest their reactions to some form of self-perceived stressful situation. Fright appears when an individual is unable to meet the expectations of his own society for a social role in which he or she has been socialized. Whether an individual will react to stress by choosing fright depends upon his or her personality.

The symptoms exhibited by a person suffering from fright vary but restlessness while asleep, listlessness, loss of appetite, disinterest in dress and personal hygiene, weakness, depression, and introversion while awake have been observed (Rubel 1964:270, 280–81) as well as vomiting, gasping, muteness, anorexia, stiffness or paralysis, coldness, unconsciousness (Cosminsky 1972:153), general apathy, fear, and fever (Méndez Domínguez 1983:280).

Fright appears to be partially an illness of pre-Columbian origin (Schendel 1968:143). Soul loss due to fright and capture of the soul are most likely to be ancient, but fright originating from stress may be a contemporary variation. In ancient Mexico it was thought that a person could lose his tonalli due to divine beings related to earth and water. It could also leave the body due to fright, or in dreams (López Austin 1980:245–46, 248).

There are no specific pre-Columbian Guatemalan treatments mentioned for fright, but the *Cruz-Badianus Herbal* contained remedies for fear or timidity (Emmart 1940:208). However, this may not have been for the same illness which exists today.

Today a patient suffering from fright is massaged and often placed in the sweatbath to relax. He or she may be "swept" or rubbed with an object to remove the illness from the body. In Guatemala, hen's eggs are often used for the rubbing (Rubel 1964:271). There may also be simulation of the "shock" which was the immediate cause of separation of the soul from the body (1964:279).

Rue (*Ruta graveolens* L.) has been used to cure fright in Huehuetenango. Rue water mixed with "spirits" from the pharmacy is a common remedy (Rodríguez Rouanet 1969:86). In some areas fright is considered to be a cold illness. (See Equilibrium-Disequilibrium below.) The patient may be given a drink of alcohol, rue, and other herbs. The curer takes some of the rue potion and spits it on the sick person's face and nude body to induce sweating. The purpose of the cure is to reestablish the heat in the body of the patient (Mendez Domínguez 1983:282).

In El Guayabo, Camotán; Nebaj, and Quiché, tobacco (*Nicotiana* spp.) was part of a mixture cast into the victim's face to startle him and remove the illness (Rodríguez Rouanet 1969:85). Among the Chortí, tobacco leaves were also used in curing fright (Wisdom 1940:348).

Another contemporary illness that is related to the concept of the tonalli is fallen fontanel (caída de la mollera). It is believed that the crown of a baby's head, or the soft part of the brain, is so soft it can fall into the mouth. If this occurs, it closes off the nasal passage and results in sore throat, coughing, and difficulty in nursing. This illness is thought to be caused by a sudden fall or rough handling of the baby or exposure to cold air (Cosminsky 1972:148; Ford 1975:5). It has been treated by putting the fingers into the baby's mouth and washing the throat with warm water where it is inflamed and pushing up on the palate (Cosminsky 1972:148). In some areas it has also been treated by turning the child upside down so that the fontanel falls back into place (Adams 1957:365–66). In actuality the depression in the crown of the head is probably the result of dehydration due to the child being ill rather than the cause of the illness (Cosminsky 1977b:93; López Austin 1980:1:250).

In pre-Columbian Mexico the head was believed to be the seat of the tonalli. Through imperfect ossification of the fontanel, the tonalli could leave the body. A person could only live for a short while without it (1980:1:224–25, 235). Specialists who recovered the tonalli applied the root of a certain plant to the fontanel of young children to return it to the head (1980:1:241).

The leaving of the tonalli was believed to create a physical hollow which was equated with the depression of the cranium. To cure fallen fontanel the child was hung upside down and shaken violently, the palate was pressed with force, perforating it, all with the intention of pushing the vault of the palate upwards until the fontanel was back in place (1980:1:250). This is essentially the same treatment that is used today. Although the relationship to the tonalli has been lost, today fallen fontanel is still considered to be dangerous to young children.

In some areas of Mesoamerica today there is a belief associated with the tonalli known as the tona. An animal is thought to be born at the same time a person is born and the two share a common fate. The animal is believed to live in a mountain that corresponds to the community in which the human lives. Part of the tonalli, or life force of the human, goes to live in the companion animal. Harm that occurs to the one will also occur to the other. As López Austin points out, there are no extant sources demonstrating that the belief in the tona was pre-Columbian although the concept of the tonalli certainly was. The belief in the tona is more common in the eastern area of Mesoamerica (1980:1:430–31), but in highland Guatemala nagualism, tonalism, and the belief in the tona appear to have fused more thoroughly than in such areas as Chiapas where the concept of the tona is still quite important (Vogt 1970:11).

In the late seventeenth century Fuentes y Guzmán discussed the relationship of a child to its tona among the Quichés:

> Having been informed of its day of birth, he [the diviner] in due time called at the residence of the parents. The mother came out with the baby in her arms and presented it. He went with her behind the house to the yard. After many ceremonies, he invoked the demon which would appear there in the form of the animal or object set opposite its birthday in the calendar, a serpent were it born on January 2nd. The diviner then addressed certain prayers to the nagual [tona] to protect the little one . . . and told the parents to take it daily at the same hour into the yard where its nagual [tona] would appear to it . . . and would finally accompany it through all its life (1969:1:280).

Fuentes y Guzmán used the word nagual, which refers to an individual who has the ability to transform into an animal or to the animal form the individual takes, incorrectly. He was really referring to the pre-Columbian practice of naming a child according to the 260-day ritual calendar, a practice that apparently existed in the Quiché area in his time. However, it appears that by the late seventeenth century, the idea of the tona, or companion animal, had been fused with ancient birthday ceremonies. Fuentes y Guzmán listed plants and objects as well as animals as naguals (tonas). This represents a melding of the concept of the tona with that of the animals, plants, and objects which appeared in the ancient divinatory calendar. Fuentes y Guzmán gave a list of the naguals (tonas) for each day in the month of January. Animals, plants, stones, and other objects such as an arrow and a broom were listed as naguals (1969:1:279). Some, but not all people, obtained the power of transforming themselves into an animal. In ancient Mexico nahualli (nagual today in highland Guatemala) referred to a person with magical powers who had the ability to transform into animals. The term was used to refer to the person or to the form he or she assumed (López Austin 1980:1:419). Where belief in the tona exists, the relationship is between one person and one animal, plant or other object, and the person does not take the form of his or her tona.

A nagual (nahualli) can also cause illness due to his evil powers (Adams and Rubel 1967:336). Various factors such as predestination, day of birth, specific knowledge, and penetential exercises were relevant in whether a sorcerer would acquire the full power of nagualism. Some used their powers for evil and others for good. Nobles as well as commoners could be naguals (López Austin 1980:1:419).

The Ihíyotl

The third animate entity was the *ihíyotl* (Nahua) which was conceived as a luminous gas which could influence human beings, attracting them to a person, animal, or object from which it emanated. One form of ihíyotl was "night air" which was given off by a corpse. Among the Aztecs many dangers were associated with emanations which came from those who led immoral lives. (See Equilibrium-Disequilibrium p. 36.) The ihíyotl was believed to be located in the liver where life, vigor, passions, and sentiments were thought to reside. The ihíyotl was an energy source and could also be used for beneficial purposes to cure and revitalize (López Austin 1980:1:257–61). In nagualism the ihíyotl was externalized and covered with another form—usually animal. The sorcerer's body, however, was not really thought to be transformed (1980:1:424, 430).

Hijillo (Spanish) is a contemporary ethnic illness probably derived from the ancient concept of the ihíyotl and is found primarily in the towns of eastern Guatemala. Swelling, diarrhea, vomiting, hair loss, marasmus, stomachache, and backache are common symptoms (Méndez Domínguez 1983:270). Among the Chortí, hijillo was believed to result in any illness, even death, but it usually caused pimples, sores, and a rash to break out all over the body, especially on the face and neck, and it produced a high fever (Wisdom 1940:329).

The cause of hijillo is often related to sexual and reproductive processes and to substances and matters associated with these processes. The patient is said to become ill by observing a birth or a sexual act, usually between dogs, by touching a newborn animal or its mother, by touching a female dog which has not been washed after having had intercourse, or by being exposed to either *vahos* (Spanish, fumes, odors, emanations) of the placenta, to animals who have recently had sexual intercourse, or to the vahos of menstruation, or the vaginal secretions of an animal in heat (Méndez Domínguez 1983:270–72).

Among the Chortí, it was believed that ritually unclean objects and persons, which included those with evil eye and strong blood, pregnant and menstruating women, corpses, sorcerers, apparitions and spirits of the dead, and all individuals who had been infected by these caused natural *aigre* (Spanish, air) to enter the body due to fright when encountering them. They also carried a special kind of aigre within themselves, which was the cause of their being ritually unclean, and infected others with it. This special "air" was called hijillo. It was considered very dangerous and likely to cause illness and death (Wisdom 1940:326–27). These agents could give hijillo at all times, but especially when angered, emotionally agitated, excited, or physically exhausted. Menstruating and pregnant women gave off hijillo that was thought to be particularly harmful to men (1940:328–29). In western Guatemala hijillo was thought to be associated with dead meat of any kind (Adams 1957:367).

Persons, animals, plants, and objects were susceptible to hijillo according to their degree of weakness at the time of contact. Those with open sores or wounds were the most susceptible, but hijillo was believed to be able to enter the body through natural openings. Infants, the aged, and the sick were particularly at risk (Wisdom 1940:329).

Hijillo may be treated by bathing in cold or warm water or by eating cold foods or drinking herbal teas (Méndez Domínguez 1983:272).

Cleansing may also be performed by using copal incense, garlic and basil, and holding unclean clothing in the fumes. The person stands naked over the incense for half an hour. The color red is also considered to be protective (Wisdom 1940:330–31). In Chamelco, a patient suffering from hijillo may be covered and rubbed with warm cow excrement to produce sweating and then take a cold bath at dawn. As an additional or alternative treatment the sick person would drink a beverage of wild pig sexual glands and take a dew bath. The treatment in most areas involves cold baths or foods (Méndez Domínguez 1983:272).

Hijillo is also thought to be prevented by avoiding corpses. In the Chortí area if a child is ill and its mother or close relative goes to the cemetery, it is believed to be necessary to protect the child against hijillo. The returning person and the child need to be rubbed down with alcohol and fumigated. If this is not done, the influence of the cemetery will worsen the child's illness (Rodríguez Rouanet 1971:152).

Among the Chortís the evil emanation coming from the dead is called *ijiyo,* a word which has been written as hijillo in the ethnographic sources, perhaps because it was believed to be derived from the Spanish word *hijo* (son). It is, however, taken from the word ihíyotl, one of the three animate entities. Foster pointed out, however, that there is a Spanish analogue to hijillo called *aire de los muertos* (Spanish, air of the dead), found particularly in Galicia (1953:210). Perhaps the belief regarding corpses is part Mesoamerican and part Spanish. This may also explain why some treatments for hijillo involve such Old World plants as garlic and basil.

In ancient Mexico a good person was said to have a clean liver while an immoral one gave off emanations which were harmful to innocent people. Corpses also gave off harmful emanations. In the Nahua of the sixteenth century the abstract of the noun for penetrating odor was *xoquíotl* or *xoquíyotl.* Among the Chortís, the word today is *xoquía* which refers in particular to hijillo which comes from a corpse (López Austin 1980:1:257–61). Hijillo, which appears to be derived from the ancient concept of ihíyotl, has persisted to a greater degree and depth in eastern Guatemala than other parts of the country. The reasons for the survival in this area are not clear.

Equilibrium-Disequilibrium

The ancient Mexicans also recognized several causes of inequality. One was sex and females were considered to be weaker. This is still believed today in Maya highland communities. For example, in the Tzutujil speaking town of San Pedro la Laguna men are considered *k'an* (aggressive, assertive, irascible) and women ideally are *nakanik* (mild, docile, submissive). The concept of blood strength is basic, and men are said to have stronger blood than women (Paul 1974:290). Age was another factor in producing inequality. The elderly were thought to be wiser and stronger with respect to their vital forces and powers than younger people (López Austin 1980:1:288). Such beliefs were also prevalent in the Quiché and Cakchiquel areas. *The Annals of the Cakchiquels,* the *Popol Vuh,* and the *Title of the Lords of Totonicapán* all mention the powers of the ancestors and deities who were sometimes said to be old (1967:76, 169; 1971:21–22). Young children and women were considered to be weak and could suffer from the glance or emanations given off by those with so much power.

Women are considered to be weaker than men particularly due to the weakening effects of menstruation, pregnancy, and the twenty-day post-partum period. Temporary debilitating conditions, such as sin, strong emotional experience, extreme envy or anger, carelessness, overwork, overexposure to heat or cold, and even certain foods can affect both sexes (Adams and Rubel 1967:335; Cosminsky 1975:189; Hinshaw 1975:118).

In ancient Mexico a sick person was thought to be in a state of disequilibrium. There were many factors that could bring about this disequilibrium such as working too hard, being overtired, and committing a sin such as a sexual transgression (López Austin 1980:1:291–92). Confession was the means of reestablishing the harmony of the individual with the gods and of restoring equilibrium (1980:1:302–303).

Those who experienced an organic change, such as menstruation, birth, and pregnancy were thought to give off a harmful force which could affect people, animals, plants, and things. For example, sexual relations with a woman who had recently given birth was said to provoke fevers and consumption. Similarly, individuals who became tired were thought to give off harmful forces and to be able to receive and transmit injuries. Being tired produced an abnormal distribution of hot and cold within the body. Fatigue was hot; rest cold. The tonalli heated up but the abdomen and feet cooled. Both the heat of the tonalli and the burden of harmful forces captured on the journey could be harmful. Travelers were accustomed to brushing off their legs and feet with bunches of herbs. These were placed on little piles of stones with the idea of leaving the tiredness there. Anyone who touched the pile felt tired or became ill in the legs (López Austin 1980:1:289–93).

According to Las Casas, there were many shrines which contained idols located along the thoroughfares in Guatemala. When people arrived at a shrine, they would strike their legs with some herbs and put the plants on the shrine and place a stone on top. It was believed that this was a good way to get rid of fatigue and strengthen the legs. They also made a small offering of something, such as cotton, cacao, pepper, or salt (1967:2:224). Today in Panajachel the Indians still remove fatigue by brushing their legs with branches and leaving them at the roadside cross (Hinshaw 1975:119).

A clear expression of the equilibrium theory is found in the strength-weakness principle in highland Guatemala. According to this belief, a strong body offers protection against illness whereas a weak body is more susceptible. The state of the body is determined by the condition of the blood—which is characterized as strong or weak and hot or cold. A person with strong blood is more immune to illness than one with weak blood. Blood is thought to be non-regenerative. A person is provided with a limited amount and any loss must lead to permanent weakness (Adams and Rubel 1967:334). Strength or weakness may be either inherent or acquired. A person is born with a strong or weak body depending upon his or her luck (*suerte,* Spanish) (Cosminsky 1975:189). As in ancient Mexico, age, sex, and organic changes also affect one's strength, with infants, women, and sometimes old people being considered weaker. Even today, however, the ancient belief that old people are stronger and more powerful than young people survives, especially if they are renowned sorcerers, healers, or town leaders (personal observation 1979: Adams and Rubel 1967:335). In Panajachel, the blood is thought to become stronger the longer one lives. The hotter the blood the stronger the person. To live to old age is possible only with strong blood or the help of evil forces (Hinshaw 1975:113, 116).

In ancient Mexico health and illness were closely related to the state of equilibrium and disequilibrium. To keep the body in a state of equilibrium, the Aztecs believed that it was necessary for an individual to maintain harmony with nature, society, and the gods. With respect to many of their medicines, the Aztecs attempted to regulate the relationship between cold and heat. The goal was to remove from the surface of the body any concentrations of heat or cold that provoked injury due to the abnormal distribution, or to carry the illness to a site of the body where it could be easily attacked. While herbal remedies were an important aspect of medical treatment, confession of any sins was also used to reestablish the individual's harmony with the gods and restoring his internal equilibrium (López Austin 1980:1:300–303).

There are some colonial and contemporary native-defined illnesses which are related to the ancient beliefs regarding equilibrium-disequilibrium. In colonial times evil or bad wind or air (*aire* or *mal aire,* Spanish) was believed to cause illness. In the sixteenth century Estrada mentioned bad airs (aires) which were thought to influence health (1955:75). Evil winds were also used to cause harm in colonial Yucatán (Roys 1965:166).

In more recent times aire has sometimes been referred to as a dusty whirlwind or other unusual movement of the air. Too much heat or cold is believed to invade the body from exposure to aires (Ford 1975:5). Aires have been thought to cause colds, coughs, fever, measles, smallpox, and whooping cough. They may attack an individual spontaneously or may be sent by a sorcerer, the ancestors, spirits, or gods (Adams and Rubel 1967:338–39; Méndez Domínguez 1983:276–77).

Today aire is known in many areas of Guatemala (Rodríguez Rouanet 1971:29–31), but the illnesses which are attributed to it differ from region to region. In Chajul, for example, cold air was thought to cause illness after a person had been heated, as before a fire, or when a person went out into the cold air with a cold. In other areas aire is thought to be associated with vahos, or emanations (Méndez Domínguez 1983:276, 279–80).

Cosminsky reviewed the various meanings of aire in Chuchexic. It was considered to be a draft, breeze, or current of air which "hit" someone who was in a weakened state and made the person ill. Aire was also used to describe the physical illness which resulted from having been hit by the aire. It was also used for the condition of internal gas or wind in the stomach. Mal aire (bad air) was seen as a particularly strong wind that resulted in paralysis, or twisting of the mouth. It also referred to air sent by black magic or witchcraft. Aire could be a vector for sorcery as sorcerers could use air as a medium for accomplishing their evil. For example, they could send an animal into the victim's body through the aire (Cosminsky 1972:117–18).

The aires play their most prominent role in illness in Yucatán and among the Chortí in Guatemala. Among the latter, aigres were the primary cause of illness, pains, aches, and malfunctioning. There were three classes of aigres. Aigres could be of natural origin entering the body in an accidental way (the least feared type), they could be acquired from contact with ritually unclean persons and objects, or they could be sent by a sorcerer (the most feared type). The natural aigres were named for the source which caused them to enter the body (the part of the body in which they were localized), or their inherent characteristics and the bodily condition they caused (Wisdom 1940:317–19). Only among the Chortí and the Yucatecos were aires considered to be self-activating. In other areas they were believed to be sent by spirits or humans and were vectors of illness, or were simply drafts of air that, being constantly around, would bother people only when they were in a special condition (Adams and Rubel 1967:340).

The ancient Mexicans spoke of an air of night (*aire de noche,* Spanish) and dead air (*aire de muerto,* Spanish), which had to be ejected from a corpse, scarifying it with a knife. This was harmful to human beings (López Austin 1980:1:257–58). Some forms of aire are probably pre-Columbian, but other aspects may stem from the Hippocratic concept of hot and cold and are Spanish beliefs. For example, in Galicia air is particularly thought of as emanations from animals, individuals, corpses, occasionally places, and even heavenly bodies (Foster 1953:209).

In ancient Mexico, malignant "airs" were thought to originate with Tlaloc, the Aztec rain god, and the Tlaloque, their mountain gods. It was believed that certain illnesses, which seem to have been those caused by the cold, came from the mountains, or that the mountains had the power of healing them (Soustelle 1974:192–93). Among the contemporary Chortí, it was the wind gods who were believed to send illness by placing aigres into the body (Wisdom 1940:397). The whirlwind was the main god of evil and was called upon by sorcerers and enemies to carry illness and misfortune to others 1940:405). Herbal cures "for one afflicted by a whirlwind or a bad wind" were mentioned in the *Cruz-Badianus Herbal* (Emmart 1940:208, 306).

Another contemporary native-defined illness which is related to the equilibrium-disequilibrium belief is evil eye (ojo or mal de ojo). Today evil eye is believed to be caused by heat, especially from a hot-blooded person who has been working hard (Méndez Domínguez 1983:285) or a menstruating woman who is thought to be in a "hot" state. It can also be caused by a pregnant woman who is envious of another's child. Children are thought to be particularly susceptible to evil eye (Cosminsky 1976:165). A dog, especially a female dog in heat, can transmit the evil eye too.

In Guatemala, evil eye is used to refer to the condition or illness of the victim rather than to the power of its owner, and it is usually, but not always, unintentional. However, the Spanish or Mediterranean concept of the evil eye refers primarily to the eye of the person with the power and is sometimes associated with willful or intentional harm, particularly stemming from envy or jealousy (Cosminsky 1976:172).

The belief in evil eye which exists today in Mesoamerica, then, is not based only on Spanish concepts but also involves ideas which originated in pre-Columbian times. In ancient Mexico tiredness (as from working and walking) was associated with heat. Sexual excitement also generated heat (López Austin 1980:1:291–92). It was believed that immoral persons, such as adulterers, prostitutes, and drunks could harm children, pregnant women, a spouse, and animals, and things. Harm was transferred by proximity to filth, and an immoral lifestyle was considered filthy. The historical sources also mentioned that people who desired someone or something intensely (especially people with strong sight) possessed negative energy and could harm others. Such a person, whose general state was bad, was sad and melancholy. This may have been related to the concept of the ihíyotl (the animate entity which was thought to be freed from the body through the sight by strong desire) (López Austin 1980:1:298–300).

In some parts of Guatemala people with eye defects, such as lesions, corneal scars, and strabismus are also regarded as having the power to cause evil eye in their gaze. This may be related to Mediterranean beliefs regarding evil eye. In other parts evil eye effects are thought to be caused by the sun or moon (Cosminsky 1976:165).

In Chinautla several types of evil eye were distinguished in Spanish. *Ojo del luna* (eye of the moon) was said to be caused by menstruating women. The victim's condition was one of general malaise. *Ojo de embarazo* (eye of pregnancy) was caused by a pregnant woman, and the illness involved pain within the body. The child was not able to sleep and was fussy. In *ojo que revienta* (eye which breaks loose), which was also caused by a pregnant woman, the child had many wounds over all its body and there was generalized pain. All of the symptoms disappeared when the pregnant woman gave birth. *Ojo del pujo* (eye which bursts forth or blows up) was caused by those with strong blood or who had been working outdoors, and it involved internal body pain (Simeon 1973:438).

Evil eye can involve a variety of symptoms; convulsion, skin eruptions, diarrhea, vomiting, anorexia, crying, listlessness, fever, being easily frightened, bad breath, throwing the shoulders and head back and forth, tossing them from side to side, or having one eye smaller or larger than the other, and screaming in one's sleep. Several of these symptoms are similar to those caused by malnutrition and intestinal parasites (Adams 1957:364–65; Cosminsky 1976:166).

Today to protect a baby, especially when many people are around, the mother usually keeps it completely covered. A red stocking cap is placed over its head or it is wrapped in a blanket. If the baby becomes ill, she may be blamed for being careless with the child and not properly protecting it (Cosminsky 1972:152; Tenzel 1970:376).

There are several cures for evil eye, and one of the most common involves passing an egg over the victim's body, making the sign of the cross (Adams 1957:365; Cosminsky and Scrimshaw 1980:269). In San

Antonio Palopó a sick infant was rubbed from head to foot with two fresh eggs in their shells, one after the other. One egg was wrapped in rue sprigs and attached to the child's abdomen by a sash. The following day the egg was removed and taken to Lake Atitlán and broken into the water. If a "boiling foam" was produced, this meant that the evil spirit that was within the infant was transferred to the egg. The second egg was then attached to the child's abdomen to remove any remains of the evil spirit (Tenzel 1970:378).

In Panajachel the following cure was administered. A cross was made of two pieces of *ocote* (Spanish, pitchpine splint) and passed over the child's body. An egg was put into its clothing. The ocote was then placed in a pan of water with two peppers. The peppers were also passed over the child's body, in the form of a cross. Then the egg was broken into the water. The eye was thought to be in the broken egg (Hinshaw 1975:177). The egg cure may be aboriginal even though hens did not exist in pre-Columbian Mesoamerica. Turkey or duck eggs have been used in some places, and both animals are indigenous to the New World (Bremme de Santos 1963:558; Simeon 1973:439). This practice is still common today in many areas of Guatemala.

Other cures for evil eye have involved herbal remedies. In Santa Lucía Utatlán when an infant is thought to have evil eye, rue (*Ruta graveolens* L.) was crushed up well and rubbed on the child's body, or two sprigs of rue were cooked and the water drunk. Rue and sugar were also taken in boiled water (Cosminsky 1976:168). In San Pedro la Laguna, rue was drunk boiled with a little *aguardiente* (Spanish, rum made from brown cane sugar) (Rodríguez Rouanet 1969:83); in San Antonio Palopó, the body of the victim was rubbed with crushed rue (Bremme de Santos 1963:558). In Huehuetenango the curer put a little rue in his mouth and sprayed it onto the child's face (Rodríguez Rouanet 1968:83). A similar cure was recorded among the Chortí (Wisdom 1940:349). In Huehuetenango after spraying the child's face, a little aguardiente and a well-crushed up pepper were applied to the child's feet. Its head would be covered and the child would be put to bed (Rodríguez Rouanet 1969:83). In San Martín Sacatépequez a cloth bag containing some grains of annatto (*Bixa orellana* L.) and some peppers (*Capsicum* spp.) were passed over the child's body. The sign of the cross was made while passing the bag, and then it was thrown into the fire (Rodríguez Rouanet 1971:177).

In San Juan Chamelco jute and the black nightshade (*Solanum nigrum* L.) were crushed up and the mixture passed over the victim's body (1971:183). Usually red pepper is one of the components passed over the body. The Mexican prickly poppy (*Argemone mexicana* L.) was another evil eye cure (Villacorta Calderón 1926:75). Fuentes y Guzmán did not mention any specific herbal cure for evil eye but did say that the rattles of the rattlesnake were good for evil eye (*fascinación,* Spanish) (1969:1:343).

There are many other ethnically-defined illnesses in highland Guatemala today. The ones included in this chapter are those that are widespread and probably of pre-Columbian origin. It is difficult, however, to determine how many of the ideas relating to any ethnic illness are purely aboriginal because European medical beliefs have combined with native explanations to produce the native etiologies existing today.

Specific Vectors of Illness

The Gods

The information in the documentary sources relating to highland Guatemala is sparse when it comes to the role of the ancient gods in illness causation and prevention. Some aboriginal deities who were believed to be responsible for illness are mentioned in the *Popol Vuh.* These were the lords of Xibalba, or the Underworld. Flying Noose (*Xik'iri Pat*) and the Blood Chief (*Kuchuma Kiq'*) were two of these lords whose job was "blood to sicken people" (*Popol Vuh* 1971:61). The vital force of the blood in many Mesoamerican towns is viewed as a conduit for receiving external harm (López Austin 1980:1:179), and that seems to be the meaning of the passage in the *Popol Vuh.* The two lords, Flying Noose and Blood Chief, caused people to become ill by tampering with their blood.

Another lord mentioned in the *Popol Vuh* was Pus Maker (*Ahal Puh*) who was responsible for causing infection. He and Bile Maker (*Ahal Q'ana*) had the power "to make people swell up. Pus comes after their feet, Bile comes after their faces, to jaundice." Edmonson also noted that, according to Adrían Recinos, the Guatemalan ethnohistorian, there were two Cakchiquel gods called *Ahal Puh* and *Ahal Canya,* and they probably had similar causative powers.

Bone Staff (*Chamiya Baq*) and Skull Staff (*Chamiya Holom*) turned people into bones and skulls. "Then one dies stretched bones or gets dropsy." Edmonson said that Recinos found evidence for the existence of two gods called *Tatan Bak* and *Tatan Holom* among the Cakchiquels (*PV* 1971:61–62). The former god in the Pokoman area was given as *Kak Tepeu* by Zuñiga in his dictionary (Miles 1957:748). Edmonson believed that "stretched bones" (*ziyah bak*) probably referred to a particular illness. The translation he gave for *xupan* was dropsy.

There were two other illness-causing lords of the Underworld called Filth Maker (*Ahal Mez*) and Wound Maker (*Ahal Tokob*).

> It is their job
> That they just come to watch people
> Whether there is alien filth,
> And whether there is want
> Behind the house
> Or before the house,
> Then when they come to be observed
> They may just stab him.

There was a Cakchiquel god called *Ahal Tecob* so this deity was known among them as well. Edmonson interpreted alien filth and want to refer to signs of withcraft and evil doing which must be punished. It may also have referred to diseases of the epidemic type introduced from outside of the Guatemala highlands and hunger.

Lord Hawk (*Ahav Xik*) and Snare (*Patan*) were resposible for those who died on the road:

> Just "sudden death" as it is called.
> Blood comes to their mouths,
> Until they die vomiting blood.
> But each of them does his job,
> Shouldering something,
> And they just smash a person in his neck
> Or his heart,
> Then he dies on the road.

There was a Cakchiquel god called *Ahal Xic* who was probably identical with the Quiché god Ahav Xik (*PV* 1971:61–64).

The illness mentioned in the passage above involved vomiting blood. This raises the possibility that yellow fever may have existed in the New World prior to the Conquest. Yellow fever is an acute disease of certain tropical areas, characterized by fever and jaundice. It is caused by a virus transmitted to humans by the *Aedes aegypti* mosquito. Symptoms include, headaches, chills, pains in the back and limbs, and rise of temperature. Vomiting, furred tongue, constipation and urinary stoppage also occur. In the final stage of the disease the patient becomes very weak and black vomiting occurs. Jaundice also appears (Thomson 1976:948–49).

Three Mexican codices provide information on an epidemic characterized by bloody vomiting. The *Selden Codex* (Roll A2) shows a period of two years of epidemic illness with blood vomit and death in section 18. The *Borgia Codex* shows a one-year cycle of an epidemic with blood vomit, and diarrhea with melena in section 13, and the *Vatican Codex* B 3773 includes bad omens forecasting another epidemic of blood vomit in section 18 (Guerra 1964:42–43). In the books of *Chilam Balam de Chumayel, Tzimin,* and *Kaua* all have exactly the same record for the events in the *Katun 4 Ahau* (1481-1500). In the first book, blood vomit was said to be coming again for the fourth time (Roys 1967:133). Bishop Diego de Landa also mentioned this epidemic (1966:41).

This illness characterized by blood vomiting was called *xekik* (Villacorta Cifuentes ·1976:50). George C. Shattuck claimed yellow fever was imported to the New World from Africa (1938:39), but the discovery of the disease among South and Central American monkeys and the transmission of it among them by indigenous carriers (such as the mosquito *Haemogogus Spegazzinii* and Vampire bat) may point to an aboriginal form of the disease (Shimkin 1973:283; Villacorta Cifuentes 1976:45). If yellow fever were present in pre-Columbian times, it may

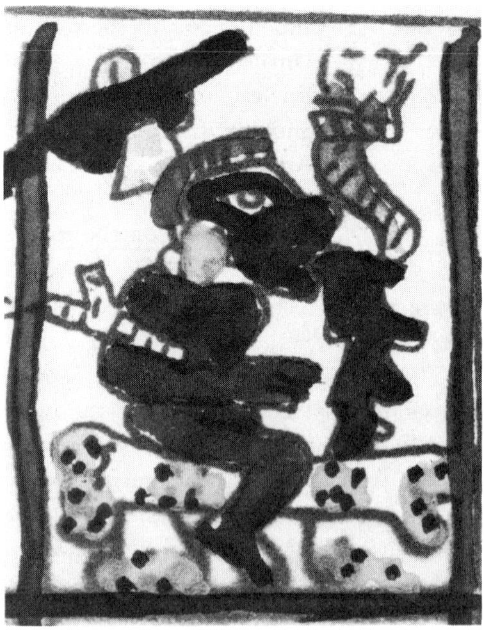

Figure 3
Tequech Mecauihni (The Throttler) from *Codex Vaticanus B* (1939:2).

have existed in a milder form than that which was brought over from Africa. Some of the tropical areas of Mesoamerica were densely inhabited prior to the arrival of the Europeans, and the lowland Indians may have developed a certain immunity to yellow fever. It is interesting to note that the Mexican codices which portray epidemics and the *Popol Vuh* of the Quichés were written by peoples not inhabiting the lowlands who were, perhaps, more seriously affected by the disease because they lacked immunity.

Other deities seem to have been more benevolent. The Quiché gods called Grandfather (*Xpiacoc*) and Grandmother (*Xmucane*) in the *Popol Vuh* (1971:22) watched over the birth of a baby (Ximénez 1967a:10). They were called *Ajk'ij* (daykeepers)—specialists who interpreted the sacred calendar. Grandfather and Grandmother were husband and wife and today in Momostenango the ideal is still that both members of a couple should be daykeepers (Tedlock 1982:85). These gods said what had to be done after a baby was born and did not permit the fire to be taken out of the house where there was a recently born child until a specified amount of time had passed (Ximénez 1967a:10). In ancient Mexico it was believed that the tonalli of a recently born child was strengthened by fire, and a fire was kept going constantly for four days in the room of a newly born baby (López Austin 1980:1:230–31; Ruíz de Alarcón 1984:43). It appears this was also a common belief in Guatemala.

Itzam Na, an important god in the Petén lowlands, was apparently worshipped by some highland Maya groups. The name was written as *Itzam* in Zuñiga and Morán and *Xtcamna* in Las Casas (Miles 1957:748). Itzam Na was a god of medicine and was invoked with *Ix Chel,* the moon goddess, and others at the feast of doctors and sorcerers during the month of Zip. In Yucatán he was known for curing the sick and bringing the dead back to life (Thompson 1972b:229).

Ix Chel was also mentioned in the dictionaries relating to the Pokoman area (Miles 1957:748) and in Las Casas (1967:2:505). In Yucatán, Ix Chel was a goddess of procreation, childbirth, and medicine, and that may have been true for the Pokomans as well. In present-day Yucatán, a group of pustule-forming diseases, including smallpox, are called "*kak* of the Virgin." As the moon goddess came to be identified with the Virgin Mary, it is likely that she was the patron of pustule-forming illnesses in ancient times (Thompson 1972b:242–43). Four incantations in the *Ritual of the Bacabs* (1965) treat of kak (Yucatec, fire) illnesses. Aboriginal syphilis was probably classed as a kak illness, and assignment of these ailments to Ix Chel, who had erotic associations, would have been logical (Thompson 1972a:50).

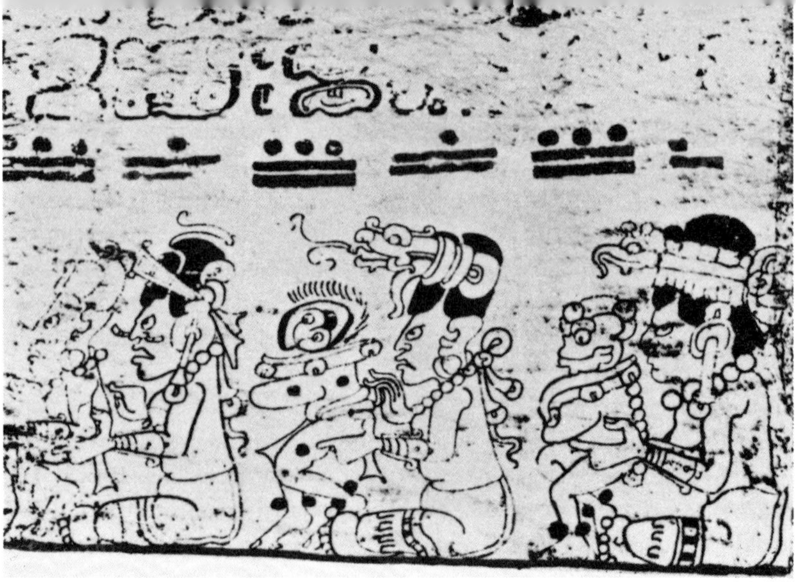

Figure 4
Ix Chel Holding Children. This drawing may tell of the effect upon children or childbirth when the conjunction of the moon with certain stars or planets fell on the days recorded, or perhaps, within the following interval (Thompson 1972a: 54–56). Courtesy of American Philosophical Society, Philadelphia, Pa.

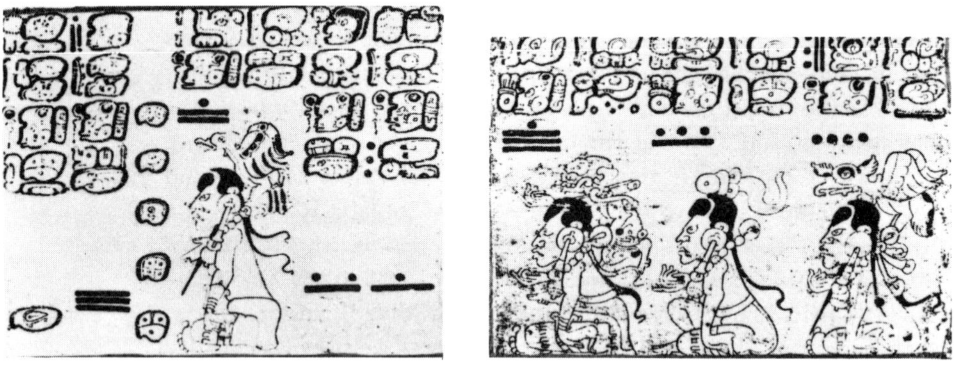

Figure 5
Ix Chel and Kak Illnesses. The goddess is shown with a vulture on her back at the left. Here vulture (*ch'om* in Yucatec) equals pock mark. Continuing to the right, the death god is shown on her shoulder. The next picture shows her with the sign for white on top of her head. In the picture to the far right a muan bird, which connotes evil, is perched on her shoulders (Thompson 1972a: 55–56). Courtesy of American Philosophical Society, Philadelphia, Pa.

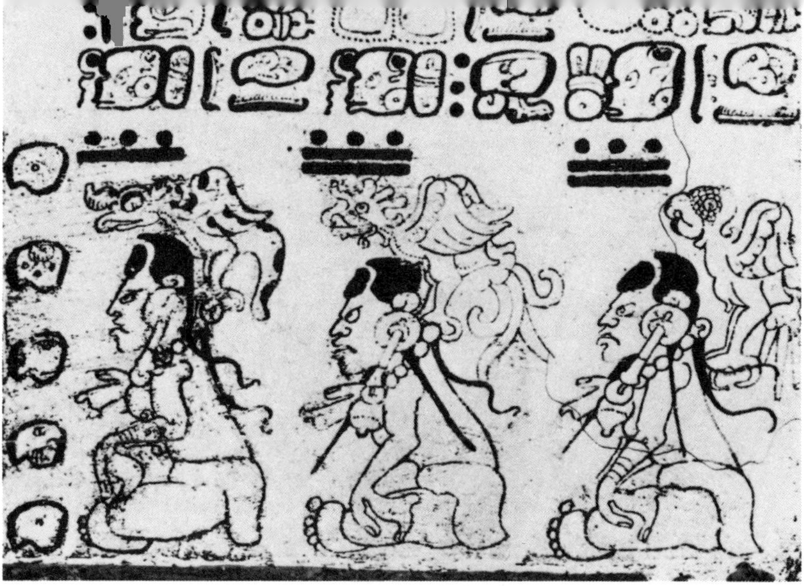

Figure 6
Ix Chel with muan bird at left, quetzal bird in middle (the bird being a metaphor for generation of children) and macaw at right, indicating macaw seizures—the generic name for a group of spasms and seizures (Thompson 1972a:57). Courtesy of American Philosophical Society, Philadelphia, Pa.

There are certain hints of a connection between *tancaz,* or *tamcaz* (Yucatec), a large body of seizures, spasms, and convulsions, and the moon. The present-day Kekchi relate epileptic fits to the phase of the moon. The Cakchiquel also believed that the moon caused illness, according to the Coto dictionary (Thompson 1972a:49–50), and the Quichés regarded Ix Chel as a goddess of procreation (Thompson 1972b:243).

Thompson also discussed the cult of the earth and thunder gods referred to as the *Tzultacah* by the Kekchis of Alta Verapaz. They were responsible for both sending fevers and illnesses and protecting people from them. Snakes were their servants and were sent to punish evildoers (1972b:274–75).

The Chortí god of remedies (*Ah Wink-ir T'sak-ar* or *Ah Wink-ir Q'opot*) is the patron of herbalists and the owner of all medicinal plants. He becomes angry if anyone wastes his medicines or uses them improperly (Wisdom 1940:401).

During the period just before the Conquest, the most important gods in the Guatemalan highlands were the gods of the most prominent lineages (Carmack et al. 1975:17). These gods were the ones who played the most important role in the documentary sources dealing with the Late Post-Classic times. What their functions may have been as far as

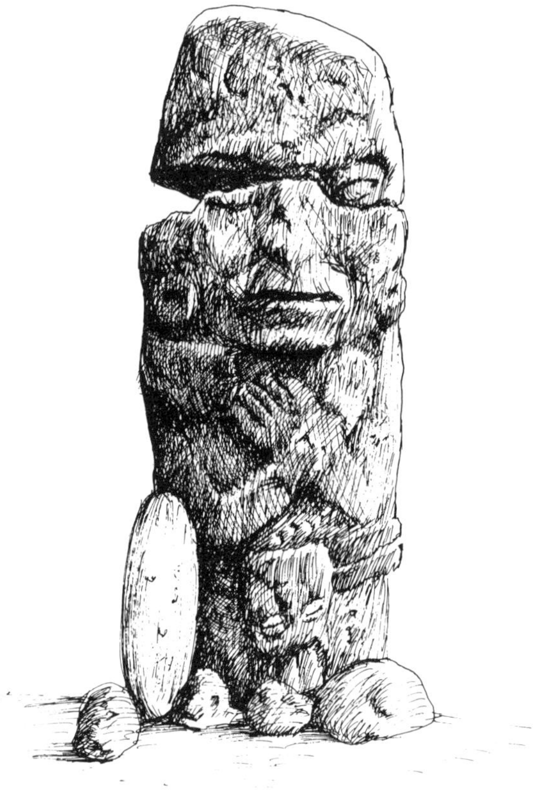

Figure 7
The Quiché Idol Ik (from Schultz Jena 1933:1, Plate IV).

medicine is concerned is not clear. Perhaps they were responsible for certain kinds of illnesses.

The idols of Chiya', the pre-Hispanic capital of Atitlán and its dependencies, were probably lineage gods who indicated when an illness would come as well as what form it would take. A more complete discussion of their role in illness is included under Community Rituals (see pp. 53–54.)

In more recent times Ruth Bunzel reported that the Quichés of Chichicastenango believed that all illness was sent by the Lord of Sickness (1967:145). No native name is given for this deity, but this may be a remnant of an ancient god who was thought to be responsible for many illnesses in earlier times.

In order to gain a more complete understanding of the role of the pre-Columbian gods in illness, it is useful to turn to the contemporary Maya highlands and look at some examples of how the causative role of deities is manifested in various Indian towns. The Judeo-Christian God plays the most prominent role in illness etiology in the western highlands (Adams and Rubel 1967:336). In the community of Santiago Chimaltenango God is held responsible for illness and punishes people who have committed such sins as engaging in sexual relations on ritual days, stealing, or quarreling with a spouse. Herbal medicines are used to aid in curing, but the only real cure is to obtain God's forgiveness. The guilt extends to the person's descendants (Wagley 1949:76). Perhaps in western highland communities like Santiago Chimaltenango where illness causation is largely seen to be the result of one deity, there was one god in pre-Columbian times who was believed to be the most important source of illnesses for those who had sinned. Serious illnesses, ordinarily of the epidemic kind, are viewed as being sent by God (Bunzel 1967:144; Douglas 1969:128). Common illnesses are not thought to be due to misconduct and are not ritually treated (Tax and Hinshaw 1969:93).

In Santiago Atitlán, William Douglas found that many aboriginal beliefs concerning illness continued to exist. Illness was viewed as either being sent by God or a sorcerer, or resulting from fright, from encountering the bad hour, or by committing a transgression against a particular spirit (1969:124–32). The Judeo-Christian God and specific saints have assumed the roles of the ancient deities and are considered responsible for certain illnesses and cures (1969:82–84, 124). As in Santiago Chimaltenango, a supernatural sanction is often thought to be necessary to effect a successful cure, and this will be done in addition to taking medicines (1969:172–73). Given the limited knowledge of pre-Columbian Tzutujil gods and their role in illness (see Orellana 1984), it is not possible to discover which saints have assumed the attributes of the various aboriginal deities. Similar beliefs exist among the Pokomans of Chinautla in the eastern highlands (Reina 1966:254–58), those of San Martín Jilotepeque (Gillin 1951:113–14), and the Mams of Todos Santos Cuchumatán (Oakes 1969:166–68).

In some towns, such as Chichicastenango and Aguacatan, many illnesses are attributed to the vengeance of ancestors who act either on their own initiative or at the behest of someone who has been wronged. The person who becomes ill as a result of the ancestors confesses and performs penance (Bunzel 1967:292–93). In Aguacatan ancestors mete out punishment to erring descendants. They may send illness, and the wrongdoer must then confess his sin and perform penance (Brintnall 1979:92). Ancestor cults were also important in pre-Hispanic times.

Important ancestors of the Quichés were mentioned in the *Popol Vuh* and of the Cakchiquels in the *Annals of the Cakchiquels*. The belief in ancestors has continued down into modern times among many highland groups.

Among the Ixil, *Q'esla Kub'a-l* is the most important god. He is a creator god who was more directly concerned with human events in the past. There are also intermediary gods who watch over humans and are the indirect cause of illness. If humans fail to serve the intermediary gods properly, they notify Q'esla Kub'a-l who sends illness to the offenders (Colby and van den Berghe 1969:96–97).

Other supernatural beings who are sometimes held responsible for illness are referred to as sprites or spirits (Spanish, *chanes, chaneka, chaneca, chaneque,* and *chancles*) and usually inhabit a specific locality. They are characterized by their dwarflike stature, light-colored skin, sometimes are bearded and blond, and generally have non-Indian or Spanish-American appearance. They may attack weak persons, or any person who has committed an offense against them. Some of these are probably of pre-Columbian derivation, but others are post-Conquest projections of ethnic social relations (Adams and Rubel 1967:337–38).

Sorcerers

Las Casas said that sorcerers (which he called *hechíceros* in Spanish) existed in Verapaz in pre-Hispanic times (1967:2:514–15). According to the *Florentine Codex,* the good sorcerer was "a wise man, a counselor, a person of trust—serious, respected, revered, dignified, unreviled not subject to insults. The good sorcerer . . . never harms anyone." The bad sorcerer, however, was "a doer [of evil]" (Sahagún 1961:10:31).

There were sorcerers who specialized solely in witchcraft, probably the hechíceros mentioned by Las Casas, who were called *ajitz* (Quiché, witch) in the Quichean area and *ah itz, ah kakzik,* and *ah var* among the Pokomans. The latter used chants called *ahalical.* Like modern witches, the ancient ajitz was probably consulted by persons of all ranks for private divination, curing, and witchcraft. Among the Pokomans, it was the only office open to women, and it may have had prerequisites similar to those experienced by witches today such as illness, a cure, and dreams (Miles 1957:750–51).

Powerful sorcerers were believed to be able to transform themselves into animals. As was mentioned previously, both the sorcerer and the animal form were called nahualli in ancient Mexico (López Austin 1980:1:419). In the *Florentine Codex* the "possessed one" was "one who transforms himself, who assumes the guise of an animal. {He is} a hater, a destroyer of people; an implanter of sickness . . . he destroys people, he burns wooden figures of them; he bleeds himself over others" (Sahagún 1961:10:31–32). Las Casas said witches were also called *balan* (*balam*) {meaning jaguar in Quiché} because they appeared to be jaguars to whomever looked at them. He said they were very harmful (1967:2:502).

In ancient Mexico the nahualli was feared because it devoured dead bodies or took advantage of sleeping victims and sucked their blood or robbed them (López Austin 1980:1:429). Today they are also thought to molest, "eat," or in some other way to cast illness or death on a victim. The nagual may eat the victim's soul and thereby kill him, or he may cast an aire or an object into the victim (Adams and Rubel 1967:341).

In Chichicastenango evil substances introduced into the body must be drawn out through the bodily eliminations, or through eruptions in order to cure the illness (Bunzel 1967:144). The belief in the introduction of a foreign body by magic to cause illness was very widespread in pre-Hispanic Mexico (Soustelle 1974:192). Sorcery was greatly feared, and Las Casas said that the punishment for sorcery was death by burning (1967:2:502).

In some areas in the Guatemala highlands where nagualism still exists, the ability to transform into different animals is attributed specifically to transforming witches. There is a separate category of sorcerers who are not capable of such transformation and therefore use other methods to harm people. In Santiago El Palmar, the transforming witch (*win,* Quiché) (who had a pact with the devil) was believed to be able to change into an animal or bird and to go stealthily into the homes of sleeping neighbors to rob them of money and goods. The win was usually male and while in animal form might take sexual advantage of sleeping women. The non-transforming sorcerer (ajitz) was also usually a male who attempted to harm others through magic. It was the sorcerer who made people ill. A sorcerer might also be a transforming witch, but it was not considered likely. In Santiago El Palmar, sorcerers (ajitz) used doll burial, exhumation of human bones, and then reburial, burial of other objects, prayers accompanied by the burning of copal incense, black candles, and incantations delivered in the cemetery (Saler 1964:312, 319, 320–21). Similar methods were used in Chuchexic (Cosminsky 1972:122). Such rituals were probably sometimes used to cause illness.

Sheila Cosminsky described two types of evil specialists—the witch and the sorcerer—who existed in Chuchexic. The witch (ajitz) had innate power and used it to harm others. He (most are males) might also be a transforming witch (*charikot,* Quiché). The other type of evil specialist, also usually male, whom Cosminsky called a sorcerer, practiced evil magic against others and learned it from other sorcerers or from books (1972:121–22). Both could make people ill.

The description of evil specialists given by Saler and Cosminsky is similar to that given by Alonso de la Peña y Montenegro, a seventeenth century observer for the Quiché area, who described two types of sorcerers of that time period. One, the true sorcerer (hechícero), had a pact with the devil and could do extraordinary things. This probably referred to a sorcerer who could transform himself. The other was said to be a cheat who claimed to understand illness and herbs and cured for payment. This could have referred to a sorcerer or to a curer who was not a sorcerer (Solano Pérez-Lila 1963:21). Today sorcerers may be called upon to treat someone if the illness is believed to be due to witchcraft (Tenzel 1970:377).

In concluding this discussion of illness causation, it may be useful to see how these factors were combined in the Quiché village of Chuchexic. The people of Chuchexic believed that there were certain conditions that made an individual susceptible to illness such as work, carelessness, diet, lack of cleanliness, luck (suerte), weak blood, ignorance, giving birth, and intense emotional experiences. Other conditions related more to ritual and social conduct and involved sins, such as lack of faith and not praying to God, not honoring the ancestors, not keeping a promise to a saint or spirit, bad thoughts, intentions, or deeds. There were also external conditions which took advantage of the factors that predisposed an individual to illness. These were environmental factors such as rain, sun, cold, wind (aire), the season (*el tiempo,* Spanish) and supernatural elements such as God, the saints, evil spirits, ancestor spirits, and sorcery.

Illness was a common punishment for violation of the moral code. Offenses could be social or ritual. Social offenses included family quarrels, gossip, or envy; ritual offenses included various types of sin. Sorcery was viewed as causing illness but usually it was the progressive nature of an illness and the failure to respond to treatment that led an ill person to suspect envy or sorcery as the cause (Cosminsky 1972:107–108; 119–21). Sorcery plays a similar role in illness causation in many highland Guatemalan towns.

CHAPTER THREE

Rituals and Medical Practitioners

RITUALS

Community Rituals

Although the gods were seen as being able to cause illness, it was also a widespread belief throughout Mesoamerica that they possessed the power to cure it as well (Schendel 1968:16). Therefore, many community-wide rituals were aimed at restoring or maintaining health. Las Casas mentioned such ceremonies which were held when illness threatened. Sacrifices were offered at these times, and the entire community participated (1967:2:214).

In Chiya' and its dependencies the major idol in each settlement indicated whether illness would come. When the lords wanted to know if there would be a pestilence, they chose persons to offer sacrifice to the idol and ask it whether illness was imminent (*RGA* 1964:99).

In one of the Tzutujil dependencies known as San Francisco during the colonial period, the idol indicated that illness was coming. It did so by appearing stretched out on the ground and bearing on its body the signs of the pestilence (*RGSF* 1952:130). In another Tzutujil settlement named Quioj (later called San Andrés), the idol appeared to the people stretched out on the ground with a rope around its neck (*RGSA* 1952:109). The most important idol in each settlement was the one that indicated the coming of major outbreaks, and this type of forecasting was probably common in other highland areas.

The Tzutujil lord selected to consult with the idol must have been a priest or someone from a prominent family attached to the temple because he had to fast for a long time, 260 days, or the full length of the sacred divinatory calendar of thirteen months of twenty days, and ate only once a day. He performed a sacrifice at the beginning of this fast and at the end—offering incense and his blood to the idol while asking it what the lords wished to know. The person chosen to consult the deity had to be ritually pure and could not go home or have sexual relations with his wife during the fast. The ruler also participated, staying in the temple on cloudy days and only going home if the day were clear (*RGAG* 1965:270). Ritual purity was considered to be very important during religious ceremonies (*PV* 1971:244), a belief that has survived down to the present in the Maya area. It is still believed that having sexual relations on ritual days causes illness (Adams and Rubel 1967:336).

Las Casas mentioned similar rituals which occurred in Verapaz but which did not specifically refer to illness. He said that men slept apart from their wives in buildings located near the temple for a period of seventy to one hundred days during ceremonial times. They sacrificed their own blood and burned incense. They also abstained from bathing and covered themselves with smoke from black torches as a sign of penitence (1967:2:214–215). Frequently, black signified death, violence, or sacrifice in Mesoamerica (Borhegyi 1959:45).

Pre-Columbian ceremonies were observed very carefully because the gods might otherwise send death to those who failed to participate or who committed serious ritual errors. The ceremonies may also have actually preserved some of the participants from contagion. Isolating from others and remaining in a room fumigated by smoke as the men of Verapaz did would have given some protection from epidemics.

Divination

Divination was the most prominent community ritual performed as a diagnostic method in pre-Hispanic times. There were several ways of performing it, but in the Guatemala highlands divination by lots was the most important. In the Tzutujil settlement of Quioj, lots were cast after the idol indicated what pestilence would occur:

> The old ones of the . . . [town] gathered and took out some ancient paintings by which they used to count the months and years, and they threw lots on the paintings and by where they fell they knew and understood the time when the . . . plague . . . was to take place (*RGSA* 1952:109).

Fuentes y Guzmán said that the most common means of throwing lots was by counting grains of maize (1972:3:400). The type of divination he described is still carried out in many highland towns today by individual curers and is used to diagnose the cause of illness. After the diagnosis is made, the curer will suggest a treatment for the illness. Tedlock described divination as performed by the diviners (aj k'ij) in the Quiché town of Momostenango. It was used to answer questions relating to illness and many other topics. Ritual purity was necessary, and diviners would not cast lots on days in which they had had sexual intercourse.

In case of illness, the first question asked was, "Does this illness have a master, an owner?" The answer will determine subsequent curing techniques used by the diviner, the patient, and the patient's family.

In Momostenango divination is carried out using *tz'ite* seeds (from *Erythrina corallodendrom* L.) and crystals. Divination involves several actions: the mixing, grabbing, and arranging of piles of tz'ite seeds; the counting and interpreting of the 260-day divinatory calendar; and the jumping and speaking of the diviner's blood (Tedlock 1982:153). In many areas of Mesoamerica blood is considered to be an animate substance, capable, in some individuals, of sending signals or "speaking." In the Guatemala highlands the diviner has a sensation within his or her body, variously described in the literature as a tingling, jumping, twitching, or twinging in the blood or muscles. This sensation conveys information about the past or the prospects of patients (Tedlock 1982:133). In Santiago Atitlán, divination does not involve the speaking of the blood but includes counting beans and/or maize kernels and the divinatory calendar:

> In many cases the *ajkun* carries as part of his divination implements a set of beans and/or a set of corn kernels which are cast on the table, then counted in sets of twos, threes, or fours . . . The count is usually, but not always, in terms of the *tzolkin* [the sacred calendar] . . . and may be repeated as many as three times to verify the count (Douglas 1969:154–55).

Momostecan diviners count the days according to the groups of seeds and crystals, beginning with the day of the divination or the day an illness began. The divination might require offerings to be made on particular days to effect a cure (Tedlock 1982:162–63, 170). Bunzel also described a similar form of divination used in Chichicastenango (1967:286–92). In the Quiché area certain days were considered to be beneficial or harmful for health. Day six was said to be good for healing, prosperity, or justice. Day nine meant pain, fighting, and chronic illness (Schultze Jena 1933:1:30).

The method of divination used in Chuchexic was similar to that used in Momostenango. The piles of maize were counted according to the day names of the 260-day calendar, and the interpretation depended on how many leftover seeds were in the last pile and on what day count this last pile fell. An odd number of seeds was a bad sign; an even number good. One number was interpreted as meaning the cause of the illness was within the family, another meant an external enemy was the cause (Cosminsky 1972:187).

Besides the aj k'ij, there were other types of diviners in ancient times. Among the Cakchiquels and Quichés, there were those who specialized in divination and were called *ajsakiwachinel* in Cakchiquel (Sáenz de Santa María 1940:39) and *hiq'vachinel* in Quiché. These were "far seers" who were prophet diviners with second sight who could "see at a distance" or scrutinize and peer into things. Among the Quiché, there were also *labahinel* or omen diviners, dream diviners (*ichiq'anel*), and *ilol,* or seers, who interpreted omens (Edmonson 1971:17). A Cakchiquel diviner, the *cholol k'ij* (probably *aj chol k'in* or "he who counts the days"), who seems to have been separate from the aj k'ij, determined if a day was good or bad for a celebration (Carmack 1973:17; Sáenz de Santa María 1940:210). Perhaps diagnosing illness was also part of the function of some of these diviners.

Another pre-Hispanic Quiché diviner was the *ah xulu,* or gleaner. These diviners asked their bodies divinatory questions and received answers by twitches in various parts of their bodies (Edmonson 1971:17; Sáenz de Santa María 1940:41). This form of divination was probably used as a method of diagnosing illness as it is today. Divination of this type involves the speaking of the blood. The role of the pre-Hispanic ah xulu has merged with that of the diviner (aj k'ij) in Momostenango.

In Chichicastenango, the diviner asks a series of questions of a client until suddenly answered by a tingling sensation in the veins of the forearms, which is said to be the voice of the blood (Bunzel 1967:290). Oakes reported that in Todos Santos the diviner touched his calf to feel twitches (1969:183). In Panajachel, Hinshaw observed that a twitching left arm, leg, or eye was a sign of impending misfortune. If the twitch occurred on the right, it indicated good luck (1975:128). Diviners in Chuchexic felt the twitch in the nerves, inside the body. One diviner referred to this method of divination as that of the movement of the blood and the body (1972:188).

In Colotenango, where most diviners were women, Leon A. Valladares described a practitioner who while sitting felt a "force" ascend her legs. This force informed her of the cause of illness and the possibility of its cure. If the force moved up the inside of her legs, the patient would live, but if it traveled up the outside, the patient would die (1957:218–19). In Santa Eulalia, diviners also received messages in their legs (La Farge 1947:182).

Among the Chortí, Charles Wisdom observed a diviner consulting a spirit believed to reside in the calf of the diviner's right leg. He chewed tobacco and rubbed the saliva on his leg. The diviner then asked his leg yes/no questions. Twitching indicated yes and no twitching indicated no. This was the most common method of divination among the Chortí (1940:344).

In Todos Santos pulsing was also used in diagnosing illness. The *pulseras* (Spanish) were mostly women, and they would tell a patient whether or not an illness would be fatal (Oakes 1969:184). Pulsing is not common in the Guatemala highlands but has been used as an additional diagnostic technique in some towns. Pulsing was used in Santiago Atitlán to determine the strength of the body's resistance to an illness (Douglas 1969:155–56). It was also practiced in the Chortí area for diagnosis. If the patient's pulse beat fast, the illness was said to be serious and was probably caused by magic. If slow, the illness was said to be probably of natural origin and easy to cure (Wisdom 1940:345). Pulsing was practiced separately from the interpretation of messages from the blood.

One final method of divination that is probably pre-Columbian and was observed by Fuentes y Guzmán was divination with tobacco. He said:

> They . . . worshipped and attributed god-like qualities to the herb they called *píziet* (*piciyetl* in Nahuatl), which is tobacco, concerning which they had superstitions. Smoking it and becoming intoxicated with it, they invoked the demon to learn of future events and to consult on the requests and petitions of others with which they had been entrusted (1969:1:281).

Some of the requests and petitions may have involved illness diagnosis and cure.

Bathing

Bathing was a common Indian therapeutic method used in all communities and was performed for purposes of personal cleanliness as well as for treatment of illness (Vogel 1973:253–59). Estrada said, "they have the custom of bathing in the rivers and still do this" (1955:73). Fray Antonio de Remesal reported that during an early post-Conquest epidemic, Indians with fevers were bathing in the rivers, and the cold water killed them quickly (1932:1:120). It was not the custom in sixteenth century Europe to bathe frequently (Schendel 1968:41–42), and the priests who came to the New World tried unsuccessfully to

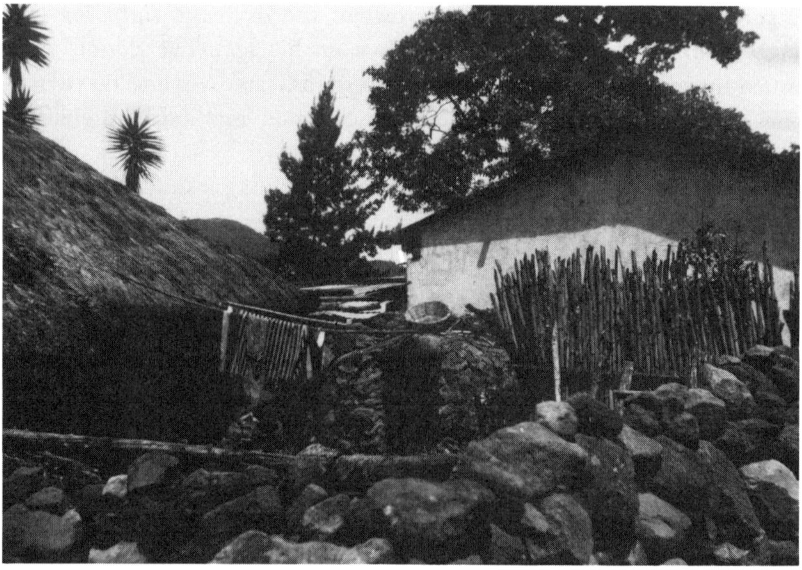

Figure 8
Sweatbath in a house compound in present-day Santiago Atitlán.

break the Indians of the habit. According to Fuentes y Guzmán, it was customary for the Indians to bathe their children often in the river, sometimes even two or three times a day (1969:1:221). This must have seemed incomprehensible to Europeans.

The sweatbath (*tuj,* Quiché) was an important feature of Indian hygiene. It was used for ritual purification, regular cleanliness, relaxation, and medicinal purposes. Among the Aztecs sweatbaths were deemed especially beneficial for soldiers, pregnant women, and new mothers (Schendel 1968:42), and this may have been the case in the highland Guatemala area as well. Today highland Indians still use the sweatbath to cure many illnesses (Tax and Hinsaw 1969:93; Virkki 1962:79). Pregnant women still bathe in the sweatbath before and after they give birth, and children are sometimes born in it (Rodríguez Rouanet 1969:57–58; Virkki 1962:79).

Samuel K. Lothrop gave a good description of a typical sweatbath located in Santiago Atitlán in 1928. It was about four feet high, had stone walls, and a wooden floor covered with clay. Inside was a pile of stones which would be heated and then drenched with water (1928:388). These structures appear to have changed little, if at all, since ancient times. Colonial observers also described them. Gage said:

> There is scarce any house which hath not also in the yard a stew, wherein they bathe themselves with hot water, which is their chief physic when they feel themselves distempered (1969:221).

Fuentes y Guzmán added:

> When a fever became strong, they entered the . . . *temazcales* [*temazcalli,* Nahua], which we call *estufas* [Spanish], or they lay out in the rays and heat of the sun, only drinking hot water and some very hot brews (1972:3:91).

Vázquez de Espinosa also mentioned sweatbaths:

> The Indians . . . have a very different system of bathing from what prevails elsewhere. Everyone makes, or has made, in his house a sort of small furnace which they heat with a fire; then the person who is to bathe strips and washes himself with hot water or they give him a good scrubbing, and then he gets into this furnace, which is hot or heated, and he sweats away there as long as he can stand it; then he comes out, wraps himself up, and gets into bed; in this way if they have tumors (syphilis) or any other trouble, they sweat it out immediately and become perfectly well (1968:219–20).

The sweatbath was also mentioned in the *Florentine Codex.* It was reputed to be most effective in treating the sick when very hot. If it was not very hot, it just gave the person a headache. It was used by pregnant women who were massaged inside the sweatbath by midwives. The newly delivered mother bathed there. Sick people were also massaged, and the bath was said to restore their nerves. Those with sores on their skin bathed and then medicines were applied to the affected areas (Sahagún 1963:11:191).

Along with the sweatbath medicinal waters were used as a cure for illness in highland Guatemala. Today Indians who live near sulphur baths continue to use the waters to cure such ailments as cramps, body pain, intestinal infection, and rheumatism (Rodríguez Rouanet 1971:327). In ancient times sulphur waters were used to treat certain conditions (Guerra 1966a:333). The medicinal waters at San Bartolomé Aguas Calientes and Totonicapán were mentioned by Fuentes y Guzmán (1972:3:46). Vázquez de Espinosa said that the hot baths of San Bartolomé Aguas Calientes were famous and the city had put up a bathhouse with rooms and compartments for invalids because the waters were very healthful (1968:220). Other healthful hot waters were located in Sonsonate (1968:228). Domingos Juarros described a vitriolic spring near Santo Domingo Mixco as being very good for curing diarrhea (1937:58).

It is clear that the Indians of pre-Hispanic and colonial Guatemala believed that water had curative powers. The sweatbath and medicinal waters were both used to treat a variety of illnesses as well as for regular personal hygiene—despite Spanish admonitions to the contrary.

Medical Practitioners

General Practitioners

Las Casas mentioned three types of medical practitioners who existed in Verapaz in ancient times. "They . . . had physicians (*médicos,* Spanish), great herbalists (*herbolarios,* Spanish), and perhaps even better sorcerers (hechíceros)" (1967:2:514–15). Among the Pokomans the physician was called *ah cut,* and this office was open exclusively to members of the nobility (Miles 1957:768). *Ajcun* was the Quiché equivalent and was derived from *cunabal,* meaning medicine (Mondloch 1978:176). This was written *ajqun* in Cakchiquel (Saénz de Santa María 1940:37) and ajkun in Tzutujil (Douglas 1969:146). Another doctor among the Cakchiquel was called the *ajkom* (Sáenz de Santa María 1949:37). This office was similar to the *ahicom* (doctor, curer) of the Pokomans and was apparently open to all (Miles 1957:768).

Las Casas described the role of the pre-Hispanic doctor (médico) in Verapaz:

> The doctor or doctors were accustomed to always be in the presence of the ruler or lord and when an indisposition came, it was not necessary to go look for them. He [the doctor] . . . applied the remedies of herbs and other natural aids that they knew from experience to be beneficial for the illness . . . After those have been given, they called the . . . diviner who had the office of casting lots, so that he might say what sacrifice would be best and most agreeable to the gods . . . Sometimes it was birds of a particular color—white, green gold, speckled, or dark, and other kinds and perhaps other animals. At other times he ordered . . . that men of a particular age or women of a particular type and manner be offered. Many times, when the illness was very grave and the sick person of high status, he ordered that a son be

> sacrificed, and usually the sons of slaves were sacrificed, and sometimes, though few, legitimate sons of the lords were sacrificed, when there were many to inherit. This was the last remedy, when every other medicine and sacrifice that could be found had been tried, and the illness was still on the increase. He [the doctor] ordered him [the lord] . . . to confess his sins . . . of adultery or fornication . . . They also confessed as a sin the breaking of any of their fasts, which were broken, according to their opinion, when they had intercourse with their wives (1967:2:525).

Perhaps this passage described the role of the Pokoman ah cut who was a noble and would be the doctor who treated other nobles. Las Casas also described another doctor, perhaps the ahicom, who treated commoners.

If anyone became ill, the first thing he did was to make sacrifices. Quail or other birds of the color appropriate to the illness were sent to the priest to be sacrificed for him. In the 260-day sacred calendar used for divination, colors were associated with each day, and certain days were responsible for certain illnesses. A doctor (médico) was also consulted:

> If he was a lord he always had a doctor in his household, but this was not true for commoners . . . The wife, if her husband became ill . . . immediately took a *manta* [blanket] or something else of value . . . to the doctor, saying, Sir, your son is ill. We pray that you will visit him, and without waiting for a reply, she put down what she had in front of him. If the doctor was free, he would go at once with her to visit the patient (Las Casas 1967:2:225–26).

According to the passage relating to treatment of the lords, the procedure followed by the doctor was to apply remedies, call the diviner to cast lots, make a sacrifice, and have the patient confess his sins. The most serious of all sins was the failure to fulfill the command of a doctor, even if it meant sacrificing all of the patient's possessions. Procedures were similar for commoners although confession could precede the casting of lots, and the doctor himself performed the divination (1967:2:226, 525).

After the Conquest, the roles of the ah cut, ahicom, and the diviner (aj k'ij) tended to merge. Curing rituals similar to those discussed by Las Casas existed in colonial times and have survived until the present. During the late eighteenth century, Archbishop Cortés y Larraz described a curing ceremony which incorporated confession. Curers (*ahcunes*) in Samayac, when called upon to heal the sick, took their patients to the mountain. There, in front of a ceiba tree, the curers lit candles, burned incense, and invoked the mountain deity to aid in the cure. Before ascending the mountain, the patient was made to confess before a candle (1958:2:268). Even today in Todos Santos, sick people are carried to the hills, and the owners of the hills are asked to help keep them alive (Oakes 1969:124).

Today in Santiago Atitlán the ajkun diagnoses and cures illnesses by means of prayers, divination, and medical treatment. Douglas said that there were two kinds of ajkuns: those who functioned primarily as priests and prayed for such things as good crops and good fortune, and those who were curers and diagnosed and treated illness. The second type of ajkun also performed the divination function formerly carried out by the aj k'ij, or pre-Hispanic Indian diviner. The two types of ajkuns existing today in Santiago Atitlán probably represent vestiges of the ancient priestly and physician curing roles (Douglas 1969:147; 154–55).

Cosminsky found that the people of Chuchexic were reluctant to consult a curer due to the expense and their fear of giving him the power to make a diagnosis. Although feared, a curer would be consulted if an illness persisted. People usually went to the pharmacy first, especially during the initial phase of an illness. This is probably precisely because the pharmacist was believed to lack supernatural power and because administering herbal and other medicines has been an early step in treatment since pre-Hispanic times.

In Chuchexic the curer is the least used means of treatment (Cosminsky 1977c:329–31). This reluctance may have existed in earlier times as well. Today curers with supernatural power are typically regarded with caution, and this was probably true in the past. In pre-Hispanic times people probably treated themselves first and then went to an herbalist or doctor if necessary. A sorcerer might have been consulted first if witchcraft were suspected.

Little is known about the way that the major treatment specialists were recruited into their calling in pre-Columbian times. Offices among the nobility were usually hereditary (Carmack 1981:157) so the ah cut probably came from a line of physicians and learned much of the lore of the profession from his relatives as an apprentice. According to Fray Pedro Morán, the ah cut was a teacher, orator, doctor, and counselor which suggests that learning was important among that group. Being nobles, physicians could read and write and study any available literature regarding medicine.

Doctors who were commoners may also have served apprenticeships although it is not known if their offices were hereditary. Probably not, as the office of ahicom was said to be open to all (Miles 1957:768). It is not likely that these curers could read since that privilege was ordinarily confined to nobility so they probably learned from observing and working with others.

Today in many Guatemalan towns individuals show a calling for the role of curer if they were continuously ill as a child or adolescent (Tenzel 1970:373). In Chuchexic one person went to a curer to determine the cause of an illness and was told that the divinatory calendar indicated that he should become a shaman. When he did, he recovered and remained well. This is an example of predestination, the belief that people born on certain days are destined for a particular role.

Among the Quichés certain days, such as Bats and Kiej, are thought to be the days of shamans (Cosminsky 1972:183). Today inborn power—which has been revealed and validated through illness and recovery, dreams and visions, special objects found, and various signs—indicates that an individual is destined to be a shaman or other type of treatment specialist (Cosminsky 1977c:328; Douglas 1969:140). This may have been the way in which commoners took up the role of curer in ancient times as well.

Specialists

Bite Specialists

Bite specialists exist today in the highlands and were probably a separate category of specialist in ancient Guatemala as well (Douglas 1969:141–43). In the *Popol Vuh* 7 Parrot asked grandfather and grandmother "What kind of poison can you make? What kind of poison can you cure?" (1971:41). This would seem to imply that bite specialists existed, but the two ancestors did not admit expertise in that area. Perhaps some general practitioners also had those skills as well as bite specialists. Among the present-day Tzutujil of Santiago Atitlán, snakebite specialists (*ruki kamats*) and spider-bite specialists (*ruki'om*) are separate, but some ajkun are also thought to be able to cure bites. In the past, bite specialists may have treated commoners while upper-class patients were treated by the doctor.

The bite specialists of Atitlán are thought to have knowledge of special prayers that must be said before, during, and after the removal of the poison. In treating a bite, the poison is removed by opening the wound with a piece of glass or obsidian blade, or a special thorn, and sucking out the blood, and presumably the poison. A tobacco poultice is then placed on the bite. This procedure may be repeated up to six times in a twenty-four-hour period. The role of bite specialist is predestined and knowledge of the necessary prayers comes to him in dreams (Douglas 1969:141–43). In Nebaj and Santa Cruz del Quiché a similar treatment is also used for snakebite. An incision is made with glass and compressed at the affected part to remove the venom (Rodríguez Rouanet 1969:84).

Diego García de Palacio, writing in the late sixteenth century, said that poisonous snakes and harmful insects were responsible for many stings and bites in the southeastern coastal region. Some of these harmful creatures were present in other coastal and highland areas, but they were more of a problem in the moist tropical zones. He also mentioned other pests such as four types of mosquitoes, many flies, and poisonous wasps whose stings made welts. If a bite was scratched, it made a sore. He reported, "I saw a boy fall down stunned from a bite, faint, and be out for two hours." Perhaps all people were not this sensitive to bites, but some individuals are more sensitive than others. There were scorpions and hairy worms which he said poisoned anything which their bodies touched, sometimes killing the victim. There were also poisonous centipedes (1927:74).

Ximénez mentioned some of the harmful and poisonous snakes existing in Guatemala in his *Historia Natural*: *mazatcuat* (*mazacoatl* in Nahua) (*Boa constrictor imperator*), *vivora* (Spanish), or rattlesnake (*Crotalus durissus*), *voladora* (Spanish), or jumping viper (*Botrops mummifer*), possibly the snake called *metlapilcoatl* in Nahua, coral snake (*Micrurus affinis*), *canti* (*Q'an tiy* in Quiché), yellow bite, or tropical water moccasin (*Agkistrodon bilineatus*) (Edmonson said that the name was also applied to the rattlesnake *Trigonocephalus specialis* 1971:14), *tamagazo* (*Botrops nasuta*), and *chichitur,* or *chinchintor* (which cannot be identified by binomial nomenclature or English). Ximénez also mentioned a snake called *buc-he,* or tail of bone, which was very poisonous (1967b:71–76). Another type of rattlesnake, *Crotalus horridus,* the timber rattlesnake, was also present in some areas and was used for medicinal purposes (Cochran 1943:7; González Sol 1939:71).

Fray Francisco Montero de Miranda, a Dominican priest who lived in Verapaz during the latter half of the sixteenth century, said that there were many poisonous snakes in that area (1954:350). In the southern piedmont the Indians feared the *tlamacaz coatl* (Nahua) which was said to be so poisonous that anyone bitten by it died within twenty-four hours (*RGAG* 1965:272). This may be the same snake called *tamagazo* by Ximénez. López Austin said that this snake was called *tlalmazacohuatl* in Mexico and inhabited hot areas, appearing when it rained (1974a:61).

Given the variety of poisonous snakes and insects, it is not surprising that the Indian medical system included bite specialists. Oakes said that shamans who cured bites in modern times in Todos Santos used loops of cord as tourniquets or employed cauterization (1969:185). Ximénez also mentioned that he experimented with burning the bitten area with a small fire brand which consumed the venom so that it did not spread (1967b:73). The curers of Todos Santos also made a poultice from water in which the skin from the snake's throat had soaked (Oakes 1969:186). Herbal cures were also used by bite specialists and will be discussed in Chapter Four.

Bonesetters

There is a passage in the *Popol Vuh* which refers to setting bones. Grandfather and Grandmother mentioned that they set bones (1971:41). This is the only reference to bone setting in the early documentary sources relating to highland Guatemala, but it does indicate that the practice existed. Fuentes y Guzmán described the treatment used by the Indians for fractures during the late seventeenth century (see Chapter Four). The main medicines were herbal, but bonesetters probably used massage just as they do today (1969:1:244; 1972:2:67–68; Rodríguez Rouanet 1969:64). The break is sometimes splintered or bandaged up (Gillin 1951:117; Paul 1976:77), and this was probably done in ancient times as well.

Today the bonesetter heals with the help of supernatural power and is predestined to the calling. The source of his or her power is usually a magical object, such as a small bone, and this item, containing supernatural power, aids the practitioner in locating the break (Girón Mena 1979:27; Paul 1976:77–78; Rodríguez Rouanet 1969:62–63). In Santiago Atitlán the bonesetter (*rukoy bak'*) uses his sacred objects (*k'ijbal* or *cuentecitos* in Spanish) to diagnose the injury. They are used as implements in a massage of the injured area and are thought to play a major part in re-setting broken or disjointed bones and in reducing the pain of the injury (Douglas 1969:143).

In ancient times the articulations of the joints were understood and sometimes portrayed in stone sculpture. Dr. Jorge Villacorta Cifuentes included one figure from the Pipil-speaking area of El Baul that showed the articulations (1976:129–30). Other earlier figurines from Kaminaljuyu also demonstrate knowledge of articulation which may have come from warfare or human sacrifice (1976:127–28).

The collection of osteological material in the National Museum of Archaeology and Anthropology in Guatemala City comes mainly from San Agustín Acasaguastlán, Kaminaljuyu, Zaculeu, and Quiché. There were not many fractures found, but the peculiar curvature of the left femur of a skeleton coming from tomb B in Kaminaljuyu may have been from a badly joined break (Villacorta Cifuentes 1976:130–31). Perhaps this was the result of ancient bone setting techniques.

Herbalists

Las Casas mentioned herbalists, and the herbalist was called *qumanel* among the Cakchiquel. The herbalist was defined by Varela as one "who cures; the doctor" (Sáenz de Santa María 1940:236). Today in Colotenango this specialist is called *kánal* and uses both plant medicines and pharmaceuticals. This occupation is usually separate from that of the *chimán* (shaman)—who treats illnessses resulting from sin which are sent as punishment by God. The chimán uses magical and religious means. Some individuals, however, appear to perform both roles (Valladares 1957:121–22).

In Santiago Atitlán, the *ajkomanel* is similar to the k'anel of Colotenango and the qumanel of the Cakchiquel and treats the sick without the use of prayer. Illness is treated as a physiological condition, and like pre-Hispanic herbalists, they treat it empirically by using herbs and, in more recent times, pharmaceuticals. The ajkun also uses herbal remedies and sometimes gets them from the pharmacy (Douglas 1969:158–59, 173).

Among the Chortí there are two general classes of curers: those who use supernatural power in curing (and are usually males), and those without supernatural resources who are said to "cure with their hands." Included in the second category are midwives, massagers, surgeons, and herbalists (Wisdom 1940:343). The latter are usually older women who also serve as midwives. The god of remedies is the patron of the herbalists (1940:354, 401). Because the herbalist does not have supernatural powers, the role is not a predestined one and can be taken up by anyone having an interest in or knowledge of medicinal plants. There is no information in the early sources as to whether the pre-Hispanic Guatemalan herbalists did formal research or whether they were primarily commoners who learned their trade by serving as apprentices to other herbalists. Herbal medicine was very important in aboriginal times, and the cures used by Indians in colonial times are given in Chapter Four.

Midwives (*iyom* in the Quichean languages) existed in pre-Columbian times and continue to practice their profession today in most highland towns. García de Palacio discussed the role of the midwife in the Pipil-speaking town of Asunción Mita in southeastern Guatemala. The Pipil allied with the Tzutujil in pre-Hispanic times (Fuentes y Guzmán 1972:2:36) and may have shared some cultural patterns with Maya-speakers. García de Palacio said that at the time of delivery, the woman confessed her sins to the midwife (*partera,* Spanish) who attended her:

> If the woman could not give birth, then they made her confess her sins. If she still did not give birth, her husband confessed his sins, and if she still could not and if he had confessed that he had been with someone, they went to the house and brought his manta and loincloth and wrapped them around the pregnant woman so that she could give birth. If this did not work, the husband sacrificed blood from his ears and tongue (1927:88).

In another passage García de Palacio related that the midwife also sacrificed her blood and sprinkled it to the four winds while making

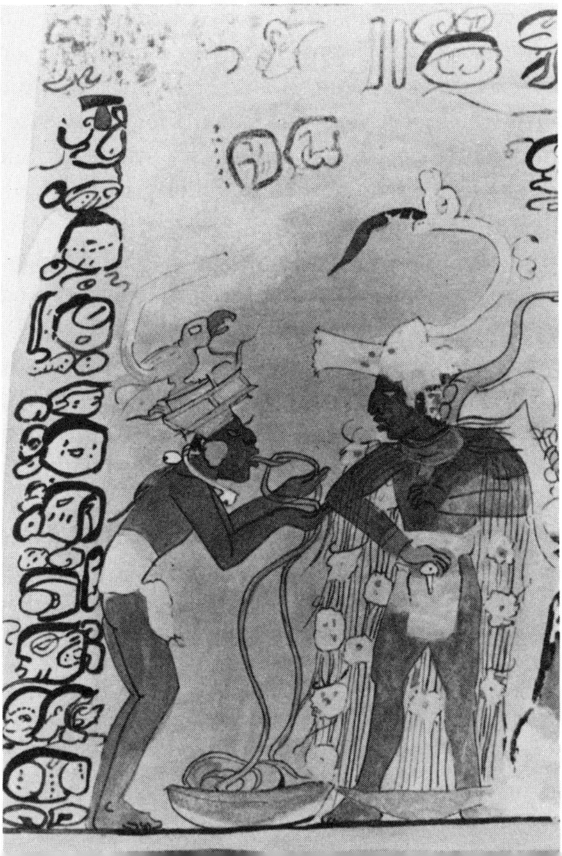

Figure 9
Self-Sacrifice Performed by Two Men. The man on the left draws a rope from a coil in a basket or bowl through his tongue, while the other man pierces his penis with a pointed bone or stingray spine, letting the blood fall to the container at his feet (Coe 1975:25 and Plate 15). Courtesy of Dumbarton Oaks Research Library and Collection, Washington, D.C.

invocations and performing ceremonies to facilitate a delayed birth (1927:76).

The clothing of the husband was said to be used to facilitate delivery. Foster pointed out that in Spain various articles of men's clothing may be used as an aid in childbirth (1960:112). Although using clothing during birth may have been adopted from Spanish custom, Landa said that it was customary in Yucatán to put an idol representing Ix Chel, the goddess of childbirth, under the bed of a laboring woman (1966:129). Ix Chel was regarded as the patroness of childbirth among some highland groups as well (Thompson 1972b:242–43).

In some modern towns a difficult delivery is still seen as an indication that the mother has behaved badly (Rodríguez Rouanet 1969:60). In Chichicastenango, if a woman is unable to give birth, a diviner is called in to discover the reason. The diviner may determine that she is being punished for her sins, and the husband will be called in to whip her to free her (Bunzel 1967:96).

The García de Palacio passage also seems to imply that the birth did not occur in the house. Babies are usually born at home today, but traditionally, birth took place in the sweatbath (Cosminsky 1972:180). In Todos Santos, on the day of a baby's birth, after delivery, the mother takes a sweatbath with the aid of the midwife, but the birth does not occur there. For twenty days, a sweatbath must be taken every second or third day (Oakes 1969:42). This is quite different, however, from Chinautla which lacks sweatbaths. There the mother refrains from all bathing for two months after birth (Reina 1966:243). In Chuchexic some midwives require extensive prenatal use of the sweatbath while others do not. After birth, the mother remains at home for the twenty-day period, and the midwife is supposed to come every three or four days and assist the newly delivered mother in taking a sweatbath (Cosminsky 1972:180–81).

The main functions of the midwife were to examine the pregnant woman during the last months of pregnancy, prescribe dietary and hygienic rules, and to attend the birth (Villacorta Cifuentes 1976:139). She probably tended the fire going in the room of the newly born baby (Ximénez 1967a:10). This may have been related to the belief in the tonalli. In the Aztec area a fire was kept going for four days, until the child was ritually bathed and named and received his definitive tonalli (López Austin 1980:231).

Benjamin and Lois Paul described the procedures used by the midwife in recent times in San Pedro la Laguna. She massaged the pregnant woman and felt the abdomen to see if the baby was in the correct position for delivery, turning it if not (Paul 1974:294). After the baby was born, the number of future births was foretold by reading the markings on the umbilical cord (Paul and Paul 1975:708; Cosminsky 1977b:86).

Las Casas described the ritual regarding the birth of a child, but he did not specifically mention the midwife. He said that when a child was born, all of the jars and things which had been used on the day of the birth and the stone used to heat the mother's abdomen were dedicated and offered in the spring or river. Lots were cast to see when the umbilical cord should be cut. They chose a day, placed the cord over an ear of maize, and used a new knife to cut it. The kernels from the ear of maize were removed and planted if it were the proper season. If not, they kept the kernels until they could be planted. After new maize grew from the planted kernels, they made gruel for the child and gave the rest of the harvest to the priest or diviner. Some kernels were kept for the child to plant when he grew up (1967:2:227–28).

Fuentes y Guzmán described a similar maize ritual. He said that after a baby was born, the Indians took a multicolored ear of maize and put the umbilical cord over it and cut it with a new knife. The ear was then smoked and planted at the appropriate time. The yield was harvested, sown again, and the increase served, after a share had been given to the priest, to maintain the child until he could plant his own *milpa* (Spanish) (1969:1:280–81). Although Las Casas and Fuentes y Guzmán did not mention the midwife in these ceremonies, she is still the one who cuts the child's umbilical cord today and probably did so in these pre-Hispanic rituals (Cosminsky 1972:181).

There is some skeletal evidence which demonstrates that birth did not always go smoothly in pre-Hispanic times. In Mound No. R22 at Finca Zunil in the piedmont an aborted fetus was buried around 800 A.D. The burial was elaborate for a fetus and the child may have been from a noble line (Villacorta Cifuentes 1976:140–43). Another burial in the tomb of Mound C at Chicol in Huehuetenango contained the skeletons of twins and a woman around thirty-five years old, presumably the mother. All three appear to have died in the birth (1976:144–45).

Fuentes y Guzmán described another unusual birth, that of Siamese twins, born in 1675 in the town of Santo Domingo Sinacao. They were taken to the capital where they were viewed by all. He said they were:

> . . . of beautiful figure, and perfectly human in the perfection and symmetry of the features. From only one abdomen two distinct perfect bodies were born, separated and divided with two bodies, each one of them with two complete arms and perfect hands, two beautiful, agreeable faces of an equal likeness, similar in every

> respect, two legs . . . and above the part that makes the waist another little leg which was very short, although it also had its foot and toenails like the others (1969:1:310).

Paul and Paul noted that the shaman had a greater role in the northwestern highlands than in the western area. His role was primarily to offer prayers, however, and the obstetrical duties of the actual birth were still performed by the midwife (1975:717–18). In pre-Columbian times the two may have shared ritual functions (Villacorta Cifuentes 1976:139). It is clear from the passage of García de Palacio that the midwife performed some ritual functions in Asunción Mita.

Today midwives are predestined for their calling, and this has probably been the case since early times. In Santiago Atitlán, such women receive signs (*señas,* Spanish) of their destiny, but are reluctant to take up the profession because it requires behavior considered inappropriate for a woman:

> They must go about at night, they must respond to the requests of almost anyone who needs their help, and since the proper pre- and post-natal care require a considerable involvement of time, they often feel, or are made to feel, that they are neglecting their own families (Douglas 1969:145–46).

In Chuchexic a woman becomes a midwife if she has a dream or finds an object that is then interpreted by a diviner as indicating that that is to be her role in life. She is born to fulfill this destiny, but does not know it until she has the dream or sign. If she fails to fulfill her role, she may be punished by God, possibly with illness (Cosminsky 1972:179). In San Pedro la Laguna many people can name women who have become ill and even died because they failed to fulfill their role (Paul and Paul 1975:710). In that town the midwife suffers a chronic and severe illness and is only cured when she has been validated by a local diviner who sponsors her:

> She learns the arts of midwifery from the spirits of dead midwives, the supernatural patronesses of childbirth, who appear in her dreams and place in her path the tangible proof of her divine power—scissors or a penknife for cutting the umbilical cord, and a conch shell or strangely shaped bone, stone, or figurine having magic power to cure sterility (Paul 1974:296).

She may have had a piece of amniotic tissue draped over her head at birth as well (Paul 1975:450). In San Pedro selection of the midwife

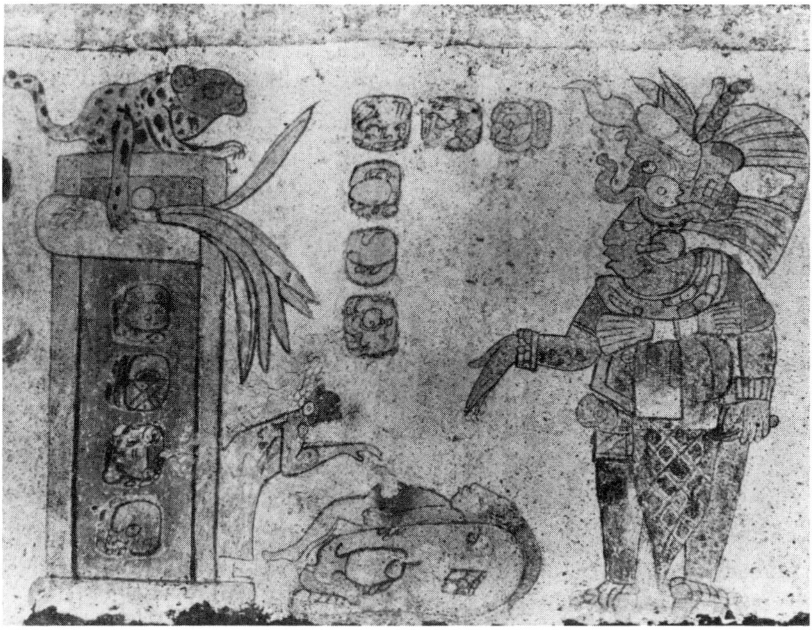

Figure 10
Heart Sacrifice. The victim, a child, lies prone. The small figure to the left, reaching toward the victim may be the recipient of the heart. The figure to the right is the executioner, carrying in his left hand a small obsidian knife with a bloody point (Coe 1982:16).

involves a series of events such as birth signs, premonitory dreams, illness, and revelation by a diviner of her destiny, discovery of magic objects, and dream instruction (Paul and Paul 1975:711).

Surgeons

The surgeon was another pre-Hispanic medical specialist. Unfortunately, little information in the colonial documentary sources for highland Guatemala refers specifically to Indian surgeons. There was a specialist among the Cakchiquel called the *ajtok'ola,* who was a surgeon who bled people and freed them from sorcery (Sáenz de Santa María 1940:40). This practitioner also existed among the Aztecs and was called *tezoc* or *teximani* but was separate from the surgeon who was called *tetecqui* or *texoxotla ticitl* (Guerra 1966a:321). The surgeon and phlebotomist (bloodletter) were probably separate in ancient Guatemala, but there is no information relating to the former. Edmonson said that the phlebotomist was called *ah hut* among the Quiché (1965:5). The ah hut was probably equivalent to the Pokoman ah cut who was a noble and a physician. Perhaps the doctor performed bleeding on the lords while the ajtok'ola treated commoners. It is not clear whether the physician generally performed surgery or whether a separate practitioner fulfilled that role as well in pre-Hispanic highland Guatemala.

Although surgery was not as highly developed as herbal medicine in Mesoamerica, Indian surgeons were probably able to perform dental extractions and mutilations, make prostheses, extract foreign bodies, drain abscesses, suture wounds, set fractures, and dislocations as well as perform amputations, bleeding, circumcision, and possibly cranial trepanation (Villacorta Cifuentes 1976:107) They may have learned much about human anatomy from performing human sacrifices and observing wounded warriors.

Obsidian knives were used as surgical instruments, and would have been adequate for simple operations (Martínez Durán 1964:33). Don Crabtree discussed the sharpness of the obsidian blade and mentioned its use as a surgical instrument. A wound made with a glass knife heals more rapidly than one made with knives of other substances (1968:470).

Ximénez noted that the Indians were very good at bleeding and were often preferred by the Spanish. He described their technique in using the obsidian blade:

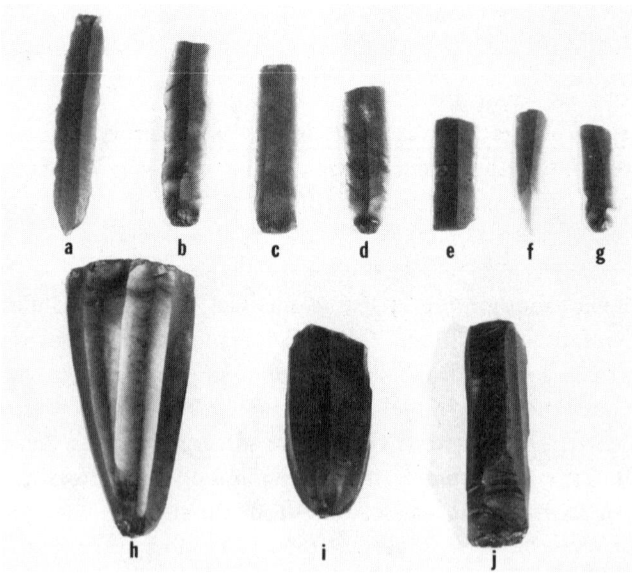

Figure 11
Obsidian blades a–g. Obsidian cores h–j.

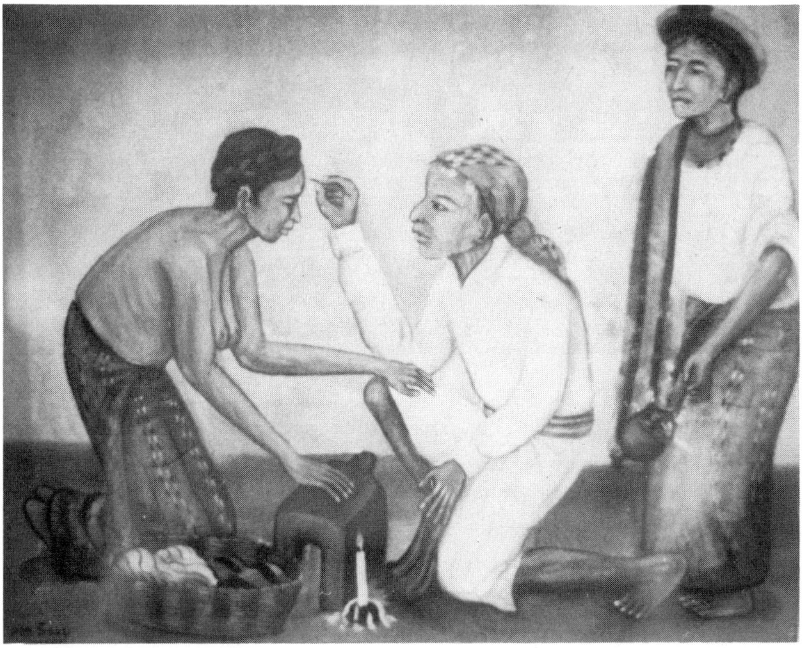

Figure 12
Curer of Santiago Atitlán treating patient with obsidian blade.

> Among the Spanish those [Indians] who bleed well are well known. They do it so deftly that they no sooner tie up an arm and extend it so that the vein shows, than they stick in the point, give it a fillip, and draw blood without cutting an artery. Because the point is so sharp and goes right to the vein, there is little risk. I have seen many Indians bleed, and all bleed without missing the vein (1967b:329).

Pedro de Alvarado, the conqueror of Guatemala, and his men also relied on Indians for bleeding (Fuentes y Guzmán 1972:3:282).

Oakes mentioned that curers in Todos Santos used phlebotomy (1969:183). Phlebotomy is also practiced in Santiago Atitlán, and paintings by local people demonstrate the procedure (see Fig. 12). Douglas said that blood letting was frequently used in conjunction with other treatment methods. A splinter of glass or an obsidian blade was used to puncture the skin, usually a number of small punctures were made, to allow "bad blood" to flow out—supposedly carrying with it the illness (Douglas 1969:157). This may be a native way of

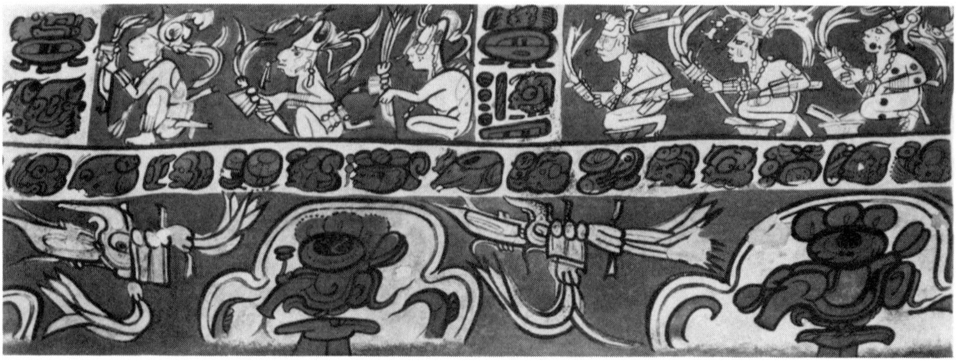

Figure 13
The Huehuetanango Vase. The upper half shows two groups of men separated by glyphs. Each holds a bone awl or knife in his hand. They are drawing blood from their penises and allowing it to drop on bark paper in a bowl (Gordon and Mason 1925–34: Plate 26). The University Museum, University of Pennsylvania.

performing phlebotomy while opening a vein was the most common European method.

Cupping is another form of bleeding practiced today which probably is not aboriginal in origin. This involves placing a cup or gourd upside down over a vessel of boiling water—rim touching rim. The cup gets hot. The curer puncture the patient's skin repeatedly with broken glass and places the cup over the skin for a few minutes so that the cup will fill with blood. Repeated applications may be carried out (Simeon 1977:26). Douglas described how cupping was performed in Santiago Atitlán. The cupping device was a large hollow gourd having a mouth about the size of a silver dollar:

> A small hole in the base of the gourd can be closed with wax. A piece of cotton, soaked in aguariente or kerosene is dropped into the gourd and ignited. The . . . [gourd] is then applied to the patient, mouth first, at the site of the "bad blood." A vacuum is created and when the gourd is removed, by puncturing the small hole in the base of the . . . [gourd] and breaking the vacuum, a large welt is left which is then punctured with . . . [a] glass sliver (1969:157–58; Cosminsky 1972:176).

Cupping, known in Spanish as *la ventosa,* was basic to classical Hippocratic therapy (Foster 1953:206) and was very likely adopted by the Indians after the coming of the Spaniards.

Surgery may have been necessary at times, especially in treating war wounds. A common weapon was the warclub which had razor-sharp blades and could cut a man in half (*RGA* 1964:99). The bow and arrow, knives, slings, and obsidian-tipped spears were also used and would have caused serious wounds (Follett 1932:380–81). Fuentes y Guzmán said that the Indians had weapons which penetrated the body deeply and, when thrown, caused fear because of the terrible wounds they could inflict (1972:2:15). The worst wounds probably killed the victims, but some men may have been saved through surgery and herbal treatment.

Zuñiga mentioned circumcision and said that it was performed on "little boys who have not the power of seed" (Miles 1957:764). The fact that circumcision was practiced and was probably part of temple routine is not surprising considering that blood sacrifice from the penis, tongue, arms, muscles, and ears was performed by all men regularly as part of religious rituals. This type of sacrifice was done by cutting the part of the body selected with a sharp obsidian blade (Las Casas 1967:2:515; *RGAG* 1965:269). A jade phallus found in the vicinity of Chichicastenango also demonstrates that circumcision was practiced in pre-Hispanic times by the Quichés (Villacorta Cifuentes 1976:107–108).

There is some debate as to whether trepanation (removing a circular piece of the skull by surgery) was ever practiced in the Guatemalan highlands. There is little information available on surgical techniques in this area so it is difficult to say if ancient surgeons could have performed the operation successfully. Examples of skulls with perforated crania have been found at Zaculeu and Tzicuai, but some authors attribute the holes to disease rather than to ancient surgery (see pages 128–29, 157 for a discussion of these crania and possible disease) (Villacorta Cifuentes 1976:108–109).

Tatooing was also performed "with the point of a blade which was very sharp." Carbon was then put into the wound so that it was colored black (Ximénez 1929:1:103). The ears and nasal septum were sometimes perforated so that ear plugs and nose ornaments could be worn (*PV* 1971:218).

In the Chortí area in recent times surgeons were observed performing many of the functions that characterized their profession in aboriginal times. They mended broken bones, treated wounds, stopped bleeding, treated gangrene and sores, and opened the flesh to let evil air escape. Wisdom said that in general, they treated all flesh conditions requiring exernal treatment and for which no ritual treatment was needed (1940:356). They were, therefore, similar to herbalists in that their role was probably not a predestined one, nor were they thought to have supernatural powers.

There were probably other types of pre-Hispanic medical specialists in the Guatemala highlands, but the ones discussed here were some of the most important. After the Conquest, native medical practices changed. This was primarily due to the decline of the nobility and the system of offices and Spanish prohibitions concerning the practice of the native medical-religious system. As pre-Hispanic written knowledge and the hereditary offices were gradually lost, the knowledge and practitioners tending to remain were primarily that of the common class. Due to these factors and the large drop in population after the Conquest (see Chapter Four) many roles were either dropped or forgotten and others merged.

CHAPTER FOUR

Illness and Herbal Medicine

This chapter will focus on illnesses mentioned by Guatemalan colonial writers which were present in the highlands and the herbal medicines used to treat them.

Arthritis, Muscle Pain, and Rheumatism

Arthritis refers to inflammation of the joints, and rheumatism is used to describe many conditions associated with diseases of the joints, tendons, muscles, or bones (Rothenberg 1968:36, 252). Remains of individuals suffering from arthritis have been found at the archaeological sites of Kaminaljuyu and Zaculeu (Villacorta Cifuentes 1976:132–33), and it may have afflicted many of the older people in ancient times. Club moss (*Lycopodium dichotomun* Jacq.) was considered to be effective in removing joint pain (Fuentes y Guzmán 1972:2:42–43). The description of this plant's curative properties given by Fuentes y Guzmán is similar to that of Hernández (Figueroa Marroquín 1957:202), so the same remedy was probably in use in both Mexico and Guatemala.

Although there is little information in the Guatemalan colonial sources for this group of ailments, several herbal treatments were mentioned by modern authors. Some of these plants were also used in earlier times as medicinal plants and probably had greater usage than those specific applications which have come down to us through the documents. Others are known only from the contemporary literature but may also have been used in earlier times.

Erwin Dieseldorff in his study of the medicinal plants of Verapaz said that the button plant (*Borreira ocimoides* DC.) was used there to treat rheumatism because the plant had a sedative effect. *Verbesina*

(Spanish) (*Salmea scandens* DC.) was also used, and jalap (*Ipomoea purga* Hayne) served to wrap up parts of the body affected by rheumatism (1940:194–95). Fuentes y Guzmán mentioned the latter plant but only discussed its purgative properties (1969:1:246). Dieseldorff said that verbesina had dark lilac flowers, and this casts some doubt on his identification because the flowers were said to be white (or greenish with age) in Morton (1981:963), a more reliable source.

Aguilar Girón discussed some plants used in contemporary times to treat rheumatism. The extract of a species of wintergreen (*Gaultheria odorata* Willd.) was applied in cases of articular rheumatism (1966:362). A decoction of yellow sage (*Lantana camara* L.) and the bark of Humboldt's willow (*Salix chilensis* Mol.) were other remedies (1966:358, 365). The latter remedy was also mentioned by Wauchope (1948:50). Bitterwood (*Trichilia havanensis* Jacq.) was used in hot baths for rheumatism (Aguilar Girón 1966:365). Other plants mentioned by Aguilar Girón as rheumatism cures were: the terebinth sumac *Rhus terebinthifolia* Schlect. & Cham.), dumbcane (*Dieffenbachia seguine* Schott), an essential oil made from the leaves of the allspice pimenta (*Pimenta dioica* Merr.), and a type of pepper (*Piper auritum* HBK.) (1966:350, 360, 364, 368).

In contemporary times in Chinautla people with rheumatism sometimes tied up the affected spot with cord taken from an old firecracker or rocket made from the century plant (*Agave americana* L.) (Reina 1966:188–89). In San Pedro la Laguna tobacco (*Nicotiana* spp.) has been used to treat rheumatism by warming up the green leaves and applying them to the painful areas (Rodríguez Rouanet 1969:84; *see also* Hernández 1959:2:82). For rheumatism and pain in the arms, legs, hips, and back cupping was reported as the standard remedy in Chinautla. It was, however, never performed on the chest and stomach because these areas housed the heart and intestines which were considered to be very delicate organs (Simeon 1977:26).

Villacorta Calderón included Florida waltheria (*Waltheria americana* L.), and jimson weed (*Datura stramonium* L.) as rheumatism remedies in his book *Monografía del departamento de Guatemala* (1926:75, 80). He also mentioned mugwort (*Artemisia vulgaris* L.), as a cure (1926:76), but this could not have been used in aboriginal times since it is a plant of Old World derivation.

Other herbal remedies have been used in recent times for muscular cramps and pains. The drug tread-softly (*Cnidoscolus urens* Anth.) was used in San Ildefonso Ixtahuacán and Huehuetenango (Rodríguez Rouanet 1969:78). Hernández said travelers used this plant on their legs to diminish fatigue (1959:2:123). In Nebaj and Santa Cruz del Quiché strips of rubber from the Panama gum tree (*Castilla elastica* Sessé) were

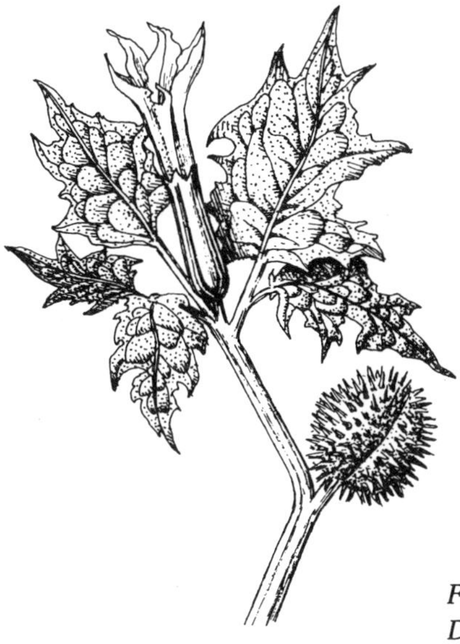

Figure 14
Datura stramonium (Thomson 1978:60).

wrapped tightly over a cramp for five to six minutes to alleviate it. In these same towns muscle cramps were treated by massaging the affected area with a cloth saturated with turpentine from the Montezuma pine tree (*Pinus montezumae* Lam.) (Rodríguez Rouanet 1969:77). The latter may be an ancient treatment because Fray Alonso Ponce, who traveled throughout Guatemala during the latter half of the sixteenth century, said that trees near Quezaltenango produced clear turpentine which was considered to be very medicinal (1873:438).

In San Pedro la Laguna and Sololá a type of hawthorn (*Crataegus pubescens* Steud.) was used to cure muscle cramps. The plant was cooked and put into a gourd which had some pieces of glass at the mouth. When it was full, they took it out and applied the mouth of the gourd to the cramp, pressing hard, and removing it quickly until blood came forth. Then the hawthorn was given to the sufferer to drink with some liquor (aguardiente) (Rodríguez Rouanet 1969:77). Here, as in Chinautla, herbal medicine was used in conjunction with cupping. Distilled liquors, such as aguardiente were not available to pre-Hispanic peoples, but perhaps beer made from maize (*Zea mays* L.) or the century plant (*Agave americana* L.) was consumed.

Although the information in the colonial sources is scant for this group of disorders, it is clear from the number of modern remedies (of which only a sample is included here) that arthritis, rheumatism, and muscle pain are common ailments. In aboriginal and colonial times

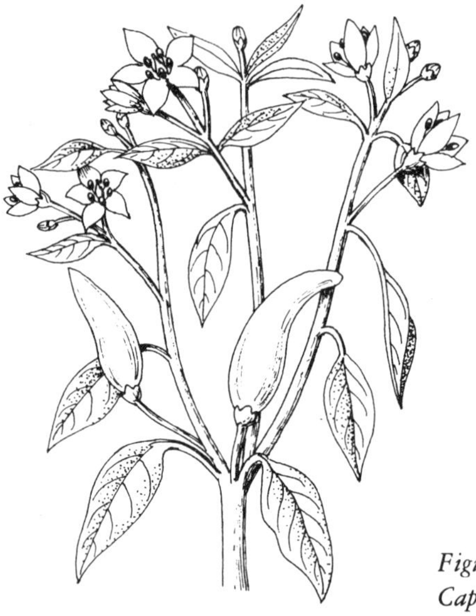

Figure 15
Capsicum annuum (Thomson 1978:49).

other sedative and analgesic drugs not specifically stated as remedies may have been used, and it is likely that some of the plants mentioned in the contemporary literature are ancient treatments. Cupping may have replaced the aboriginal method of bleeding. Wrapping up the affected area and/or massaging it are probably native practices.

BITES

There were many biting animals and insects in Guatemala, but the ones that were most dangerous were poisonous. Several herbal remedies were used in colonial times to cure such bites.

Red pepper (*Capsicum annuum* var. *minimum* Heiser) was considered to be effective against poison (Fuentes y Guzmán 1972:3:32). The yellow oleander (*Thevetia peruviana* Schum) was another widely regarded antidote (Ximénez 1967b:253). The roots of thicket hawthorn (*Crataegus intricata* J. Lange) (Fuentes y Guzmán 1969:1:244), *Curarina* (Spanish) (*Cissampelos pareira* L.) (1969:1:229), and the contrayerva torus herb (*Dorstenia contrajerva* L.) (*RGA* 1964:104; *RGZ* 1955:77) were ground and drunk against all types of venom. Contrayerva was also used in Yucatán against poison (Ossado 1944:567). Curarina has been used in contemporary times as well to counteract poison and for

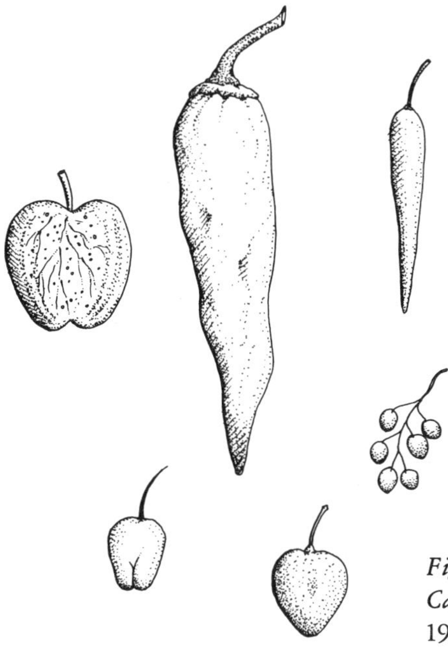

Figure 16
Capsicum annuum (Fuentez y Guzmán 1932–33:8:76).

snakebite (Rodríguez Rouanet 1971:112, 189; Villacorta Calderón 1926:74). Dieseldorff also said that it was considered good for bites of poisonous animals in Verapaz and that a popular medicine called curarina was made from it (1940:194). Fuentes y Guzmán said that cups made from the coconut (*Cocos nucifera* L.) were thought to be good for poison (1972:2:115). A species of hura (*Hura polyandra* Baill.) when put on a bite, was said to prevent venom from continuing its action (Ximénez 1967b:250).

Two species of tobacco (*Nicotiana rustica* L. and *Nicotiana tabacum* L.) were also used in curing bites. The juice of the former was squeezed into the wound and the leaves were then placed over it (*RGAG* 1965:273). The latter was carried in the mouth against snake or insect bites. The nicotine content of rustica is greater than that of tabacum and it is the hardier of the two species (Furst 1976:25). The Indians of San Bartolomé, or Xeoj, as it was known in ancient times, told how tobacco was used prior to the Conquest:

> One {type} . . . is used for all swellings and to remove any chill . . . The leaves are heated and placed on the part where required, and they remove chill and reduce pain. The other {type} is more lively and strong, and the natives call it Mexican tobacco. This one, ground and dried, and mixed with a little lime is generally

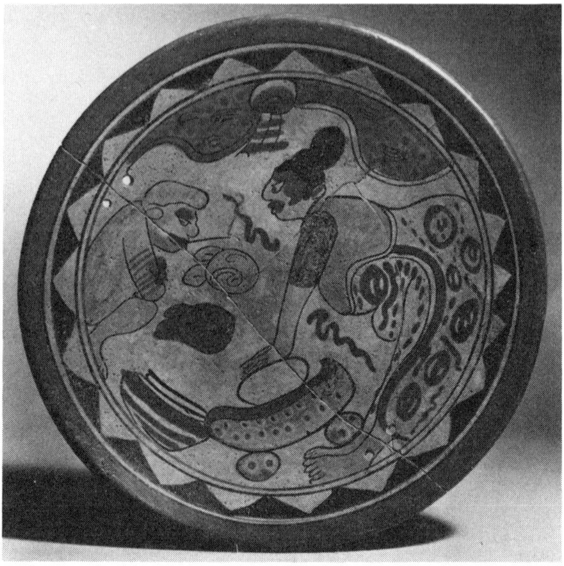

Figure 17
Man Smoking and Woman Grinding. The scene takes place in a palace, indicated by the swagged curtain above. A woman grinds corn. Across from her crouches a male smoking a cigar or cigarette (Coe 1982:94).

> carried in the mouth by Indians and Negroes who say that it gives them strength and takes away their thirst . . . they carry it in little gourds and in their mouths to defend themselves against any snake or poisonous insect bite. They also make small pipes (*cañutillos,* Spanish) which they light and suck the smoke. They find this very healthful for any illness (*RGAG* 1965:273–74).

According to Francisco Hernández in Mexico tobacco also was put on the bite of a poisonous snake (1959:3:376).

Several other medicinal plants which were reputedly good for poison are known from contemporary native practice. A decoction of the bark of a type of acacia (*Acacia hindsii* Benth.) has been used to alleviate the pain of spider bites, and a species of Dutchman's pipe (*Aristolochia maxima* L.) has been employed as an antidote for snakebite and bites of other harmful animals (Aguilar Girón 1966:361–62). The juice of the roots of *rehilete de floras rojas* (Spanish) (*Mesechites trifida* Muell. Arg.) and a powder made from the seeds of the cedron simaba (*Simaba cedron* Planch.) were used to treat stings and bites (1966:356, 366). Dumbcane (*Dieffenbachia seguine* Schott) is another contemporary remedy (1966:350), and *hierba mata cucaracha* (Spanish) (*Hapophyton cinereum* A.DC.) has been used to make a lotion which is a common insect repellent (1966:356). Villacorta Calderón said that the avocado (*Persea americana* Mill.) was used to cure bites in Guatemala and Chinautla (1926:74).

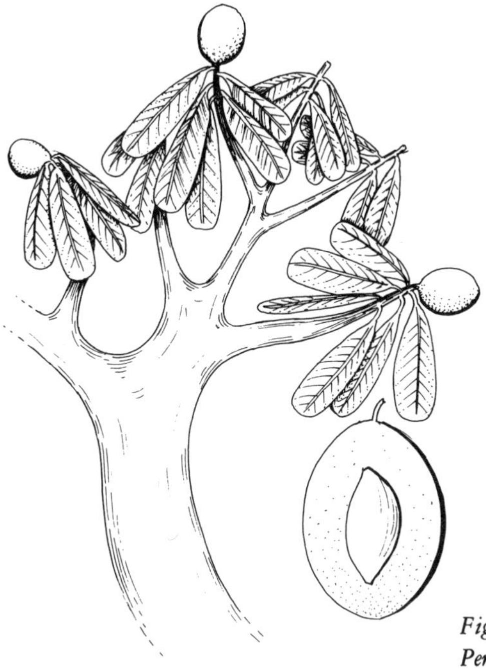

Figure 18
Persea americana (Figueroa Marroquín 1957:91).

Although bezoar stones may not have been used by the Indians in pre-Hispanic times in the same manner as by Spaniards, after the Conquest, they were popular antidotes for poison in the colonial period and will be discussed here.

Bezoar (from Persian *pad-zahr,* or anti-venom) stones were calcareous concretions which sometimes appeared in the organs of such animals as the deer and were thought to have curative properties (Monardes 1925:1:xxii; Schendel 1968:63; *RGZ* 1955:78). They were very popular in Europe, especially as poison indicators, and the use of the stones for this purpose was begun in the New World by the Spaniards. The gasplant dittany (*Dictamnus albus* L.) was food for the deer and was thought to engender the stones (Fuentes y Guzmán 1969:1:244). Hernández also mentioned them and said that the bezoar was called lord of venom (1959:3:307).

Monardes, writing in the sixteenth century, said that the stones were also used as a heart remedy and as an aid in curing pestilent fevers. They were reputed to be good for leprosy, elephantiasis, scabies, quarternary ague (malaria), and worms (1925:2:27–29). Bezoar stones were used when ordinary medicine did not work, but there is no evidence that the stones had any effect either.

Among the pre-Hispanic Cakchiquels, the dentist was called *aj guaré,* or he who is doctor of the mouth (Cifuentes Aguirre 1963:81). Two deities of the *Popol Vuh* seem to have had some dentistry capabilities because they said, "we just remove jaw bugs" (1971:41). Perhaps the main role of the dentist in ancient times was more cosmetic and involved filing and inlaying teeth for ornamental purposes, but they may have filled cavities as well (1971:42; Villacorta Cifuentes 1976:116–17). Teeth were probably extracted too, but there is no information on how it was done in Guatemala. In Mexico rattlesnake venom and vinegar were used to extract teeth painlessly (Roys 1931:188; Schendel 1968:51). Perhaps this method was also known in Guatemala. Jade dental prostheses were also made (Villacorta Cifuentes 1976:117).

During the colonial period several plants were used as toothache remedies. The sap from the branches of the deer fig (*Ficus glabrata* HBK.), the yellow oleander (*Thevetia peruviana* Schum) (Fuentes y Guzmán 1972:2:56, 117; Hernández 1959:2:417), and the fruit of pepper (*Capsicum* spp.) (Fuentes y Guzmán 1972:3:32; Farfán 1944:193) were put on a piece of cotton and applied directly to a painful tooth.

The leaves of the dividivi (*Caesalpinia coriaria* Willd.) were chewed like tobacco to stop a toothache (Fuentes y Guzmán 1969:1:244–45). Loose teeth were strengthened by rubbing the sap of the cut shoots of the Barbados nut (*Jatropha curcas* L.) on them (Fuentes y Guzmán 1972:3:305). In contemporary times in Tactic (Rodríguez Rouanet 1971:100) and in San Raimundo (Villacorta Calderón 1926:78) the Barbados nut was observed being used for a toothache. The false hellebore (*Veratrum sabadilla* Retz.) was said to alleviate pain when the grain was put on a cavity, but it also blistered the gum due to its caustic nature (Fuentes y Guzmán 1969:1:243). Hernández said it tightened teeth very well (1959:3:12).

Tobacco (*Nicotiana* spp.) was another toothache remedy. The tooth was washed with a small cloth wet with the juice. Next, a little ball of tobacco was applied directly on the tooth (Monardes 1925:1:80). Hernández said that warmed tobacco mitigated toothache when it was wrapped around the painful part or when placed mashed into a cavity (1959:2:82).

Other toothache remedies are found in the contemporary literature. The southern maidenhair fern (*Adiantum capillus-veneris* L.), which was mentioned by Fuentes y Guzmán as a medicinal plant (1969:1:243–44), has been used as a toothache remedy (Simeon 1977:39). Cocoa, or *cacao* in Spanish (*Theobroma cacao* L.), another plant with medicinal uses in earlier times, has been used to cure a painful tooth. A piece of

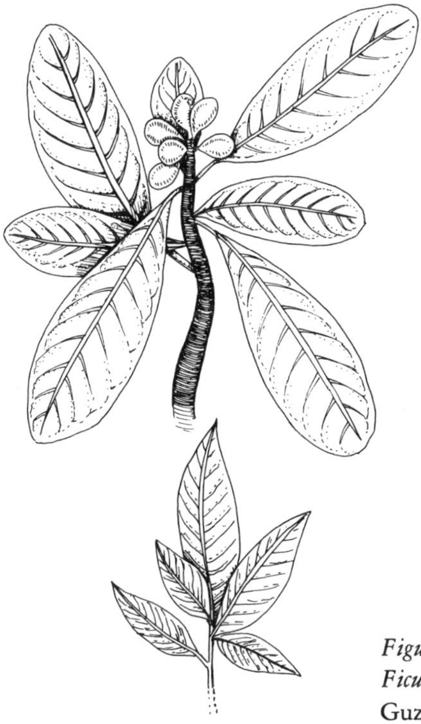

Figure 19
Ficus glabrata (Fuentes y Guzmán 1932–33:7:87).

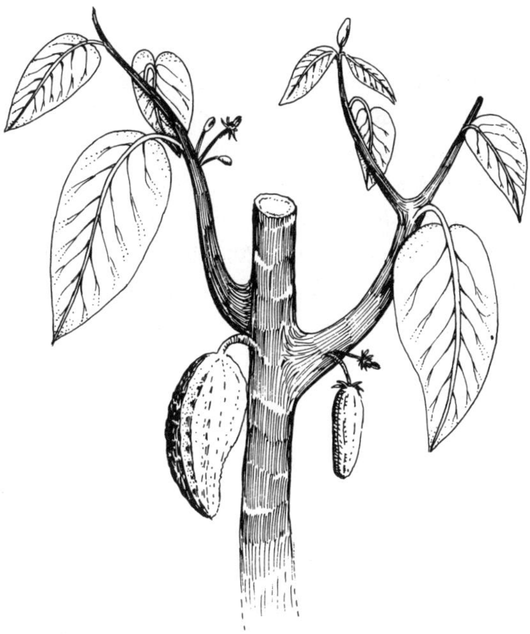

Figure 20
Theobroma cacao (Figueroa Marroquín 1957:99).

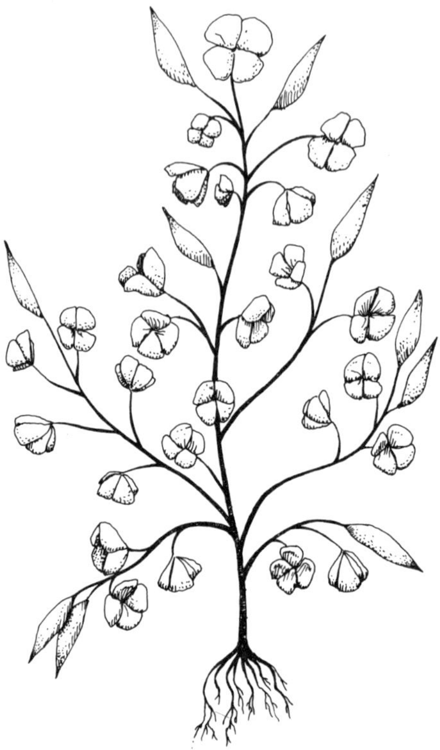

Figure 21
Oxalis corniculata (Fuentes y Guzmán 1932–33:8:184).

cacoa flower served as a toothache remedy when put into a cavity (Rodríguez Rouanet 1971:99–100). The sap of the Florida waltheria (*Waltheria americana* L.) soaked into a piece of cotton and put on the painful tooth two or three times a day was another contemporary cure (Rodríguez Rouanet 1969:82). Another remedy used was the Jamaica fishfuddle tree (*Piscidia piscipula* Sarg.). The bark of this tree contains piscidin which has narcotic and analgesic properties (Aguilar Girón 1966:100). A drop of the latex of copey clusia (*Clusia rosea* Jacq.) put on cotton and stuffed into a tooth cavity has also been used to allay toothache (Morton 1981:566).

Fuentes y Guzmán also said that the creeping oxalis (*Oxalis corniculata* L.) was used to make a mouthwash for sores in highland Guatemala in his time. It was also cooked between banana shoots (*Musa sapientum* L.) and applied as a paste on inflamed or injured gums (1972:3:112). It is not clear whether this identification is correct, however. *Oxalis corniculata* L. may be an Old World plant, but there were several species

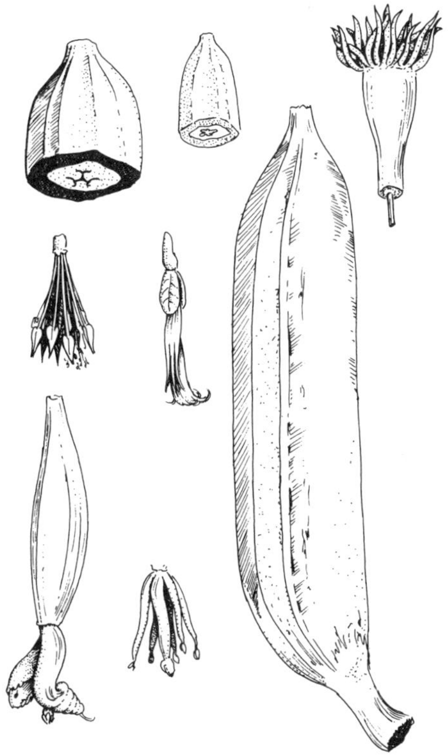

Figure 22
Musa sapientum (Figueroa Marroquín 1957:181).

of oxalis that had medicinal uses (see for example Hernández 1959:3:18–20). In the *Cruz-Badianus Herbal* it was stated that a species of *Oxalis* was used as a medicine to bring saliva when the mouth was dry. A drink was made from the leaves (Emmart 1940:116, 235–36).

Cocoa butter made from cacao (*Theobroma cacao* L.) was another remedy used to alleviate the pain of a burning mouth or other parts (Ximénez 1967b:250). Dieseldorff said that a species of stonecrop (*Sedum dendroideum* Moc. & Sessé ex DC.) was used for burning mouth in Verapaz and that polygala (*Polygala floribunda* Benth.) was used to fortify the teeth (1940:196). According to Aguilar Girón, the extract of white clary (*Heliotropium angiospermum* Murr.) was another remedy used to cure gum infections (1966:358).

There are a few other plants which have been used for mouth disorders in general: the bark of the Mexican cedar (*Cedrela mexicana* M. J. Roem), the Guiana crabwood (*Carapa guianensis* Aubl.), and a type of oxalis (*Oxalis corniculata L.*) (Mellen 1974:128–29).

Recent epidemiological surveys have demonstrated that digestive problems are endemic and continue to be the leading cause of illness and mortality, especially in early childhood, in highland Guatemala (Logan 1973a:537). Such ailments have probably characterized the area for a long time. This also seems to have been true in Yucatán. In the lexicon of Fray Pedro Beltrán, which contains information on anatomy and organic syndromes in that area, the frequent incidence of intestinal disorders is indicated by the variety of terms for dysentery (Guerra 1964:39).

Several cures for bloody flux were mentioned by colonial writers, but this vague label may have been applied to several conditions (Vogel 1973:199). Dysentery was one of these and may have been caused by contaminated water or food. Dysentery is an acute form of diarrhea with spasms in the bowels and bloody excretion. It is caused by either the dysentery bacilli or amebas. The specific causative amoeba is *Entamoeba histolytica* (Ackerknecht 1972:47, 49).

In bacillary dysentery the first symptoms are usually pain in the abdomen followed by diarrhea. There may also be nausea, aching pain in the limbs and shivery feelings. There is always fever. In amoebic dysentery the amoebas settle in the wall of the large intestine, where they cause inflammatory changes and then ulceration. Symptoms may appear within a week of infection or be delayed for months or years. In dysentery caused by bacilli, the mortality rate may be considerable if sulfa drugs are not used (Thomson 1976:278–79).

According to the *Relación Geográfica Aguacatepec,* bloody flux (*camaras de sangre* in Spanish) was dangerous and few who were young or old escaped it (1965:272). It was considered to be more serious among young people than in older ones (*RGA* 1964:101). Dysentery may have been more common in the piedmont and coastal area than in the highlands as is true today (Shattuck 1938:21).

There were several herbal medicines used in colonial times to treat digestive ailments, and knowledge of these was probably passed down from pre-Hispanic times. The roots of cambray (*Cosmos sulphureus* Cav.) were ground up with cacao (*Theobroma cacao* L.) and dissolved in warm water for the sick person to drink (*RGSA* 1952:113). In ancient Mexico, this plant was taken as a drink by those who could not eat or who were tired (López Austin 1971:131).

A powder made from the outer husk of the coconut (*Cocos nucifera* L.) was toasted, dissolved in hot water, and given to people who had dysentery (*disentería,* Spanish), according to Fuentes y Guzmán

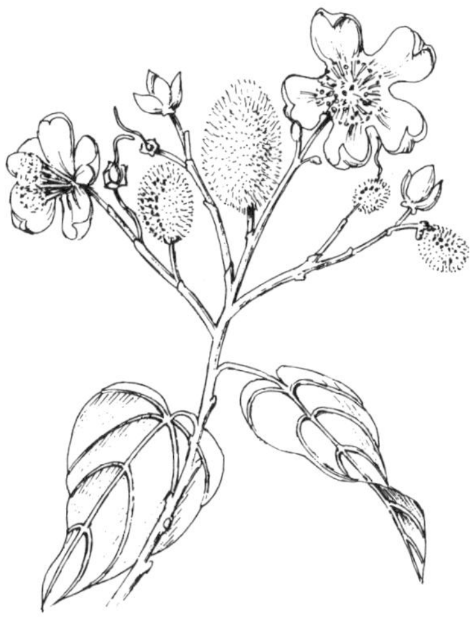

Figure 23
Bixa orellana (Chickering 1973:37).

(1972:2:115). Hernández also said that the husk was good for diarrhea, cured indigestion, and that it was a stomach tonic (1959:2:168). The Mexican earflower (*Cymbopetalum penduliflorum* Baill.) was a remedy considered good for any abdominal flux. It was toasted into a powder and as much of it as would fit on a coin (*real,* Spanish) was taken by the sick person (Fuentes y Guzmán 1972:2:117). In Mexico the plant was said to be taken by those who were unable to eat (López Austin 1971:133).

Fuentes y Guzmán mentioned another plant, the resurrection selaginella (*Selaginella lepidophylla* Spring), which was considered to be a plant with many useful properties (1972:1:243), and this same plant has recently been used in some areas for diarrhea (Rodríguez Rouanet 1969:65). Fuentes y Guzmán also mentioned that *cumalatole* (from Nahua *comalatolli*), a maize beverage, was good for dysentery (1969:1:228). More recently, purple maize was boiled and the liquid taken in San Pedro la Laguna for relief of diarrhea. The liquid obtained from maize dough was sweetened and also used (Rodríguez Rouanet 1969:80).

Many of the medicinal plants used today in highland Guatemala are digestive remedies. The plants included below were used in colonial times for other illnesses and may also have been taken for digestive problems.

Annatto (*Bixa orellana* L.), which was used in ancient times in the esteemed cacao beverage, has been taken with vinegar and sugar for dysentery (Rodríguez Rouanet 1969:80). One glass was taken warm every three hours. Hernández said that in Mexico annatto was used to alleviate dysentery (1959:2:28).

The custard apple (*Annona reticulata* L.) was used for the same purpose in Verapaz with the cooked shoots being drunk (Rodríguez Rouanet 1969:81; Wauchope 1948:50). The dried, powdered fruit has also been used in the highlands (Logan 1973a:541). Fuentes y Guzmán mentioned a type of *annona* (Spanish) but did not mention it as being used for dysentery or diarrhea (1972:2:42–43). Hernández, however, said that the custard apple cured diarrhea (1959:2:92). Perhaps it was used in this fashion in Guatemala too.

Fuentes y Guzmán also mentioned a species of eryngo (*Eryngium carlinae* Delar.) as being medicinal (1972:2:116), and Dieseldorff reported that it was used for diarrhea in Verapaz (1940:192). Villacorta Calderón claimed it was used as a purge and as a diarrhea remedy (1926:75). Another medicinal plant described in Fuentes y Guzmán was the banana (*Musa sapientum* L.) (1972:3:112). In Chinautla the banana has been used for dysentery (Wauchope 1948:50; Villacorta Calderón 1926:76).

A tea made from the root and bark of the black cherry (*Prunus capuli* Cav.) was another cure mentioned in the contemporary literature (Aguilar Girón 1966:86; Mellen 1974:152). This cure was also mentioned by Hernández as having been used in Mexico (1959:2:301). In the *Florentine Codex,* however, the black cherry was said to cause diarrhea when many were eaten (Sahagún 1963:11:121). The Mexican elder (*Sambucus mexicana* Presl. ex A.DC.) is another modern cure for diarrhea (Mellen 1974:157), and Ximénez said that it was considered to be a good purge and emetic during the colonial period (1967b:277; see also Hernández 1959:3:218–19).

The dried, powdered fruit of the guava (*Psidium guajava* L.) has been used in recent times for cramps, diarrhea, and indigestion (Logan 1973a:541). It was also used in ancient Mexico for dysentery (Ortíz de Montellano 1975:218).

A syrup made from the bark of the American storax (*Liquidambar styraciflua* L.) has been considered good for diarrhea and children's dysentery (Aguilar Girón 1966:86). This plant was mentioned by Ximénez as a colonial medicinal export (1967b:245), and it was part of the Aztec medicinal corpus (Ortíz de Montellano 1975:218, 219). The avocado (*Persea americana* Mill.) has also been used in recent times for diarrhea (Villacorta Calderón 1926:74). Hernández (1959:2:29) mentioned this same use for sixteenth century Mexico.

A type of hawthorn (*Crataegus pubescens* Steud.), (Villacorta Calderón 1926:77), *gumbolimbo* (*Bursera simaruba* Sarg.) (1926:78; Logan 1978:185), a type of cudweed (*Gnaphalium attenuatum* DC.) (1976:78), asthma weed (*Euphorbia hirta* L.), the garlic guineahen weed (*Petiveria alliacea*

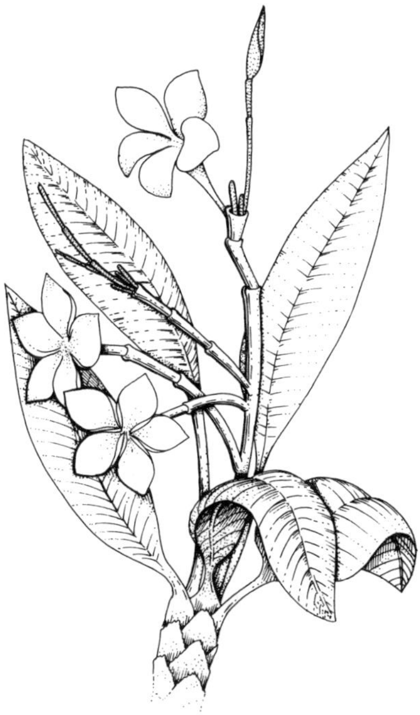

Figure 24
Plumeria rubra (Chickering 1973:91).

L.) (Morton 1981:198), and a type of stonecrop (*Sedum dendroideum* Moc. & Sessé ex DC.) (Cosminsky 1972:369; Hernández 1959:3:14) were other cures.

Constipation was another common digestive ailment, and many cathartics were employed to treat it. Purging was a very important aspect of Spanish medical doctrine (Foster 1953:206), but purges were probably important in pre-Columbian times as well. The gum of the wood of the Mexican frangipani (*Plumeria rubra* var. *acutifolia* Poir.) (Fuentes y Guzmán 1972:2:114; Hernández 1959:2:268), and the seed of the Mexican prickly poppy (*Argemone mexicana* L.) were considered good purges (Hernández 1959:2:267; Ximénez 1967b:302). The latter has also been used in recent times for constipation (Villacorta Calderón 1926:75).

Pepper (*Capsicum* spp.) was used to purge the stomach and intestines (Fuentes y Guzmán 1972:3:32). It was also taken by Indian women after birth as a purge (1972:3:32). *Elotatole* (from Nahau *eloatolli*), a beverage made from unripe maize, was another common purge (Fuentes y Guzmán 1969:1:228) as was the goldenshower senna (*Cassia fistula* L.) (Hernández 1959:2:56; *RGZ* 1955:75).

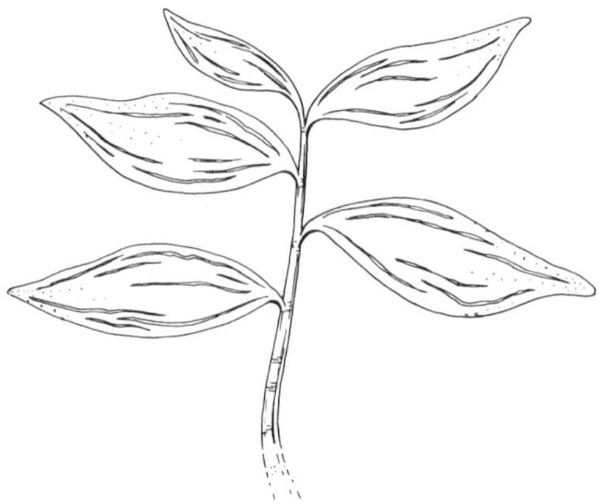

Figure 25
Zebrina pendula (Fuentes y Guzmán 1932–33:7:98).

Ximénez said that *pulque* (Spanish), a drink made from the century plant (*Agave americana* L.), was also a purge but could be taken for any illness (1967b:256; Farfán 1944:7v). The seeds of the Barbados nut (*Jatropha curcas* L.) had purgative properties (Ximénez 1967b:252; Farfán 1944:30v), and the plant has been used in Tactic in modern times (Rodríguez Rouanet 1971:23) and in San Raimundo (Villacorta Calderón 1926:78) as a purge. A type of ruellia (*Ruellia geminflora* HBK.) was used in Santa Catarina Pinula as a purge, and its action was said to be drastic (1926:78). The Old World tamarind (*Tamarindus indica* L.) was used in El Progreso as a laxative and purge (1926:79; *see also* Hernández 1959:3:173).

Jalap (*Ipomoea purga* Hayne) (Fuentes y Guzmán 1969:1:246; Hernández 1959:2:423; Farfán 1944:8) and vanilla (*Vanilla planifolia* Andr.) (Farfán 1944:210; Gage 1969:155) were two other purges important in colonial times. Hernández said that vanilla toned up the stomach and dissipated flatulence (1959:2:161). The wandering Jew (*Zebrina pendula* Schnizl.) has been used as an enema for constipation, and it was also used for dysentery (Hernández 1959:2:30; Logan 1973a:542; Simeon 1977:35). Oil from the seeds of the fruit of the sandbox tree (*Hura crepitans* L.) was another purge (Aguilar Girón 1966:118; Hernández 1959:3:109). This plant was also mentioned by Ximénez as a purge (1967b:252). Yellow sage (*Lantana camara* L.) and the billywebb sweetia (*Sweetia panamensis* Benth.) were other remedies for constipation (Villacorta Calderón 1926:75). When ground up and drunk, tobacco (*Nicotiana* spp.) was said to be a good purge (*RGSF* 1952:138).

Stomach and intestinal pain often accompanied diarrhea and constipation or occurred without those complaints. Fuentes y Guzmán

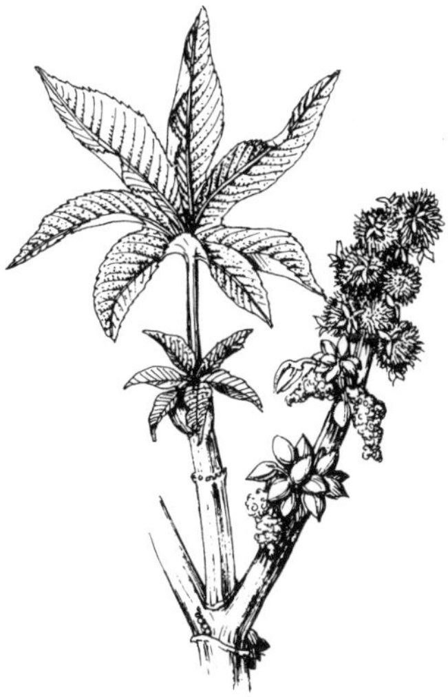

Figure 26
Ricinus communis (Thomson 1978:94).

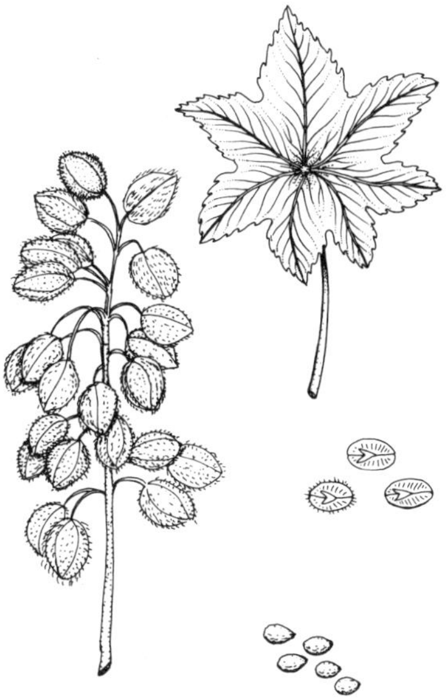

Figure 27
Ricinus communis (Fuentes y Guzmán 1932–33:8:82).

said that the sap of the ground-up flowers of the Aztec marigold (*Tagetes erecta* L.), when dissolved in wine or water, remedied the abdomen (1969:1:246). The description of the curative properties of this plant are similar in Fuentes y Guzmán and Hernández (1959:2:220) so it is possible that the former borrowed in this instance from the latter (Figueroa Marroquín 1957:188–89). Fuentes y Guzmán also said that the bark of Mexican frangipani (*Plumeria rubra* var. *acutifolia* Poir.), when made into a syrup, was a good remedy for pain in the side as was drinking continuously from cups made of coconut (*Cocos nucifera* L.) (1972:2:114–15). *Cihuapahtli* (Nahua) (*Montanoa tomentosa* Cerv.) was also considered to be good for pain in the side (Fuentes y Guzmán 1969:1:241; Hernández 1959:2:294). Ximénez said that a type of pepper (*Piper aduncum* L.) was taken by women in his time "to compose the stomach" (1967b:292). Cacao (*Theobroma cacao* L.) was also considered to be good for the stomach (Gage 1969:157).

Fuentes y Guzmán mentioned two Old World plants, the Chinabox jasmine orange (*Murraya paniculata* Jack) and the castor plant (*Ricinus communis* L.) which were considered to be good for colic and stomach and abdominal pain. The affected part was rubbed with castor oil and

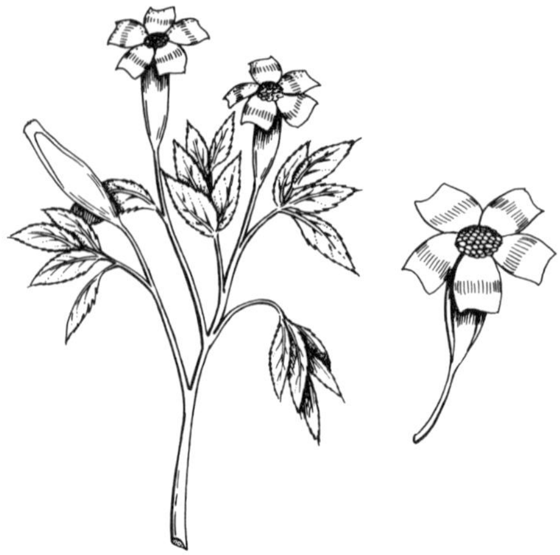

Figure 28
Tagetes spp. (Fuentes y Guzmán 1932–33:6:251).

the sick person drank a few drops of it as well (1969:1:242; 1972:3:35; Farfán 1944:47–47v). In recent times the leaves of the castor plant have been used for indigestion and cramps (Logan 1973a:542), and the seeds have been used as a purge in San Raimundo and San Pedro Sacatepéquez (Villacorta Calderón 1926:76).

Recently the sweet marigold (*Tagetes lucida* Cav.), a plant mentioned by Fuentes y Guzmán as being good for urine suppression (1969:1;241) and by Hernández as good for indigestion (1959:2:324), has been taken in Sololá for stomachache (Rodríguez Rouanet 1969:81). It has also been used for stomachache and inflammation in Chuchexic (Cosminsky 1972:367). Logan said it was used for stomachache, indigestion, gas, and diarrhea in the highlands (1973a:542).

Contrayerva (*Dorstenia contrajerva* L.) had many medicinal uses in colonial times (Martínez 1944:80–81) and was still being used for the stomach and dysentery or diarrhea in recent times (Aguilar Girón 1966:349; Logan 1973a:541). Several other plants have been used in contemporary times for stomach problems. The shoots of a species of ironweed (*Vernonia deppeana* Less.), a plant mentioned by Ximénez (1967b:307), were used for gastric illnesses (Mellen 1974:145). Wormwood (*Artemisia absinthium* L.), an Old World plant mentioned by Fuentes y Guzmán (1969:1:244), was used for stomachache (Rodríguez Rouanet 1971:92). Another plant he discussed was the jointed flatsedge (*Cyperus articulatus* L.) (1969:1:237) which in modern times has been taken for stomachache (Rodríguez Rouanet 1971:95) and which Hernández said was used to fortify the stomach (1959:2:123). A type of

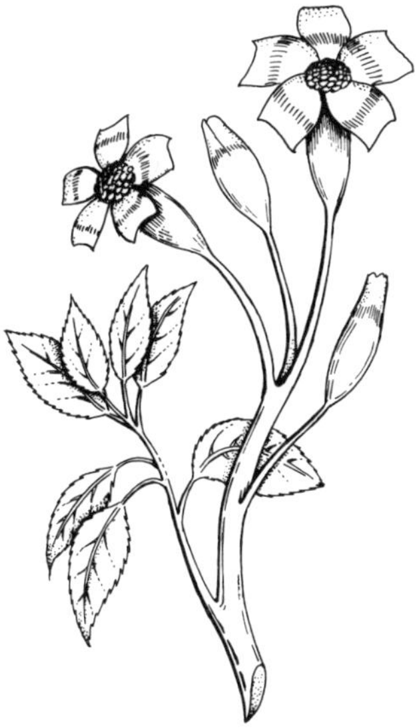

Figure 29
Tagetes spp. (Fuentes y Guzmán 1932–33:6:251).

dill (*Anethum foeniculatum* L.) was used as a stimulant and gastric in Canalitos, and mugwort (*Artemisia vulgaris* L.) was used as a stomach remedy in several other towns (Villacorta Calderón 1926:75–76). The cedron simaba (*Simaba cedron* Planch.) was used for stomach problems (Aguilar Girón 1966:366). Verbesina (*Salmea scandens* DC.) was used for stomach inflammation (Dieseldorff 1940:195).

Fuentes y Guzmán mentioned the Mexican gianthyssop (*Agastache mexicana* Benth.) along with other medicinal plants (1969:1:244). It has recently been used for curing stomachache. Three branches of the plant were cooked, strained, and sweetened, and then the liquid was taken in small amounts. This cure was also used for menstrual problems (Rodríguez Rouanet 1971:91, 251). Ruellia (*Ruellia geminflora* HBK.) has been used for intestinal inflammation in Santa Catarina Pinula (Villacorta Calderón 1926:78). The Old World rosemary (*Rosmarinus officinalis* L.) and vervain (*Verbena litoralis* HBK.) were taken for stomachache (Cosminsky 1972:367–68). Mexican eupatorium (*Eupatorium ligustrinum* Lag.) has been used for stomach and intestinal inflammation (Morton 1981:933).

Bunzel reported an interesting remedy used in Chichicastenango to cure children's stomach problems. The stomach was rubbed with ashes or a stick of pitchpine from the Montezuma pine tree (*Pinus montezumae* Lam.) (1967:144). Rodríguez Rouanet described many cures employing the pine tree (1971:306). In the sixteenth century white resin was extracted from pines and used to make poultices for fractures (*RGA* 1964:103).

During the colonial period, flatulence was remedied by smoking the tassel of an ear of maize (*Zea mays* L.) according to Fuentes y Guzmán (1969:1:227). Cambray (*Cosmos sulphureus* Cav.) was drunk in powder form as a cure for wind (1972:2:116). Tobacco (*Nicotiana* spp.) was used in the Tzutujuil area in pre-Hipanic times to cure indigestion, constipation, and flatulence (*RGSA* 1952:116). Hernández (1959:2:82) mentioned similar uses in Mexico. It has also been used in recent times to cure stomachache (Rodríguez Rouanet 1969:81).

Dropsy

Dropsy (*hydrops,* Eng.; *hidropesía,* Spanish) itself is not a disease but is caused by heart and other disorders. Heart disease produces increased pressure in the veins and also impurity of the blood due to defective pumping action of the heart. Blood pumped from a damaged heart returns by way of the vena cava vessel at low pressure, allowing fluids to leak out of the capillaries into surrounding tissues. The kidneys are prevented from functioning at the level of efficiency necessary to excrete the fluid. The body becomes swollen, there is stress on the heart, and ultimately congestive heart failure results (Lewis 1977:172–73, 177). Cirrhosis, tumors, and other diseases of the liver may, by interfering with the circulation through it, cause dropsy of the abdomen and later of the lower limbs (Thomson 1976:266).

There were a few plant remedies mentioned specifically for curing dropsy. According to Fuentes y Guzmán, the Aztec marigold (*Tagetes erecta* L.) was used in colonial Guatemala to treat dropsy (1969:1:246). This cure may have been based on that described by Hernández (1959:2:220). Ximénez said that the Mexican elder (*Sambucus mexicana* Presl. ex A.DC.) was very medicinal, and that its young shoots were cooked and made into a salad which was a good purge for those suffering from dropsy (1967b:277).

A type of club moss (*Lycopodium dichotomun* Jacq.) was another remedy. The plant was boiled and the liquid drunk (Fuentes y Guzmán 1972:2:42–43). In the *Cruz-Badianus Herbal* it was stated that a plant (club moss) called *tzonpilihuizpahtli* (Nahua) was used in cases of dropsy:

> Water under the skin comes out through cutting and all the purulent matter is to be removed; when this has been done, the leaves of brambles and *tzonpilihuizpahtli* are to be ground and

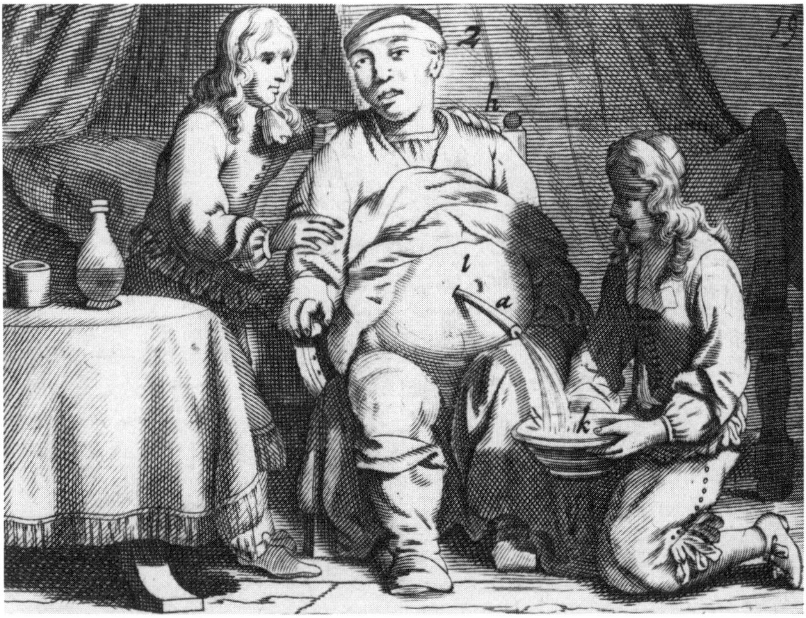

Figure 30
Man Being Treated for Dropsy (Schultetus 1693:134).

> cooked in water with wine incense to which is to be added Indian wine. The medicine thus prepared let it be put repeatedly on the festering part, which also is to be covered (Emmart 1940:126, 246).

Perhaps the disorder was not common as few plant remedies are mentioned in the early sources. It is not known if Indian surgeons in highland Guatemala punctured the affected areas to drain the fluid away as was done in Mexico and Europe.

Ear and Throat Disorders

When the young shoots of the castor plant (*Ricinus communis* L.) were cooked lightly and put into the ears, they were thought to cure deafness in colonial times. The leaves were used to cure earache (Fuentes y Guzmán 1972:3:35).

Fuentes y Guzmán said that gargling with a solution made from the creeping oxalis (*Oxalis corniculata* L.) was good for inflammation and

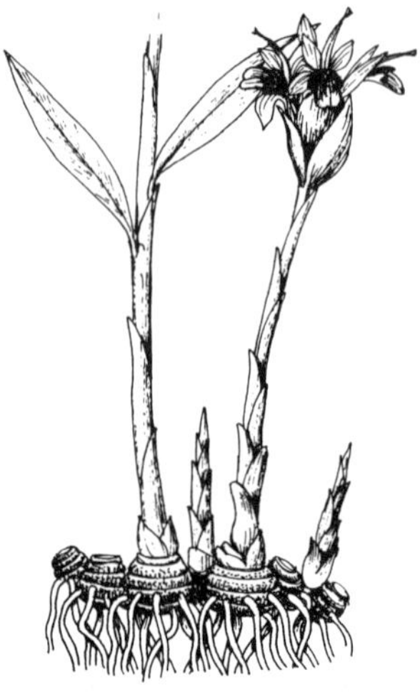

Figure 31
Zingibre officinale (Thomson 1978:111).

sores of the throat (1972:3:112). In aboriginal and colonial times some of the remedies used for mouth disorders were probably used for throat problems as well.

Several teas have been used for throat ailments in contemporary times. These were made from the leaves and stems of the garlic guineahen weed (*Petiveria alliacea* L.) (Villacorta Calderón 1926:74), the flowers of the roseleaf sage (*Salvia involucrata* Cav.), the stems and roots of the chaw-stick (*Gouania lupuloides* Urb.), the leaves of a species of martynia (*Proboscidea triloba* Schlect. & Cham.), the bark of the azure ceanothus (*Ceanothus coeruleus* Lag.), and the rhizomes of ginger (*Zingiber officinale* Rosc.) (Mellen 1974:146–47).

Goiter (*bocio,* Spanish; *guëguëcho,* from Nahua *quechquemitl*), an enlargement of the thyroid gland, may develop into a mechanical obstruction to breathing and swallowing at an advanced stage. It affects women two to three times as frequently as men and is due to iodine deficiency or possibly to infection, with the agent being very sensitive to iodine (Ackerknecht 1972:153, 156–57). The exact means of transmission of the disease is not clear. Parasites infesting certain waters or lack of sunlight may combine with the effect of the water in the development of goiter. Simple goiter is usually found in deep valleys in mountainous districts. Exopthalmic goiter may be due either to an increase of the normal secretion of the thyroid gland, or to perversion in quality of this secretion. People having it also have such symptoms as extreme nervousness, muscular tremors, throbbing of the great vessels, heart palpitations, and protrusion of the eyeballs (Thomson 1976:385–87).

Healthful waters were located at several places throughout the Guatemala highlands, and such waters were considered to be an important cure for goiter. Fuentes y Guzmán noted the location of warm springs near Lake Amatitlán which were believed to be beneficial for many illnesses, particularly goiter (1969:1:249). Medicinal waters near Santiago Atitlán were collected in containers and taken away to be used for goiter, kidney stones, and urinary suppression (1972:2:41). An exception to the belief that medicinal waters cured goiter was noted by Gage who reported that the people of Sacapulas thought goiter was caused by the water of the river. The priest of Sacapulas had goiter as did many others in the town during Gage's travels in the early seventeenth century (1969:166).

Goiter, often referred to as a tumor in colonial sources, appears to have existed at Kaminaljuyu in aboriginal times (Villacorta Cifuentes 1976:94). In colonial times goiter was treated with a plant remedy as well as heathful waters. The seeds of a species of cowitch (*Mucuna argyrophylla* L.) were hung around the neck for a few months. This was said to destroy the swelling so that no trace of it remained (Fuentes y Guzmán 1972:2:158).

Elephantiasis

Elephantiasis is a disease characterized by gross overdevelopment of the skin and subjacent textures. It is caused by repeated attacks of inflammation of the skin and subcutaneous tissues and concurrent obstruction of the lymphatic vessels. The common cause in the tropics is infection with threadlike worms (*Wuchereria* or *Filaria bancrofti*), which are transmitted by certain mosquitoes. The worms invade the lymphatic vessels and may attack any part of the body, but most commonly the legs, which become very enlarged and disfigured by the great thickening of the textures so as to resemble those of an elephant. Pressures on the muscles of the legs causes them to atrophy and become weak. During the early stages of the disease, the lymphatic glands are enlarged. Repeated inflammation of the lymphatic vessels ultimately leads to their blockage, and this is responsible for the later stage of the disease, elephantiasis (Thomson 1976:295–96, 651–52).

Most of the information in the colonial sources regarding this disease refers to Spanish priests who contracted it, due to their habit of walking barefoot. Elephantiasis was endemic to the warm, coastal areas, and there were some Indians who also suffered from it. Spaniards who contracted the disease used native remedies to treat it.

Fray Francisco Vázquez de Herrera, writing in the late seventeenth century, noted that elephantiasis was called *ychancicat* (from the Nahua word *tzicatl* meaning ant) because the sores, usually on the feet and legs, were connected inside the affected areas like ant holes. Fray Alonso Bustillo, a Franciscan, contracted ychancicat and was treated with Indian herbal medicines. False hellebore (*Veratrum sabadilla* Retz.) was also used to treat his sores. Bustillo was not cured and died from elephantiasis in 1551. Another Franciscan priest, Fray Agustín de Avila, also contracted it. His legs swelled up so much that his foot and leg seemed to form a thick, round trunk (Vásquez de Herrera 1938:2:153; 1940:3:19).

There were no remedies for elephantiasis mentioned in the colonial sources other than false hellebore, lemon juice, and onion, but a type of palm (probably *Acrocomia vinifera* Oerstd.) has been used in recent times to treat it (Rodríguez Rouanet 1969:65). The nipplefruit (*Solanum mammosum* L.) has also been used in the initial phase of the disease as well as for scrofula and skin problems (Aguilar Girón 1966:352). Perhaps these and other plants were the medicines used by the Indians in the sixteenth century.

Epilepsy

Epilepsy (*gota coral,* Spanish) is a collective term for a group of chronic convulsive disorders which have in common the occurrence of brief episodes, or seizures, associated with loss or disturbance of consciousness, usually but not always with characteristic body movements, or convulsions, and sometimes autonomic hyperactivity. Abnormal and excessive EEG discharges are always correlated. There are more than a dozen distinguishable forms of epilepsy (Goodman and Gilman 1970:204). Epilepsy can also be caused by injuries to the head and organic diseases of the brain (Thomson 1976:309).

The only cure mentioned in the colonial literature for epilepsy is club moss (*Lycopodium dichotomun* Jacq.) (Fuentes y Guzmán 1972:2:42–43), but there is no evidence that it really alleviated the symptoms of an epileptic attack (*alferecía* in Spanish).

Today rue (*Ruta graveolens* L.), an Old World plant, is used to treat epileptic seizures. A piece of rue leaf is cut and placed over the victim's nose so that the aroma can be inhaled (Simeon 1977:27). Jimson weed (*Datura stramonium* L.), which has sedative properties, was another remedy used in modern times for epilepsy (Villacorta Calderón 1926:80).

According to Fuentes y Guzmán, the young shoots of the thicket hawthorn (*Crataegus intricata* J. Lange) were ground up into a fine paste which was then applied lukewarm to swollen eyelids. This treatment reduced the swelling and took away the painful burning sensation as well. A decoction of the Old World fennel (*Foeniculum vulgare* Mill.) was used in colonial times as an eyewash (1969:1:244).

A species of oxalis may have been used to treat eye injuries in pre-Columbian times. According to a passage in the *Popol Vuh,* Hawk's wounded eye was cured by putting a little of the covering of a rubber ball into it. This remedy was called acid gum and may have referred to the acid plant, *xoxocoyolin* (Nahua), a species of oxalis (1971:106). Hernández mentioned several species of xoxocoyolin and said that one called *totoncaxoxocoyollin* appeared in the *Cruz-Badianus Herbal* and was said to cure glaucoma (probably cataracts):

> Pierce with a needle a fleshy growth in the eye, loosen it and draw it out, and sprinkle the white of the eye with burnt human excrement and salt, a little at a time. Then, next day apply to it sun-dried and ground roots of native acid herbs (Emmart 1940:101, 221).

The eye cure mentioned in the *Popol Vuh* could also refer to the Panama gum tree (*Castilla elastica* Sessé), or rubber. Zuñiga said that it was used for medicinal purposes in the colonial period (Feldman 1971:190). In the *Florentine Codex* rubber was mentioned as a remedy for all ailments including eye problems (Sahagún 1963:11:112). Farfán said that when a mixture containing melted rubber was put on the eyes it removed pain and burning (1944:193v).

Fuentes y Guzmán said that the Mexican prickly poppy (*Argemone mexicana* L.) was useful in treating cataracts (*nubes,* Spanish). The stems and leaves exuded a yellow liquid which was used to dissolve them quickly. He said that he saw an Indian use such an eyewash twice and be cured, but that people with delicate natures could not use it due to its caustic action (1969:1:240). Ximénez also said that the sap of this plant was good for eye ailments and that it was very medicinal (1967b:302). Hernández said the milk of the Mexican prickly poppy, when mixed with mother's milk and applied to the eyes, cured inflammations. The distilled juice was used as one constituent of a medicine that was said to dissolve cataracts (1959:2:267). In the *Florentine Codex,* the plant was said to cure eye pains (Sahagún 1961:10:143).

Another cure for cataracts involved using banana (*Musa sapientum* L.)

skins cooked lightly in hot ashes and placed on the eyelids. Fuentes y Guzmán observed a Negro slave using this cure and said that the slave was cured (1969:1:244). The banana is still used for medicinal purposes today in Guatemala but not specifically for eye problems (Rodríguez Rouanet 1971:273).

Ximénez told how Fray Tomás de la Torre, a Franciscan priest, was cured of blindness by an Indian doctor (médico). The native advised the priest to eat such things as chicken, fish, and vegetables but to avoid honey and cacao. The priest was told to wash his head every day, especially his forehead, with cold water and to press his temples until one or two tears started and then to wash his eyes with plain water at night. Fray Tomás was still blind after three days, and the curer told the priest that when he said he would be cured in three days, he had thought the illness had begun recently. He predicted that in nine days Fray Tomás would say Mass, and after twelve days, he would see the sun. In that time the priest was cured, and the Indian said that he would have died in three or four months without the cure (1929:1:422–23). It is not clear what form of blindness Fray Tomás had, and Ximénez did not say what medicines, if any, were used other than water. The Indian may have employed an eyewash as well made from such a plant as the Mexican prickly poppy, or the priest may have had temporary blindness.

Several teas for eye problems have been reported in the modern literature: the juice of *tatascamite* (Spanish) (*Perymenium grande* Greenman) (Mellen 1974:120), the juice of the stalk of the wild grape (*Vitis tiliifolia* Humb. & Bonpl.) (1974:119; Wauchope 1948:50), and the sap of the stem or a decoction of the root of a species of glorybush (*Tibouchina longifolia* Baill.) (Mellen 1974:119). The gum obtained from the bark of the marmalade box genipa (*Genipa americana* L.) has also been used to cure eye disorders (Aguilar Girón 1966:365), and the Florida waltheria (*Waltheria americana* L.) has been used for inflammations of the eyes (Vilacorta Calderón 1926:75).

Fatigue and General Body Discomfort

Tonics were used to stimulate the body and to promote health. Mexican chía (*Salvia hispanica* L.) was taken as a refreshing, healthful drink. Both Fuentes y Guzmán and Cortés y Larraz mentioned it (1969:1:228; 1968:2:281). Hernández mentioned several types of *chían* which were used in Mexico for medicinal purposes (1959:2:67–

74). Farfán attributed several medicinal uses to chía (see for example, 1944:79v, 158v). In recent times chía has been used in some highland towns as a general stimulant (Villacorta Calderón 1926:78). Fuentes y Guzmán said that the medicinal uses of the Old World fumitory (*Fumaria parviflora* Lam.) were well known (1969:1:243). Martínez said that it was taken as a bitter tonic in Mexico in contemporary times so it may have been used that way in Guatemala too in colonial times (1944:134).

Several tonics have been used in the Guatemala highlands in modern times. Ironweed (probably *Vernonia deppeana* Less.) was used in Verapaz (Dieseldorff 1940:193; Morton 1981:978), and it may have been used as such in earlier times as well. Wormwood (*Artemisia absinthium* L.) was also a tonic and stimulant (Aguilar Girón 1966:372; Villacorta Calderón 1926:74). Curarina (*Cissampelos pareira* L.) (1966:348) and the Old World ginger plant (*Zingiber officinale* Rosc.) (1966:354) were also used. According to Hernández, a species of ginger was taken as a healthful drink in Mexico (1959:2:153), and Fuentes y Guzmán mentioned ginger among medicinal plants used in colonial Guatemala (1972:2:116). He did not, however, specifically say it was a tonic. Mexican cedar (*Cedrela mexicana* M. J. Roem) (Morton 1981:401), the leaves of a type of walnut (*Juglans pyriformis* Liebm.), the Mexican prickly poppy (*Argemone mexicana* L.), contrayerva (*Dorstenia contrajerva* L.), hawthorn (*Crataegus pubescens* Steud.), vanilla (*Vanilla planifolia* Andr.) (Villacorta Calderón 1926:75, 77–78, 80), and the cedron simaba (*Simaba cedron* Planch.) (Aguilar Girón 1966:366) were other tonics and stimulants mentioned by twentieth century writers.

Anemia was one cause of fatigue, and there are plants mentioned in the contemporary sources that were used specifically to treat it. These were: the leaves and fruit of the purple mombin (*Spondias purpurea* L.) (Mellen 1974:141), the juice of the ground-up shoots of the yellow mombin (*Spondias mombin* L.), and the juice of the fruit of the *sapodilla* (Spanish) (*Manilkara zapota* Van Royen) (Mellen 1974:141). These remedies for anemia were consumed as teas and may also have been used in earlier times for this disorder.

Tobacco (*Nicotiana* spp.) was another general remedy and Mexican tobacco (*Nicotiana tabacum* L.) was said to give people strength and to take away thirst (*RGAG* 1965:273; Hernández 1959:2:81–82). In the *Florentine Codex* the uses of tobacco were described:

> He who suffers fatigue rubs himself with it . . . And it is chewed . . . It intoxicates one, makes one dizzy, possesses one, and destroys hunger and desire to eat (Sahagún 1963:11:146).

Fever

People suffered from fevers in pre-Hispanic as well as in colonial times, but those occurring in aboriginal days were not as virulent and devastating as those which accompanied the introduced epidemic diseases. Fever may also occur with food poisoning, infection, and colds. There were some New World endemic fever-producing disorders such as parrot fever (*psittacosis*), a viral disease contracted from tropical birds in lowland areas (Villacortes Cifuentes 1976:59), but it was rare among highland populations, and possibly a native form of yellow fever.

Fuentes y Guzmán said that the plant called *raíz de la estrella* in Spanish (now called *alcotán* or curarina) (*Cissampelos pareira* L.) healed those touched by fever (1969:1:229). It has also been used to treat it in contemporary times (Rodríguez Rouanet 1969:79; Dieseldorff 1940:194). Ximénez said that the *granadilla* (Spanish) (*Hyperbaena guatemalensis* Standl.) was good for any sick person but especially for those suffering from fever (*tabardillo,* Spanish) and pneumonia or pleurisy (*dolores de costado,* Spanish) (1967b:271–72). Certain strains of pneumonia were present in the New World prior to the Conquest (Shattuck 1938:47).

Pulque, a fermented drink made from the century plant (*Agave americana* L.), was frequently taken for fevers and other illnesses (Fuentes y Guzmán 1969:1:218, Hernández 1959:2:349) as was maize (*Zea mays* L.) (Fuentes y Guzmán 1969:1:227; Hernández 1959:2:290; Sahagún 1963:11:142). For those suffering from chills and fever the Aztec marigold (*Tagetes erecta* L.) was applied externally as an ointment to destroy the violence of the affliction (Fuentes y Guzmán 1969:1:246). Hernández said that the same plant was good for fever (1959:2:220).

There are many modern herbal remedies used for fever, usually taken in the form of teas. The leaves of the coffee senna (*Cassia occidentalis* L.) have been used as a febrifuge in recent (Mellen 1974:142) times. Hernández said that a related plant was used for fevers in Mexico (1959:2:362).

The sweet-pea tree (*Gliricida sepium* Steud.), a tree used to shade the delicate cacao plants in pre-Hispanic and colonial times, was another fever remedy (Rodríguez Rouanet 1969:78); annatto (*Bixa orellana* L.) (Aguilar Girón 1966:361; Hernández 1959:2:28), the black cherry (*Prunus capuli* Cav.) (Farfán 1944:245v), and the leaves of wormwood (*Artemisia absinthium* L.) (Rodríguez Rouanet 1971:124–25) were others. Wormwood was mentioned by Fuentes y Guzmán and may also have been an ancient remedy for fevers (1969:1:244).

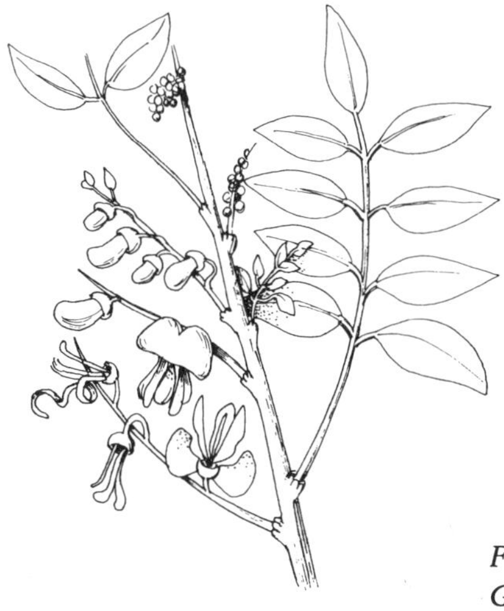

Figure 32
Gliricida sepium (Chickering 1973:66).

The bark of the Mexican talauma (*Talauma mexicana* Don.), a contemporary febrifuge (Mellen 1974:142), was also described as a fever medicine in the *Florentine Codex* (Sahagún 1963:11:201). The golden-shower senna (*Cassia fistula* L.), renowned for its medicinal properties in colonial times, has been taken for fever today in several places with barley (*Hordeum vulgare* L.) (Rodríguez Rouanet 1969:78). An infusion of eucalyptus leaves (*Eucalyptus globulus* Labill.) has been used for fever in Chichicastenango (Bunzel 1967:144) and other areas of Guatemala (Cosminsky 1972:367; Villacorta Calderón 1926:76). The black nightshade (*Solanum nigrum* L.) (Cosminsky 1972:369), the gumbolimbo (*Bursera simaruba* Sarg.) (Villacorta Calderón 1926:78), hawthorn (*Crataegus pubescens* Steud.) (Cosminsky 1972:367; Villacorta Calderón 1926:77), the garden polypody (*Phlebodium aureum* John Smith 1926:74), Humboldt's willow (*Salix chilensis* Mol.) (Wauchope 1958:50), and Mexican cedar (*Cedrela mexicana* M. J. Roem) (Morton 1981:401) were other contemporary febrifuges. Hernández said that hawthorn was used to reduce the heat of fever and to cure epidemic fevers (*exantemas,* Spanish) (1959:3:31).

John Gillin described two cures for fever used by the Pokomans of San Martín Jilotepeque, and these contemporary practices may indicate rituals which formerly accompanied the use of herbal remedies. In one ritual the curer passed a live bird or chicken over the sick person's body while massaging him. The curer then stood up, letting the bird fall to the ground. If the bird died, this meant that the fever had been absorbed into the bird's body, and the person would recover. The second cure involved taking a small chicken which had been stripped of its feathers, cutting it open alive, and removing the viscera. The warm, bloody flesh was then divided into thirds and tied to the patient's wrists and back of the neck. The flesh was thought to absorb the fever and facilitate recovery (Gillin 1951:113).

Fractures

Fuentes y Guzmán described the treatment used for fractures during the late seventeenth century. The most important remedy for broken bones and dislocations was an ointment made from a species of meadowrue (*Thalictrum hernandezii* Tauch.). The branches and leaves of this plant were ground up, combined with beef fat, and applied to the injured part (1969:1:244; Hernández 1959:2:320–21). When children suffered from broken bones, the cooked meat of the gourd of the crossleaf calabash tree (*Crescentia alata* HBK.) was placed on the break as hot as the child could tolerate. This supposedly strengthened and mended the break so well that the child would never be bothered by it again (1972:2:67–68).

Contemporary bonesetters have used methods similar to those described by Fuentes y Guzmán. Using their secret, magic bone, they locate the break (Rodríguez Rouanet 1969:64). The magic bone is a special small bone which magically appears to those called to the bonesetter role. It is then concealed in the hand by the healer during diagnosis and aids in locating the break in a patient's body (Paul 1976:77–78). According to the severity of the break, the bonesetter massages the area, sometimes using hot fat. Fresh tobacco leaves might then be placed against the break and the bone set (Paul 1976:77; Rodríguez Rouanet 1969:64). Hernández spoke of the ability of tobacco juice to clean wounds and promote the growth of new tissue (1959:2:82). Balsam or glycerine might also be used, and avocado leaf (*Persea americana* Mill.) was used in Chuchexic (Cosminsky 1972:369). In Momostenango the illness referred to as "dislocated bone" was treated by a specialist known as a bone dresser who was also a calendar diviner. As treatment, he bathed the affected area in a certain herb, arranged the bone in its proper place, wrapped it with leaves from the tz'ite tree (*Erythrina corallodendron* L.), and tied it with tz'ite splints (Tedlock 1982:57). In Chuchexic the bonesetter treated fractures, sprains, and bruises but was not thought to have special divine powers that aided in the cure (Cosminsky 1972:182). Cosminsky also reported the use of stonecrop (*Sedum dendroideum* Moc. & Sessé ex DC.) to treat fractures

(1972:369). Among the Chortí the surgeon took care of broken bones but also treated other problems such as wounds, sores, and cancer. Broken bones were bound with a splint and a mixture of plants was used to make a plaster which was placed all around the break. Leaves were then wrapped around it and the splints were tied on (Wisdom 1940:356).

In Camotán the leaves, bark, and fruit of the Barbados nut (*Jatropha curcas* L.) were crushed up and placed on a fracture. The area was then wrapped up with the bark of the same plant (Rodríguez Rouanet 1971:135). This plant was reputed to have medicinal properties by Fuentes y Guzmán (1972:3:305), Ximénez 1967b:252–53), and Monardes (1925:1:51–52), but it was not specifically cited as being used for fractures.

In contemporary times many plants have been used to cure broken bones. In San Raimundo and San Pedro Sacatepéquez the leaves of the castor plant (*Ricinus communis* L.) were used to cure fractures, and in other towns mugwort (*Artemisia vulgaris* L.) was used (Villacorta Calderón 1926:76). A species of epiphyllum (*Epiphyllum strictum* Brit. & Rose) was used for broken bones in Verapaz. The hot leaves were tied over the injured bone (Dieseldorff 1940:196). Another remedy used elsewhere was made from the leaves and stem of the vegetable pear (*Sechium edule* Sw.). These were boiled, and the liquid was used for fractures. A large cloth immersed in the water was applied to the area for one hour twice daily (Simeon 1977:42). The copey clusia (*Clusia rosea* Jacq.) is another plant which has been used in contemporary times to aid in the healing of fractures (Aguilar Girón 1966:368). The custard apple (*Annona reticulata* L.) has also been used for fractures and dislocations (Wauchope 1948:50; Villacorta Calderón 1926:74).

Headaches

Fuentes y Guzmán mentioned one plant that was commonly used to cure headaches in his time. The leaves of the Mexican frangipani (*Plumeria rubra* var. *acutifolia* Poir) were applied to the temples of a person suffering from a headache and were said to cure it quickly. As this remedy was applied externally, it was considered safe medicine (1972:2:114). The leaves of the castor plant (*Ricinus communis* L.) were used in the same fashion (1972:3:35); however, this plant is of Old World origin and would not have existed in pre-Hispanic times.

In the Tzutujil area tobacco (*Nicotiana* spp.) was used for headaches (*RGSA* 1952:116; *RGSF* 1952:138). Hernández also said that it calmed pains of the head, fortified it, and produced repose (1959:2:81). In the *Florentine Codex* tobacco was also mentioned as a headache remedy (Sahagún 1961:10:140), and it has reportedly been used in recent times to cure headaches (Rodríguez Rouanet 1969:81).

In contemporary times Verapaz, the leaves of *hormiguillo* (Spanish) (*Siparuna nicaraguensis* Hemsl.) were applied to the forehead of a person who had a headache (Dieseldorff 1940:194). The crossleaf calabash tree (*Crescentia alata* HBK.) has also been used to treat headaches (Simeon 1977:38). Cihuapahtli (*Montanoa tomentosa* Cerv.) was another headache remedy (Rodríguez Rouanet 1971:81–82, 84). These last two plants were both mentioned by Fuentes y Guzmán but not specifically as headache cures. Eucalyptus (*Eucalyptus globulus* Labill.) was used in Chuchexic to treat headaches (Cosminsky 1972:367).

Heart Disorders

Club moss (*Lycopodium dichotomun* Jacq.) was considered to be good for persons suffering from a bad heart. An infusion of the plant was taken with meals (Fuentes y Guzmán 1972:2:42–43). The leaves of the gasplant dittany (*Dictamnus albus* L.) were eaten during breakfast by those "touched by passions of the heart" (1969:1:244). During the late sixteenth century Fray Francisco Montero de Miranda, who resided in Verapaz, said that annatto (*Bixa orellana* L.) was medicinal and good for the heart (1954:354). Vázquez de Espinosa, who wrote during the seventeenth century, said that annatto was a heart stimulant (1968:238).

Fuentes y Guzmán also mentioned a plant which he called *yulpactli*. He was probably referring to *yollohxochitl* (Nahua), the Mexican talauma (*Talauma mexicana* Don.) (1969:1:229), which was a common heart medicine in ancient times as well as today (Ortíz de Montellano 1975:219; Aguilar Girón 1966:369). Hernández also mentioned this plant and said that it strengthened the heart (1959:3:5).

In contemporary times hawthorn (*Crataegus pubescens* Steud.) has been used to treat heart ailments and so has rue (*Ruta graveolens* L.) (Villacorta Calderón 1926:77–78). The shieldleaf pumpwood (*Cecropia peltata* L.) was also used as a cardiac tonic in Guatemala (Morton 1981:144).

Helminthic Infections

The tapeworm (*taenia*), called *tepulcuat* (from Nahau *tepolcoatl*) by Fuentes y Guzmán, afflicted the people of highland Guatemala and was believed to enter a person's body while he was relieving himself, making its way into the intestines. The remedy for expelling the parasite was for the sufferer to sit over a vessel containing warm milk as the smell was thought to attract the worm (1972:2:62). In modern times Oakes recorded a description of the death of a man from tapeworm: "He died because of an animal inside him that was jumping about in his stomach." This was the explanation given by an Indian woman of Todos Santos when her brother died (1969:47).

There are other types of worms which are endemic in Guatemala today, but these are not specifically mentioned in the colonial sources. Shattuck discussed several types of these worms, and some of them, such as *Ascaris lumbricoides* (roundworms) and *Mansonella ozzardi* (filaria) are probably native to the New World (1938:209–21). *Necator americanus* (American hookworm) was another common parasite. *Ancylostoma duodenade* is another type of hookworm. Both may cause severe anemia and sometimes the urge to ingest earthy substances. These worms enter through the soles of the bare feet (Ackerknecht 1972:130, 133).

There were two cures for worms mentioned in the colonial documents. A type of bromelia (*Bromelia karatas* L.) was eaten as a cure for abdominal worms (Fuentes y Guzmán 1972:2:116). If a child's intestines were rubbed with an ointment made from castor oil (*Ricinus communis* L.), this was thought to expel the worms (1972:3:35–36). False hellebore (*Veratrum sabadilla* Retz.) was toasted, made into a powder, and given to animals suffering from worms (Fuentes y Guzmán 1969:1:243; Hernández 1959:3:12).

Contemporary vermicides have included teas made from the leaves of Salvador cedar (*Cedrela salvadorensis* Standl.), the entire tridax plant (*Tridax procumbens* L.), and the seeds of the spigelia plant (*Spigelia humboldtiana* Schlect. & Cham.) (Aguilar Girón 1966:355; Mellen 1974:139; Dieseldorff 1940:196). The ripe fruit of the green sapota (*Pouteria viridis* Pitt.) (Mellen 1974:139), the oil of American wormseed (*Chenopodium ambrosioides* L.) (Dieseldorff 1940:195; Valladares 1957:119; Villacorta Calderón 1926:74), mugwort (*Artemisia vulgaris* L.) (Villacorta Calderón 1926:76), and the bark of the West Indian locust (*Hymenaea courbaril* L.) (Aguilar Girón 1966:92) taken in decoction were remedies for worms. Hernández said that a decoction of the roots of *epazotl* (Nahua), or American wormseed, expelled harmful animals from the abdomen (1959:3:369).

Taken orally, the juice of the papaya (*Carica papaya* L.) was said to be a strong vermicide (Aguilar Girón 1966:361). Among the Chortí basil (*Ocimum basilicum* L.) and the garlic guineahen weed (*Petiveria alliacea* L.), were two plants which were inhaled in a mixture said to

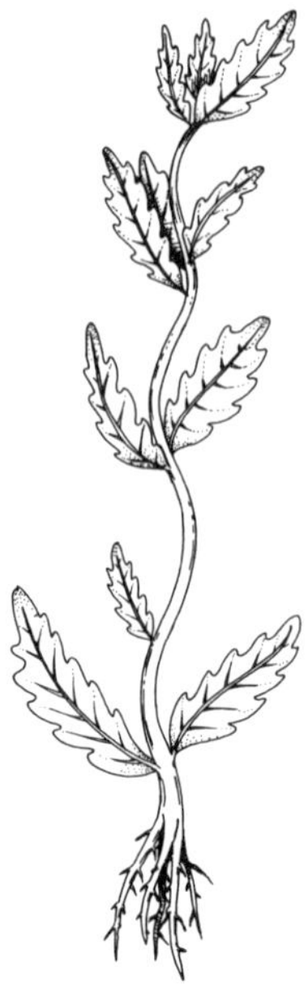

Figure 33
Chenopodium ambrosioides (Figueroa Marroquín 1957:131).

cause the sick person to vomit the worms (Wisdom 1940:351). Basil has also been used as a vermicide in other parts of Guatemala (Villacorta Calderón 1926:74).

HEMORRHOIDS

Hemorrhoids (*almorranas,* Spanish) were treated with ointments and baths. Fuentes y Guzmán said that a decoction of snakeroot eryngo (*Eryngium campestre* L.) was used to stop the pain of hemorrhoids, reduce the swelling, and, upon continued application, to open them. A decoction of the treebeard tillandsia, or Spanish moss (*Tillandsia usneoides* L.), was also thought to aid hemorrhoid sufferers (1969:1:243). An ointment made from the juice of the flowers of the Aztec marigold (*Tagetes erecta* L.) was another remedy. The juice was fried in strained oil to which a little wax was added. This condensed and thickened to form the ointment (1969:1:246).

Contemporary cures have included teas and baths made from the juice of the leaves of the erect spiderling (*Boerhaavia erecta* L.), the flowers, bark, and leaves of the monkey hand tree (*Chiranthodendron pentadactylon* Larr.) (Mellen 1974:148)—which was used in ancient

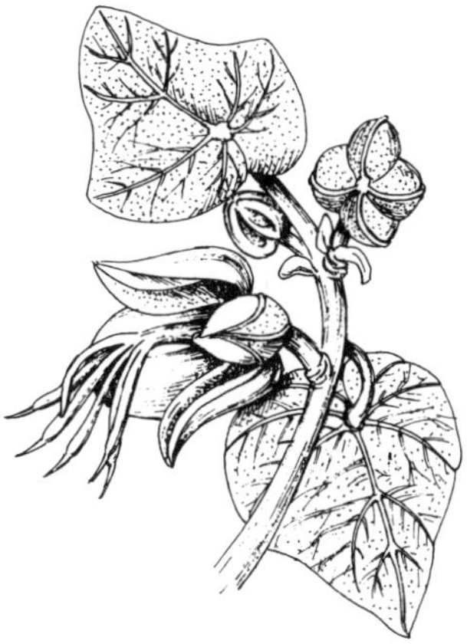

Figure 34
Chiranthodendron pentadactylon
(Chickering 1973:52).

times for the same purpose in Mexico (Martínez 1944:395), and the juice of the leaves of a type of stonecrop (*Sedum dendroideum* Moc. & Sessé ex DC.) (Mellen 1974:148). The bark and shoots of ironweed (*Vernonia deppeana* Less.) were another remedy (Villacorta Calderón 1926:79).

Liver Disorders

In colonial times the strap polypodium (*Campyloneurum phyllitidis* Presl.) was boiled and the liquid drunk to purify the liver (Fuentes y Guzmán 1972:2:117). A cacao beverage or cocoa butter (*Theobroma cacao* L.) eaten with sugar and cinnamon were taken for "heat of the liver" (1972:2:65; Hernández 1959:2:305).

In modern times the bark of the West Indian locust (*Hymenaea courbaril* L.) has been used to make a drink for liver ailments. The garden polypody (*Phlebodium aureum* John Smith) has been used for the same purpose (Rodríguez Rouanet 1969:82). Teas made from the roots of two species of greenbrier (*Smilax aristolochiaefolia* Mill. and *Smilax spinosa* Mill.) were considered good for hepatitis (Mellen 1974:117). The guava (*Psidium guajava* L.) has also been used as a hepatitis cure (Wauchope 1948:50).

The leaves and stems of the garlic guineahen weed (*Petiveria alliacea* L.) were made into a tea which was also used for liver problems. Another was made from the sprouted bark and unripe fruit of the Guinea chestnut pachira (*Pachira aquatica* Aubl.). Small branches of wormwood (*Artemisia absinthium* L.) were cooked in half a liter of water to make a remedy for liver pain in San Juan Ostuncalco. Two glasses of this liquid were taken daily until the person was cured (Rodríguez Rouanet 1971:98). In Cobán five small leaves of Mexican eupatorium (*Eupatorium ligustrinum* Lag.) were boiled and the liquid drunk for liver ailments. This treatment was continued for nine consecutive days (1971:21). Humboldt's willow (*Salix chilensis* Mol.) has also been used for liver problems (Wauchope 1948:50). Ruellia (*Ruellia geminflora* HBK.) was used in Santa Catarina Pinula for liver problems (Villacorta Calderón 1926:78).

Some plants have also been used in recent times as cholagogues to stimulate the flow of bile which aids in the absorption or digestion of fats. These remedies were usually taken in the form of teas. The leaves of wormwood (*Artemisia absinthium* L.) (Mellen 1974:140) were used as a cholagogue. Since Fuentes y Guzmán mentioned this plant but did not give any specific remedies for it (1969:1:244), perhaps this medicine was a colonial remedy. The leaves of the tread-softly (*Cnidoscolus chayamansa* McVaugh), the leaves and fruit of tridax (*Tridax procumbens* L.), the leaves of mugwort (*Artemisia vulgaris* L.), and the roots of tartago nettlespurge (*Jatropha podagrica* Hook) were other cholagogues used in recent times (Mellen 1974:140).

Neurological Disorders

Fuentes y Guzmán mentioned two remedies for neurological disorders, both of which were specifically used for pinched nerves. The site of pain was rubbed with castor oil (*Ricinus communis* L) (1972:3:35). Another remedy was the Aztec marigold (*Tagetes erecta* L.) (1969:1:246). Perhaps ointments and drinks used for wounds and pain were taken for pinched nerves as well.

Some contemporary remedies for neurological problems have been mentioned in the more recent sources. The flowery tops of the sweet marigold (*Tagetes lucida* Cav.) have been used to make a tea for neuralgia (Mellen 1974:126). Fuentes y Guzmán mentioned this plant as a cure for urinary problems, but it probably had other medicinal uses in colonial times (1969:1:241).

The yellow oleander (*Thevetia peruviana* Schum) was considered to be a good remedy for paralysis (*perlesía*, Spanish) during colonial times (Ximénez 1967b:253). A variety of anil indigo (*Indigofera suffruticosa* Mill.) was also used to cure *hosa* (Spanish), which Ximénez also said was paralysis. The branches were broken up, and the leaves were crushed into small pieces and put into boiling water. The drink had to be given quickly or it had no effect. It induced vomiting and sweating and supposedly cured the patient (1967b:294, 296). Fuentes y Guzmán also mentioned indigo but did not give any specific cures (1972:3:294). A decoction of jimson weed (*Datura stramonium* L.) was used as a bath by those who were crippled and trembled (1969:1:246). Today the juice of fleabane leaves (*Pluchea odorata* Cass.) has also been used to cure paralysis (Aguilar Girón 1966:362).

Respiratory Disorders

Coughs, colds, and chest ailments are common today in highland Guatemala, and given the number of remedies given by colonial writers, these complaints must have been rampant in earlier times as well.

The hot sap of the Mexican frangipani (*Plumeria rubra* var. *acutifolia* Poir) was rubbed into a sore chest to reduce the pain and cure it according to Fuentes y Guzmán (1972:2:114). Hernández also noted that Mexican frangipani was used to cure chest pain (1959:2:268). Cocoa butter (*Theobroma cacao* L.) was used to make an ointment thought to have cooling properties and to be good for the lungs (Fuentes y Guzmán 1972:2:65). For a painful, tight chest an ointment made from the flowers of the Aztec marigold (*Tagetes erecta* L.) (Fuentes y Guzmán 1969:1:246) or the billywebb sweetia (*Sweetia panamensis* Benth.) might be used (Fuentes y Guzmán 1972:2:116–17; Hernández 1959:2:192–93). When taken as a drink, pepper (*Capsicum* spp.) was said to clear the chest (Fuentes y Guzmán 1972:3:32). Hernández, however, said that immoderate use of pepper could cause illness of the pleurae and pneumonia (1959:2:138). A decoction of the adder's tongue fern (*Ophioglossum vulgatum* L.) was also used to clear the chest (Fuentes y Guzmán 1969:1:242). *Istatole,* or white *atole* (*iztacatolli* in Nahua), was a maize (*Zea mays* L.) beverage which was used as a decongestant (1969:1:227). Hernández reported that maize soothed the chest (1959:2:290); Farfán said that it was good for sufferers of colds (1944:62v). He also said that the century plant (*Agave americana* L.) loosened the chest and facilitated spitting (1944:71). Sahagún said that pulque, a drink made from the century plant, was taken for coughing (1961:10:149–50).

When drunk in powder form, cambray (*Cosmos sulphureus* Cav.) was said to act as a cold remedy (Fuentes y Guzmán 1972:2:116). Hernández said that it was very favorable to the chest (1959:3:220). A decoction of the cudweed (*Gnaphalium attenuatum* DC.), which caused sweating,

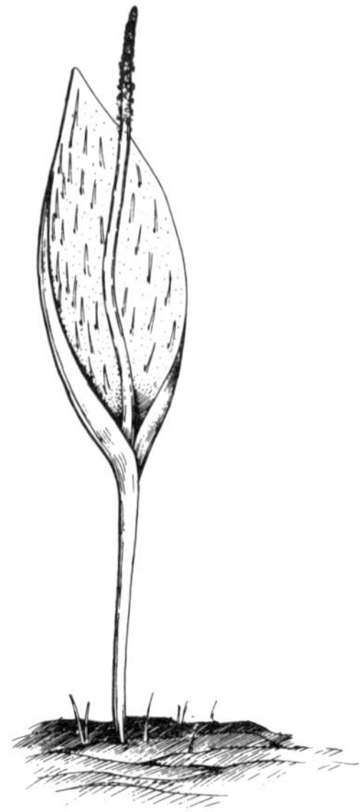

Figure 35
Ophioglossum vulgatum (Figueroa Marroquín 1957:153).

was also thought to be good against colds (Fuentes y Guzmán 1969:1:242) as was curarina (*Cissampelos pareira* L.) (1969:1:229). Pine resin from the Montezuma pine (*Pinus montezumae* Lam.) was considered good for removing cold from various illnesses among the sixteenth century Tzutujil (*RGA* 1964:103). More recently, the pine has been used as an expectorant (Villacorta Calderón 1926:78). Contrayerva (*Dorstenia contrajerva* L.) was also used for colds during the colonial period (Vázquez de Espinosa 1968:237).

Many cold remedies have been used by the modern peoples of the Guatemala highlands. Peru balsam (*Myroxylon balsamum* var. *pereirae* Harms.) was used for colds and bronchitis (Aguilar Girón 1966:366). Hernández said that Peru balsam cured respiratory difficulties and was good for many illnesses (1959:2:186). The goldenshower senna (*Cassia fistula* L.) (Rodríguez Rouanet 1971:276), a tea made from slices of the stems of the Montezuma pine (*Pinus montezumae* Lam.), and the mucilage of the cochineal cactus (*Nopalea cochenillifera* Salm-Dyck) have been used for colds and coughs (Mellen 1974:130–31). Hernández said the *nopal* (Spanish) was good for many illnesses (1959:2:312).

In recent times in Chichicastenango adults with colds went to the mountains where there were lots of pine trees because the odor of the trees was thought to kill coughs. For children, twigs of green pine were boiled in water with cinnamon and given to them to drink. If this did not cure them, then the curer was called in. Cathartics were

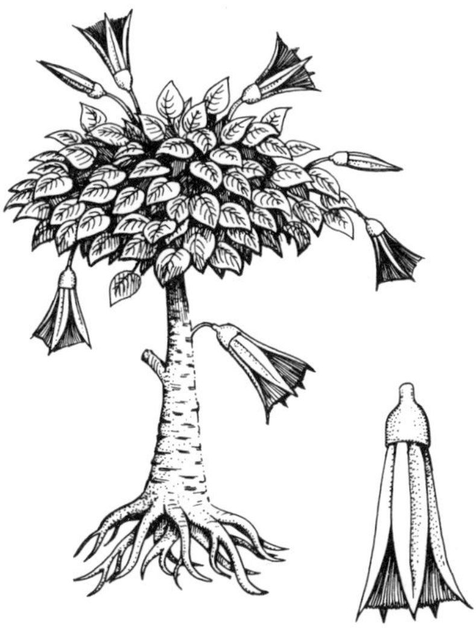

Figure 36
Bombax ellipticum (Fuentes y Guzmán 1932–33:8:443).

also used in Chichicastenango to treat colds. A good purge was said to be made by taking a little chocolate (cacao) (*Theobroma cacao* L.), without the butter, and cooking it in water (Bunzel 1967:144–45). Farfán also mentioned the use of purges as a cold treatment (1944:63v–64). Infusions of creeping oxalis (*Oxalis corniculata* L.) were also taken in Chichicastenango for colds, and a poultice of crushed leaves warmed in ashes was put around the throat (Bunzel 1967:144–45).

Recently, the bark of a species of bombax (*Bombax ellipticum* HBK.) has also been used as a cold remedy (Mellen 1974:137). A plant which may be bombax was included in the *Cruz-Badianus Herbal* where its virtues for treating coughs were noted:

> One troubled with a cough is to drink frequently the juice of the root of *tlaco-xiloxochitl* peeled and ground in water, with part of which, mixed with honey, the throat is to be smeared. But if he spits blood, he is to take this same drink before the midday meal. And it would be somewhat useful if he would merely nibble the same root in honey and chew it (Emmart 1940:119, 240).

Bombax was also mentioned by Fuentes y Guzmán but not specifically as a remedy for repiratory problems (1972:3:308). Hormiguillo (*Siparuna nicaraguensis* Hemsl.) has been used in modern times for colds and influenza (Morton 1981:230). Ginger (*Zingibre officinale* Rosc.) has

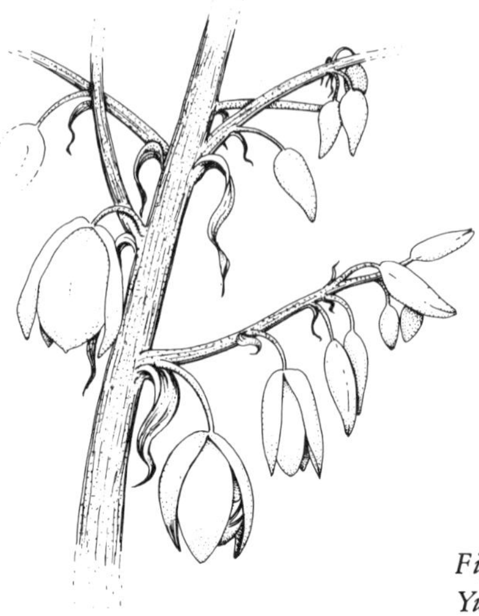

Figure 37
Yucca elephantipes (Chickering 1973:123).

been used for colds and polypody (*Phlebodium aureum* John Smith) as an expectorant, (Villacorta Calderón 1926:74, 76). The cedron simaba (*Simaba cedron* Planch.) (Aguilar Girón 1966:366), vervain (*Verbena litoralis* L.), and eucalyptus (*Eucalyptus globulus* Labill.) (Cosminsky 1972:367) are other modern cold remedies.

Another contemporary remedy, the black insides of the crossleaf calabash tree (*Crescentia alata* HBK.) was put into boiling water with a sweetener, and the liquid was drunk as a cough syrup (Simeon 1977:29). This plant was used in colonial times for treating fractures and blows (Fuentes y Guzmán 1972:2:67–68). White horehound (*Marrubium vulgare* L.) has also been used for coughs in recent times (Villacorta Calderón 1926:78) as has a warm drink made from the Mexican elder (*Sambucus mexicana* Presl. ex A.DC.) and a small stem of bulbstem yucca (*Yucca elephantipes* Reg.) boiled with a small leaf of hawthorn (*Crataegus pubescens* Steud.) (Simeon 1977:29). Ximénez said that the Mexican elder was very medicinal but did not say it was used for coughs (1967b:277). The shieldleaf pumpwood (*Cecropia peltata* L.) has been used as a remedy for whooping cough (Morton 1981:144).

Fuentes y Guzmán said the *epasoatole*—a beverage made from maize (*Zea mays* L.)—and American wormseed (*epasote* or epazotl in Nahua) (*Chenopodium ambrosioides* L.) aided those suffering from asthma (1969:1:228; Hernández 1959:2:369). A tea made from the latex, herb, and flowers of asthma weed (*Euphorbia hirta* L.) has been used in contemporary times for asthma (Mellen 1974:131), and Fuentes y Guzmán also reported that asthma weed was a remedy for many illnesses (1969:1:245).

Other modern asthma remedies are the following: a species of coralbean tree (*Erythrina folkersii* Krakoff & Moldenke) was used in Verapaz to treat asthma and hysteria. The bark, flowers, and leaves produce a hypnotic sleep. This remedy is one which must have been used with caution as the plant is poisonous (Dieseldorff 1940:196; Morton 1981:318–19). The garlic guineahen weed (*Petiveria alliacea* L.), the resurrection selaginella (*Selaginella lepidophylla* Spring), Dutchman's pipe (*Aristolochia maxima* L.), the century plant (*Agave americana* L.) ironweed (*Vernonia deppeana* Less.), and jimson weed (*Datura stramonium* L.) (Villacorta Calderón 1926:74–76, 79–80) were other plants used to relieve spasms and alleviate asthma.

Tobacco (*Nicotiana* spp.) was used to cure respiratory problems (*RGSA* 1952:116; *RGSF* 1952:138). Fuentes y Guzmán reported that curers used Mexican tobacco because the smoke was believed to be good for people suffering from asthma. The curers used it for medicinal purposes in the form of cigarettes which were wrapped using leaves of the guava tree (*Psidium guajava* L.) (1969:1:341–42). In the *Florentine Codex* tobacco was said to be inhaled for catarrh:

> Small tobacco is inhaled; and the gullet is massaged, and there is vomiting. And one is not to drink cold things; only tepid [or] hot things is one to drink [and] eat. And one is to take care not to expose himself to the sun (Sahagún 1961:10:144–45).

Tobacco was also used for respiratory disorders in Yucatán during the eighteenth century (Ossado 1944:541).

Pneumonia (mal or dolor de costado, Spanish) was another pre-Hispanic disease which existed in the highlands (Shattuck 1938:47). New strains, however, may have been brought over by the conquerors. Pneumonia was probably not a major cause of death in aboriginal times, and some of the remedies given for colds were probably used to treat it. In contemporary times ruellia (*Ruellia geminflora* HBK.), which is known for its use as a cathartic, has been used to alleviate the symptoms of pneumonia as well (Aguilar Girón 1966:350). In several other towns, hawthorn (*Crataegus pubescens* Steud.) was used for lung illnesses (Villacorta Calderón 1926:77). Although Villacorta Calderón does not specify pneumonia, that is probably what he meant by lung illnesses.

Skin Disorders

There were several endemic skin diseases, and remedies for these were given in the colonial sources. Although highland peoples probably suffered from common skin ailments, they were more of a problem on the coast. Captain Juan de Estrada, an official living on the coast during the latter half of the sixteenth century, spoke of skin illnesses:

> The Indians of this coast have an illness . . . called *jiotes* [*jiote,* Spanish; *xiyotl* in Nahua; scabies?] which is a type of sharp itch over all the body and others which wound the throat like scrofula, and they say that these two illnesses come from a certain fruit they eat (1955:75).

Jiote was prevalent in some coastal and highland towns and was probably an aboriginal disorder (Fuentes y Guzmán 1972:3:42; *RGSA* 1952:113; *RGSF* 1952:134). Scabies or itch is caused by the parasite *Sarcoptes scabiei.* The female burrows into the skin, particularly that on the front of the wrist, the web and sides of the fingers, the buttocks, genitals, and feet, forming small tunnels in which she lays her eggs. The larvae hatch in the burrows in four to five days, and it is the movement of the larvae which causes the intense itching and gives scabies its common name of itch. The main symptoms are itchiness and heat. Infected parts of the body become red and scabbed as the result of scratching, or the surface of these places may be inflamed (Thomson 1976:471; 645). Among the Aztecs xiyotl meant mange (*sarna,* Spanish), scalp ringworm (*tiña,* Spanish), leprosy, and perhaps herpes (Arriola 1973:78, 304).

Besides jiote, ringworm (*tinea*; *empeines,* Spanish) and other skin afflictions existed in various parts of the country. Ringworm is the name given to inflammatory problems of the skin produced by molds. Scalp ringworm, a childhood disease, is usually due to a species of fungus (*Microsporon audouini*) (Thomson 1976:732).

The most important therapeutic method for treating skin problems in Guatemala was bathing the affected area with herbal decoctions. Ointments were sometimes used in conjunction with the bath.

Due to its caustic nature, the rusty paullinia (*Paullinia fuscescens* HBK.) was thought to be very effective against jiote, ringworm, and *sarna antigua* (Spanish, old mange). Sufferers bathed with a decoction of the plant which stung cruelly but quickly left them free of their

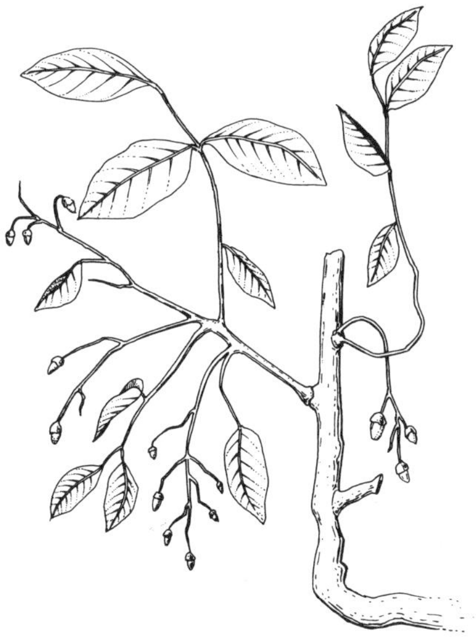

Figure 38
Rourea glabra (Figueroa Marroquín 1957:103).

illness (Fuentes y Guzmán 1969:1:240). A bath prepared from a decoction of false hellebore (*Veratrum sabadilla* Retz.), cooked until the liquid took on the color of wine, was said to be good for healing ringworm, sarna antigua and *reciente* (Spanish, recent) whether limited or extensive. It was not as effective as rusty paullinia in treating jiote, however (1969:1:243). A decoction of the bark of the sweet-pea tree (*Gliricida sepium* Steud.) was used to cure ringworm and jiote. A bath made from the white flowers of a species of strongbark (*Bourreria huanita* Hemsl.) was applied fresh or dried to treat any burning, rash, or blisters on the face or parts of the body (Fuentes y Guzmán 1969:1:245). A species of rourea (*Rourea glabra* HBK.) was another remedy for jiote, but it almost poisoned the patient. The same plant was used in colonial times to poison coyotes and was not the favored cure for skin ailments due to its danger (Fuentes y Guzmán 1972:2:117).

The sap from the cut branches of the deer fig (*Ficus glabrata* HBK.) was used to treat scalp ringworm. The head was scraped with a broken ear of maize, and the sap smeared on with a feather. The head was covered with a cloth, and this was reputed to cure ringworm very well (Fuentes y Guzmán 1972:2:56). An ear of maize (*Zea mays* L.), when carbonized, was also considered a caustic remedy for ringworm (Fuentes y Guzmán 1969:1:227). Most ringworm remedies are New World plants, but one Old World plant was mentioned for skin problems in general. During the colonial period the oil of the castor plant (*Ricinus communis* L.) was used to make an ointment employed by women to remove marks from the skin, especially from the face, and to cleanse facial pimples (1972:3:36).

Monardes said that balsam was used by Spaniards and Indians during the sixteenth century to cure wounds. It was applied externally just as in modern times and was said to be an aboriginal remedy (1925:1:23, 25–26). Balsam may also have been used in Guatemala to treat skin illnesses. Today the liquid of the stems of the tolu balsam (*Myroxylon balsamum* Harms.) has been used as a tea or an ointment against scabies and other skin parasites (Mellen 1974:133).

Another skin disorder endemic in Guatemala is *pinta* (*mal de pinto* or *carate* in Spanish), which may have originated in Chiapas (Villacorta Cifuentes 1976:71). It is caused by a fungus or spirochete (*Treponema carateum*) and consists of pigmented patches of skin. It is disfiguring but not dangerous (Ashburn 1947:206; Wood 1978:49–50) and may be white, black, gray, brown, purple, or violet in color. Pinta is characterized by rough, itchy scaly lesions (Shattuck 1938:70). Although there are no specific cures mentioned in Guatemalan colonial documents for this disease, the treatments used for itch and ringworm may also have been applied to pinta.

Leishmaniasis, a disease native to certain parts of Central America, is due to infection with a number of parasites of the genus *Leishmania*. The parasite is transmitted to humans by the bite of certain sand flies of the *Phlebotomus* type. Leishmaniasis is characterized by lesions which are similar to those produced by leprosy. Victims often have their mouth, nose, and ears eaten away, but the forearms and lower portions of the legs are other favored sites for the disease. Lesions may appear on the skin or mucous membranes (Shattuck 1938:113–15, 132).

Leishmaniasis occurs in two forms, either as a debilitating general affliction, visceral leishmaniasis, commonly known as *kala azar,* characterized by enlargement of the spleen; or as a skin disease referred to as cutaneous leishmaniasis (Ackerknecht 1972:136). In Central America leishmaniasis, in its milder cutaneous form, is often called *chiclero's* (Spanish) ulcer, and it is most common in tropical areas, especially where chicle is gathered (Shattuck 1938:120, 132). Cutaneous leishmaniasis tends to be diffuse, involving the nose and throat, and leads to widespread erosion of the nasal cartilage. It may terminate in a fatal broncho-pneumonia (Thomson 1976:501).

Highland Indians who traveled on expeditions to Alta Verapaz and the Petén may have contracted leishmaniasis. There was some traffic between the inhabitants of the tropical and highland areas in pre-Columbian times, especially for trade. Like pinta, leishmaniasis may not have been categorized as a specific illness in ancient or colonial times as no specific remedies are given for it. Treatments for other skin ailments, or those used for sores, may have been used to treat pinta and leishmaniasis as well.

An insect which was particularly bothersome to those living in tropical areas was the sand flea (chigger), which was called *nigua* in Spanish. These entered the soles of the feet, causing them to burn and itch. When scratched, the feet festered. It was customary to remove the chigger immediately, but as they were often difficult to extract, some sufferers waited until after the chigger had laid a bag of eggs. Thomas Gage described how they were commonly removed:

> Then with the point of a pin they dig around the bag, till they can take it out whole with the pin's point . . . They put in a little ear wax or ashes where the bag lay, and with that the hole is healed up again in a day or two (1969:267).

The site where the eggs were deposited could render the victim open to infection, particularly tetanus (Crosby 1972:209). No specific remedies were given for treating the wound caused by sand fleas, but wound medicines such as balsam may have been applied.

There are several contemporary remedies for skin illnesses. The latex, herb, and flowers of asthma weed (*Euphorbia hirta* L.), which was a colonial remedy for many ailments (Fuentes y Guzmán 1969:1:245), has been used to make an ointment for scabies and other skin parasites (Mellen 1974:133). The leaves of the coffee senna (*Cassia occidentalis* L.), which Hernández said was good for skin ailments (1959:2:131), have also been used to treat ringworm in Guatemala (Morton 1981:298). The *Cruz-Badianus Herbal* included this plant and said that it was used in a mixture with two other plants and dove's excrement to heal a scabby face (Emmart 1940:243). The red part of the seeds of annato (*Bixa orellana* L.) was used to prevent skin eruptions and scars (Aguilar Girón 1966:361; Villacorta Calderón 1926:74). The Mexican sunflower (*Tithonia diversifolia* Gray) was applied externally on eczema and sores of domestic animals (Morton 1981:973–74). Yellow sage (*Lantana camara* L.) was another eczema cure (Villacorta Calderón 1926:75). In eastern Guatemala the leaves of tridax (*Tridax procumbens* L.) was placed on the flesh to kill carnivorous insect larvae (Morton 1981:974). Among the Chortí rue (*Ruta graveolens* L.) was used to treat an affliction that was probably pinta (Wisdom 1940:352). Cudweed (*Gnaphalium attenuatum* DC.), cihuapahtli (*Montanoa tomentosa* Cerv.), a type of walnut (*Juglans pyriformis* Liebm.) (Villacorta Calderón 1926:78–79), and American wormseed (*Chenopodium ambroisoides* L.) (Cosminsky 1972:368) are other plants which have been used to treat skin problems.

Sores (Also Burns, Contusions, and Wounds)

Tonics for contusions were prepared in colonial times from boiled avocado shoots (*Persea americana* Mill.) (Fuentes y Guzmán 1969:1:239) and the gourd of the crossleaf calabash tree (*Crescentia alata* HBK.). The hot liquid from the boiled avocado shoots and the heated juice of the crossleaf calabash gourd were thought to be good for any blow received from a fall (Fuentes y Guzmán 1972:2:67). It has also been used for this purpose in Colotenango and Jacaltenango in contemporary times (Rodríguez Rouanet 1971:137, 139). The drink prepared from avocado shoots provoked sweating and was said to keep the injured individual from catching cold. It was administered in diminishing proportions for eight to nine days and was said to expel through the urinary tract all the blood collected internally, preventing it from becoming infected and forming an abcess. Fuentes y Guzmán said that this cure was widely known and used (1969:1:239). Hernández said that the oil of the avocado seed cured rashes and scars (1959:2:29). The avocado was also used by those who suffered blows and bites in colonial Yucatán (Ossado 1944:544). In recent times the avocado has been used to treat many illnesses (Rodríguez Rouanet 1971:267). Another contemporary cure for blows observed in Santa Catarina Pinula was ruellia (*Ruellia geminflora* HBK.) (Villacorta Calderón 1926:78).

For minor bruises such as bruised knuckles, an ointment made from the ground and boiled seed of the castor plant (*Ricinus communis* L.) was considered effective (Fuentes y Guzmán 1972:3:35), but this remedy was not pre-Hispanic. It has also been used in modern times for blows and fractures (Wauchope 1948:50).

In daily life people working in their fields or around their homes would certainly have received cuts and wounds. Warfare was common during the period preceding the Conquest, and wounds, especially those made with obsidian tipped spears and arrows, were frequent (*Annals* 1967; Fuentes y Guzmán 1972:2; *PV* 1971).

The avocado seed (*Persea americana* Mill.) was a caustic used to heal and close old sores. This remedy was said to act even more quickly on fresh ones (Fuentes y Guzmán 1969:1:239). An ointment made from the Peru balsam (*Myroxylon balsamun* var. *pereirae* Harms.) was considered to be very effective in healing cuts. Hernández said that it closed wounds and healed old ones (1959:2:187). Fray Alonso Ponce who received a deep cut in his finger while on his way to the piedmont town of Patulul claimed that after he applied balsam ointment the flow of blood ceased quickly and his wound closed (1873:430).

A species of cowitch (*Mucuna argyrophylla* L.) was said to be useful in stanching the flow of blood due to a wound or from natural causes (Fuentes y Guzmán 1972:2:158). False hellebore (*Veratrum sabadilla* Retz.) was also reputed to have a strong curative effect on old wounds and festering sores (*RGZ* 1955:78). Hernández said that it was used to cure sores in Mexico (1959:3:12). American storax (*Liquidambar styraciflua* L.) has been used to treat wounds in recent times (Villacorta Calderón 1926:77) and it was prized as a healing agent in earlier times as well. Hernández said that it cured rashes when the skin was torn off with the fingers (1959:2:112).

A decoction of wandering Jew (*Zebrina pendula* Schnizl.) was used to treat sores (Fuentes y Guzmán 1972:2:65). Hernández mentioned it as a cure for mange (1959:2:30). A species of beautyleaf (*Calophyllum brasiliense* var. *rekoi* Standl.) was considered to be very medicinal, especially for wounds (Ximénez 1967b:245). The balsam of the Aztec marigold (*Tagetes erecta* L.) (Fuentes y Guzmán 1969:1:246), and the leaves of the century plant (*Agave americana* L.) were said to be good remedies for wounds. The liquid from the latter when pressed on a wound was said to cure it quickly (1969:1:218; Hernández 1959:2:349), and the century plant has been used in recent times to cure wounds (Rodríguez Rouanet 1971:149, 150).

In the *Florentine Codex* cooked sap from the century plant was described as being used to treat skull wounds. If the skull was broken, the break was joined with a bone awl and covered with the sap or grated green leaf (Sahagún 1961:10:140–41; 1963:11:179). The dried, powdered leaf was also packed into incisions when cysts were removed or were used as a poultice. The white wine made from the sap was added to many kinds of medicines and was considered good for those who had fallen down (1961:10:162). It was used for sores of the lips as well (1961:10:146). Farfán also said that the century plant was used to cure head wounds as was the Aztec marigold (*Tagetes erecta* L.) (1944:288v–289, 290).

The ground-up leaves of the spearleaf saltbush (*Atriplex hastata* L.) were applied to sores and Fuentes y Guzmán said they healed them quickly. It was even said to erase scars (Fuentes y Guzmán 1972:3:306). The skin of the roots of bombax (*Bombax ellipticum* HBK.) had astringent properties and was used to heal sores on any part of the body (1972:3:308).

The jointed flatsedge (*Cyperus articulatus* L.) was applied to bad sores to close them. If a plaster made out of this plant was put on any healthy part of the body, however, it would apparently have the opposite effect and open a deep and horrible sore (1969:1:237). Recently, in Santa Catarina Pinula this plant was still used for sores and mange (Villacorta Calderón 1926:74).

The creeping oxalis (*Oxalis corniculata* L.) was used as a bath for sores

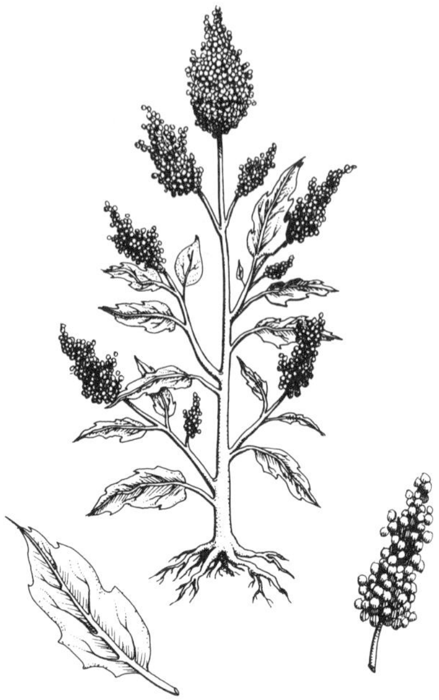

Figure 39
Atriplex hastata (Fuentes y Guzmán 1932–33:8:442).

(Fuentes y Guzmán 1972:3:112). Hernández said that a type of acid plant was used to cure burns in Mexico (1959:3:20) so perhaps they referred to the same plant. The castor plant (*Ricinus communis* L.) was used for sores and scabs on the head (Fuentes y Guzmán 1972:3:35), and the sap of the Old World plant called *arbol de María* in Spanish (*Verticillaria acuminata* Ruiz et Pavon) was said to close wounds quickly from one day to the next (1972:2:54). Tobacco (*Nicotiana* spp.) and jimson weed (*Datura stramonium* L.) were used for swellings (*RGA* 1964:104). Hernández said that tobacco juice was good for wounds (1959:2:82). In the *Florentine Codex* lime with tobacco was said to be spread on head abscesses (Sahagún 1961:10:140) and jimson weed (*toloa,* Nahua) was used on knee swellings (1961:10:158).

Cures for sores and wounds were also mentioned in the contemporary sources. A species of ironweed (*Vernonia deppeana* Less.), a plant mentioned by Ximénez (1967b:307), was used in Verapaz to reduce inflammation (Dieseldorff 1940:193) and elsewhere as a hemostatic (Villacorta Calderón 1926:79). A powder made from the leaves of cudweed (*Gnaphalium attenuatum* DC.) has been used as a general healing agent and hemostatic (Mellen 1974:123, 129; Villacorta Calderón 1962:78). The oil obtained from annatto (*Bixa orellana* L.) was used to treat burns (Rodríguez Rouanet 1971:217). A species of coralbean tree (*Erythrina berteroana* Urb.) (Aguilar Girón 1966:361), eucalyptus (*Eucalyptus globulus* Labill.) (Villacorta Calderón 1926:76), and the garden polypody (*Phlebodium aureum* John Smith) (1926:74) were other hemostatics. The leaves of tridax (*Tridax procumbens* L.) have been used as a poultice, usually fried with lard, for inflammations (Morton 1981:974). Mugwort (*Artemisia vulgaris* L.) has been used for sores, and bulbstem yucca (*Yucca elephantipes* Reg.) and gumbolimbo (*Bursera simaruba* Sarg.) for scars (Villacorta Calderón 1926:76, 78). The raw fruit of the vegetable pear (*Sechium edule* Sw.) was said to heal wounds, leaving no scar, and hormiguillo (*Siparuna nicaraguensis* Hemsl.) was used for cuts (Dieseldorff 1940:194, 197).

Tumors

Cihuapahtli (*Montanoa tomentosa* Cerv.) was said to destroy tumors of the intestines and veins (Fuentes y Guzmán 1969:1:241). Bombax (*Bombax ellipticum* HBK.) was used to destroy obstructions of the abdomen (1972:3:308), and a bath made from a decoction of the jimson weed (*Datura stramonium* L.) was used by those suffering from intercutaneous tumors. Put on a tumor, it supposedly reduced the inflammation and opened it up (1969:1:246). Hernández said that a species of jimson weed (*tlapatl,* Nahua) was used against tumors. The crushed leaves were applied to it (1959:3:180). In the *Cruz-Badianus Herbal* a type of jimson weed (*tolohua* or toloa) was used in a mixture with another plant for glands or swellings (Emmart 1940:246).

Two Old World plants were also used to treat tumors. Hormiguillo (*Verticillaria acuminata* Ruiz et Pavon) was said to destroy them and was considered to be good for many other illnesses (Fuentes y Guzmán 1972:2:54, 56). An ointment made from castor oil (*Ricinus communis* L.) was used for the same purpose (1972:3:35). Recently the root of ruellia (*Ruellia geminflora* HBK.) was used for tumors in Santa Catarina Pinula (Villacorta Calderón 1926:78).

Urinary Disorders

Urinary stoppage was a common affliction and was treated with various plant remedies. Stoppage may have been due to obstruction of the urinary passage, inflammatory irritation of the urinary tract, certain nervous conditions, or trauma to the back of the abdomen (*Barefoot Doctor's Manual* 1974:380).

Native legend said that a tiger once suffered from urine retention and taught the Indians to drink a brew made from the leaves of a plant called *chulbalam* (Quiché). This remedy was said to have an immediate diuretic effect (Fuentes y Guzmán 1969:1:243; *Annals* 1967:79). An excellent white wine was made from a type of palm tree (*Acrocomia vinifera* Oesrtd.) which was tasteful and good for human health. It was also a good diuretic (1972:2:115). The sweet marigold (*Tagetes lucida* Cav.) was boiled, dissolved in water, and taken for urine retention. It was said to cure it quickly (1969:1:241). Hernández mentioned several species of *Tagetes*. He said that some had the ability to provoke the flow of urine (1959:2:220, 324).

The maize (*Zea mays* L.) beverage *jactole,* sour or acid *atole,* was another remedy for urine retention (Fuentes y Guzmán 1969:1:227–28). Jacatole is probably the same as the *xocoatolli* (Nahua) mentioned by Hernández. He said that it was taken in the morning by sick people to cleanse the body, provoke urine, and purge the abdomen (1959:2:290). The skin of bombax roots (*Bombax ellipticum* HBK.) (Fuentes y Guzmán 1972:3:308; Hernández 1959:2:145) and the maize beverage *tlamiztatole* were both mentioned as remedies (1969:1:227). Hernández said that *tlatonilatolli* (Nahua) provoked urine flow (1959:2:291). Maize has also been used as a diuretic in contemporary times in Guatemala (Villacorta Calderón 1926:77).

The juice of the ground-up flowers of the Aztec marigold (*Tagetes erecta* L.) dissolved in water or wine (Fuentes y Guzmán 1969:1;246) was a seventeenth century diuretic as was the pineapple (*Ananas comosus* Merr.). In colonial times the pineapple (Fuentes y Guzmán 1972:3:29) and bombax (*Bombax ellipticum* HBK.) (1972:3:307–308; Hernández 1959:2:145) were used to flush out the kidneys.

Gage said that annatto (*Bixa orellana* L.) stimulated urine flow and was good for any stoppage (1969:154–55), and Ponce said that it was good for *mal de orina* (Spanish), which may refer to diabetes or some other urinary disorder (1873:392). Hernández also said that it provoked the flow of urine (1959:2:28), and Vázquez de Espinosa mentioned it as being good for urinary complaints and other troubles (1968:238). Ximénez also said that annatto was good for the urine (1967b:277), and Ossado mentioned that it was used for urine in Yucatán (1944:541).

The drug tread-softly (*Cnidoscolus urens* Anth.), which grew abundantly in Guatemala, was considered to be good for urine retention (Ximénez 1967b:300). It was used to treat gout in ancient Mexico according to the *Florentine Codex* (Sahagún 1963:11:146). It has been used in modern times to treat and dissolve urinary stones (Mellen 1974:148). Vázquez de Espinosa said that guaiacum (*Guaiacum sanctum*

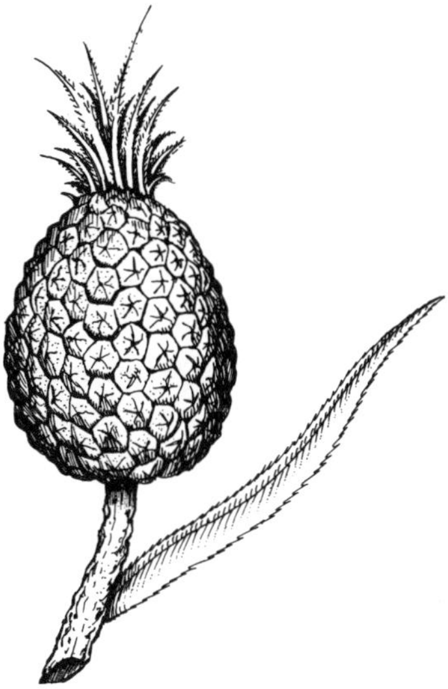

Figure 40
Ananas comosus (Fuentes y Guzmán 1932–33:8:74).

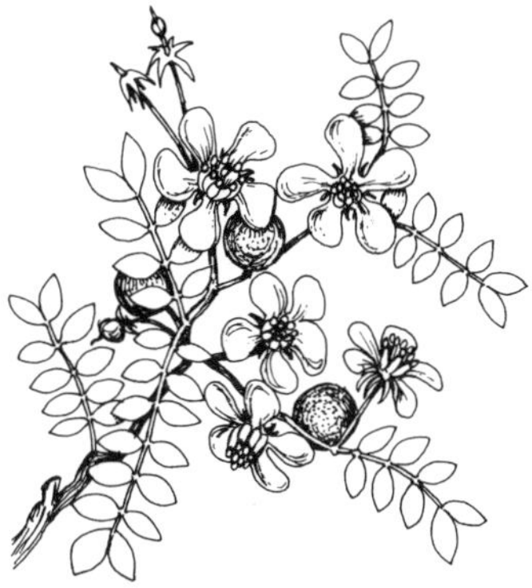

Figure 41
Guaiacum sanctum (Chickering 1973:68).

L.) was used to make cups, and that water poured into them turned blue and was a great help in urinary troubles and other illnesses (1968:210). The Barbados nut (*Jatropha curcas* L.) was another remedy used for gout. To gain relief three seeds were eaten (Fuentes y Guzmán 1972:3:305).

Several contemporary remedies have been used for urinary stoppage. A tea made from the flowers of the Mexican prickly poppy (*Argemone mexicana* L.) was used for urinary stones (Mellen 1974:148). The goldenshower senna (*Cassia fistula* L.) was used for urinary problems in Tucurú (Rodríguez Rouanet 1971:186), and Farfán said that it was used as a purge by those who had urinary blockage (1944:99–100). A decoction of the new shoots of shieldleaf pumpwood (*Cecropia peltata* L.) was used as a diuretic (Morton 1981:144). The purple mombin (*Spondias purpurea* L.) (Wauchope 1948:50), American wormseed (*Chenopodium ambroisoides* L.), the garden polypody (*Phlebodium aureum* John Smith), and the resurrection selaginella (*Selaginella lepodophylla* Spring) were used as diuretics (Villacorta Calderón 1926:74–75). In colonial Yucatán selaginella was also used for mal de orina and kidney problems (Ossado 1944:570). Bulbstem yucca (*Yucca elephantipes* Reg.) and the century plant (*Agave americana* L.) were other diuretics (Hernández 1959:2:349; Villacorta Calderón 1926:76, 77). Herb vendors also said that a type of eryngo (*Eryngium carlinae* Delar.) was boiled and the decoction taken to relieve urinary troubles (Morton 1981:646).

Several plants have been used in modern times to treat kidney ailments. Teas made from the goldenshower senna (*Cassia fistula* L.) and the nipplefruit (*Solanum mammosum* L.) were used for this purpose (Mellen 1974:128). Farfán said that the goldenshower senna was used as a purge by those suffering from kidney pain (1944:198v). Anil indigo (*Indigofera suffruticosa* Mill.) has been used in contemporary times in Verapaz for kidney infection and inflammation of the bladder (Dieseldorff 1940:196). The vine decoction of *bejuco chirriarte* (Spanish) (*Disciphania calocarpa* Standl.) was taken in Huehuetenango as a remedy for kidney ailments (Morton 1981:218). The century plant (*Agave americana* L.) was taken in Chuchexic for kidney pain, inflammation, and urinary pain (Cosminsky 1972:369). Hernández said the juice was a diuretic (1959:2:349).

Venereal Disorders

There has been some controversy as to whether venereal disease was native to the New World (see for example Crosby 1972:139–40; Goff 1967:279–94), and present evidence points to its existence among the Indians in aboriginal times. In the following passage *bubas* (Spanish) appears to refer to a form of venereal disease:

> In their gentility it [bubas] was considered by the lords to be a sign of greatness to have it because it was an indication of more power to cohabit with many women from whom it could be contracted, something ordinary people could not do (Ximénez 1967a:10).

However, as mentioned by Figueroa Marroquín, the Indians seem to have called many ailments bubas (1957:21).

Goff examined skeletal remains from Zaculeu and found two crania which may have exhibited syphilitic osteitis. These skulls dated from the latest chronological phases right before the Conquest. He performed tests which demonstrated that the skulls could have been syphilitic, but this could not be positively determined. The crania were compared with bones from other areas showing similar characteristics, and Goff

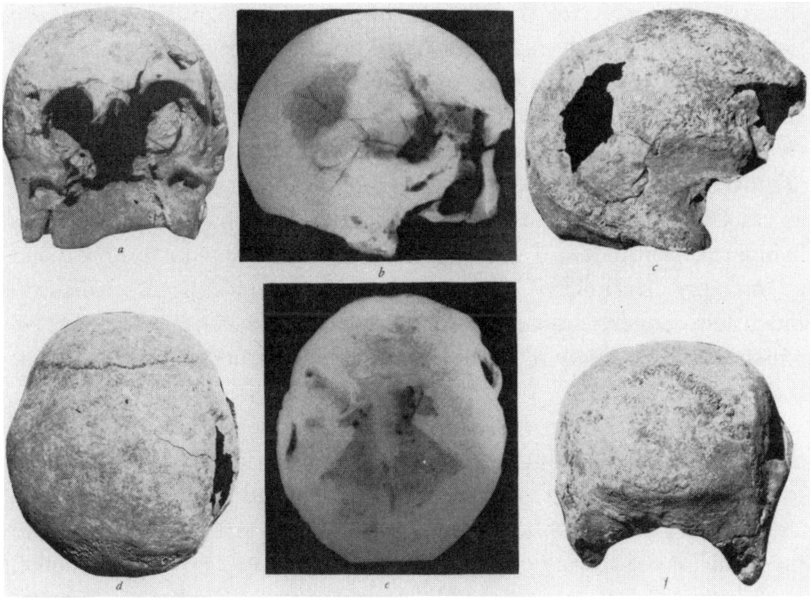

Figure 42
Syphilitic Skulls (Woodbury and Trik 1953:459).
a. Frontal view, showing extensive right-sided osteitis and edentulous fragment of mandible.
b. Roentgen lateral view, showing bone density of syphilis and gummatous defect of right parietal region.
c. Right lateral view, showing roughening of outer table of bone, gummatous defect with thinning of margins and loss of sequestra from area of diseased parietal bone.
d. Vertex view. Note bulging of right parietal with defect plus thinning of margins and over all roughening of surface-syphilitic osteitis.
e. Roentgen view.
f. Occipital view, showing extension of osteitis over practically entire outer surface.

felt that they were syphilitic lesions. Other skeletal material from Mexico support this interpretation (1953:318–19; 1967:288–89). The Aztecs had many gods connected with venereal disease, and the syndromes given by Sahagún's informants clearly support the belief that syphilis-like lesions existed in pre-Columbian Mesoamerica (Guerra 1966a:320). However, the holes could also have been caused by onchocerciasis (see p. 157).

Corinne Shear Wood reviewed the theories on the origin of venereal syphilis and the question of whether it originated in the Old or New

Worlds. She concluded that the absence of pre-Columbian, Old World skeletal remains with signs of syphilis and the growing proportion of ancient syphilitic bones from the New World supports the position that the disease originated in the Americas. It is possible, however, that the Old World had a milder form of the disease caused by organisms (*Treponema*) with which we are no longer familiar (1978:55).

Las Casas personally asked the Indians if they had known syphilis before the Conquest and was told that they had suffered it from beyond all memory. Both Las Casas and Oviedo reported that syphilis was much less dangerous for the infected Indians than for the Spaniards—which would be likely if syphilis were endemic among the Indians but the Spaniards had had no prior contact with the disease (Crosby 1972:139).

The fact that it affected Spaniards more strongly probably indicates that the Indians had built up an immunity due to long contact with the disease. According to Goff, syphilis increased in virulence around 1495–96 (1967:279–80; see also Lewis 1977:309). This may have been the result of the introduction of a new strain or to a powerful mutant. Syphilis was at least new in the Old World in the sense that the venereal mode of transmission and the symptoms that resulted therefrom were new (McNeill 1977:193). The disease was most likely found in Europe at low incidence since primeval times, but the first major epidemic occurred among the sailors returning from Columbus's first voyage to the New World. The disease was then passed onto the Spanish soldiers fighting for the king of Naples and finally reached the French troops of Charles VIII who had forced Naples to surrender after a three-week siege. As his army returned north, the Italian peninsula was inundated with syphilis which became known as *morbo gállico* in Spanish (Lyons and Petrucelli 1978:376).

Today the first stage of syphilis is often so mild as to escape detection, but when it reached Europe during the late fifteenth century, the lesions progressed rapidly to painful, massive sores and often to gaping wounds, loss of limbs, and facial disfigurations (Wood 1978:47). By the eighteenth century, the disease had probably assumed its modern form.

An illness called *cancro* (chancre), which may have been syphilis, was present in colonial times in Guatemala. Cancro may refer to the sore or chancre developed by syphilis sufferers. San Cristobal de Amatitlán came to the attention of the Spaniards in 1780 because of the Indian remedy for this problem. It involved eating a certain kind of lizard found in the area. Although this remedy would not affect a cure if the cancro was advanced, it never failed at least to alleviate it, according to Domingos Juarros. The Indians were said to have used this remedy "from the earliest periods," but it had only come to the attention of the Spaniards in the late eighteenth century (Juarros 1937:58).

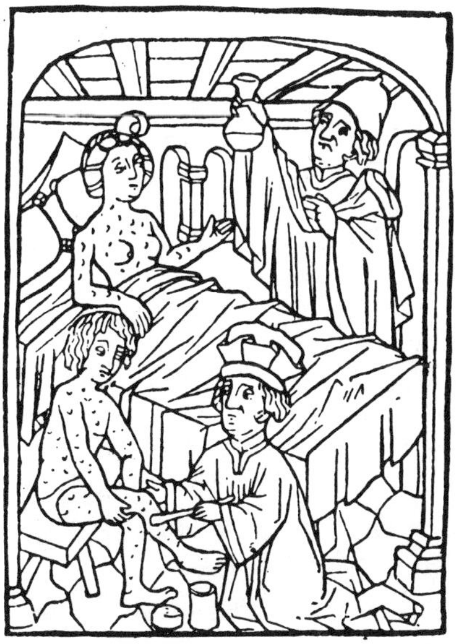

Figure 43
Treatment for Syphilis (1497). A scene from a pamphlet warning people of the disease (Jeanselme 1931:187).

Some of the cures taken for venereal disease in the colonial period were probably aboriginal remedies. Ximénez said that guaiacum (*Guaiacum sanctum* L.) was good for *mal gálico* (Spanish) and other pains (1967b:260). Farfán also said that guaiacum was used to cure bubas (1944:90). It was used for the same purpose in colonial Yucatán (Ossado 1944:533).

Fuentes y Guzmán said that the trunk of the Chinabox jasmine orange (*Murraya paniculata* Jack) was used for mal de bubas (1969:1:242) and also reported that a type of club moss (*Lycopodium dichotomun* Jacq.) easily and quickly exhausted morbo gálico (1972:2:42–43). The common groundsel (*Senecio vulgaris* DC.), called *nanahuapahtli,* or medicine of bubas in Nahua, was also used for syphilis (Fuentes y Guzmán 1972:2:116). Hernández mentioned several species of nanahuapahtli which were used to cure syphilitic sores (1959:3:62–63, 71).

Ximénez said that a decoction of the gumbolimbo (*Bursera simaruba* Sarg.) was used to wash sores of the "shameful parts which came from heat" (1967b:255). It has recently been used to treat venereal disease (Rodríguez Rouanet 1969:82). In modern times the greenbrier (*Smilax officinalis* L.) has been used as a cure for syphilis (Dieseldorff 1940:197; Villacorta Calderón 1926:80) and was used to treat a variety of illnesses in colonial times (Ximénez 1967b:302; Monardes 1925:1:39, 42). It is, therefore, possible that greenbrier, or sarsaparilla, served as an aboriginal remedy for syphilis as well. Hernández said that a species of greenbrier called *quauhmecatl* in Nahua was useful in reducing pain of the joints and other parts caused by syphilis (1959:2:250). The

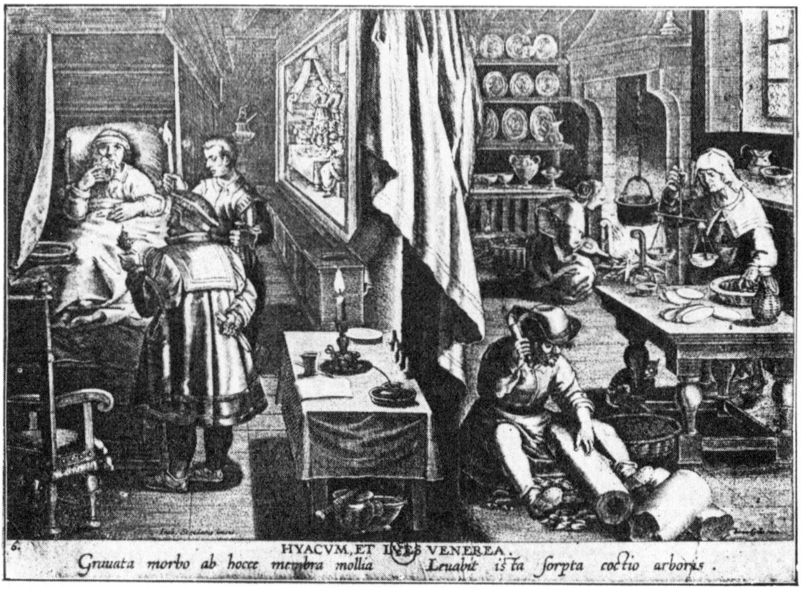
HYACVM,ET VENEREA.
Grauata morbo ab hocce membra mollia
Leuabit ista sorpta coctio arboris.

Figure 44
Guaiacum Cure for Syphilis. The middle of the illustration shows a picture of a bordello where the patient contracted syphilis. The extreme left shows the patient drinking a portion of guaiacum as the doctor stands before him holding an evergreen rod, the symbol of recovery. On the right side, a servant is chopping guaiacum wood which will be prepared by the two women. The original is in *Nova Reperta* by Stradanus (Jeanselme 1931:193).

billywebb sweetia (*Sweetia panamensis* Benth.) has also been used in contemporary times to treat syphilis (Morton 1981:350) as has cihuapahtli (*Montanoa tomentosa* Cerv.) (Villacorta Calderón 1926:79).

Fuentes y Guzmán mentioned that American wormseed (*Chenopodium ambroisiodes* L.) was used in colonial times as a blood purifier (1969:1:228). Impurity of the blood was associated with venereal disease. Several plants have been made into teas and used in contemporary times as blood purifiers: the entire bejuco chirriarte (*Disciphania calocarpa* Standl.), the leaves of a type of tread-softly (*Cnidoscolus chayamansa* McVaugh), the leaves and stem of the black nightshade (*Solanum nigrum* L.), the entire Siberian motherwort (*Leonurus sibericus* L.), and the fruit of the pigeon plum (*Coccoloba diversifolia* Jacq.) (Mellen 1974:150–51).

None of the plant remedies used in the colonial period were effective against syphilis. Prior to the discovery of penicillin, salts of mercury

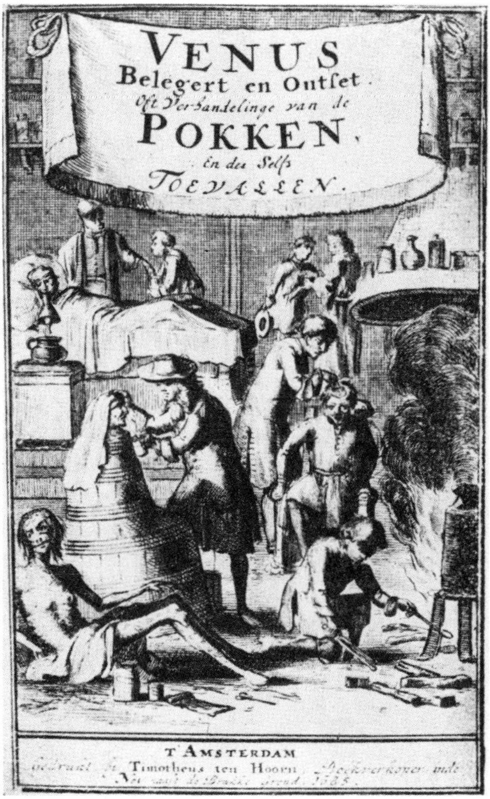

Figure 45
Treatments for Syphilis. The patient at the right receives a mercury-salve massage. The woman at the left takes a sweatbath in a barrel. In the background the man in bed inhales mercury vapors. The woman in the front of the illustration is in the terminal phase of the disease. Her nose and limbs have been eaten away. The original is from *Praxeos medicae* by S. Blankaart (Jeanselme 1931:188).

were used to treat syphilis. Salts of mercury are highly poisonous and probably led to the death of many sufferers. In 1910, Paul Ehrlich discovered the anti-syphilitic action of organic arsenical preparations, and these were used to treat the disease in conjunction with bismuth salts. For nearly forty years organic arsenic preparations were the primary treatment for syphilis (Thomson 1976:560, 824). Not until penicillin was used against it in the 1940s was a reliable cure available (Wood 1978:48).

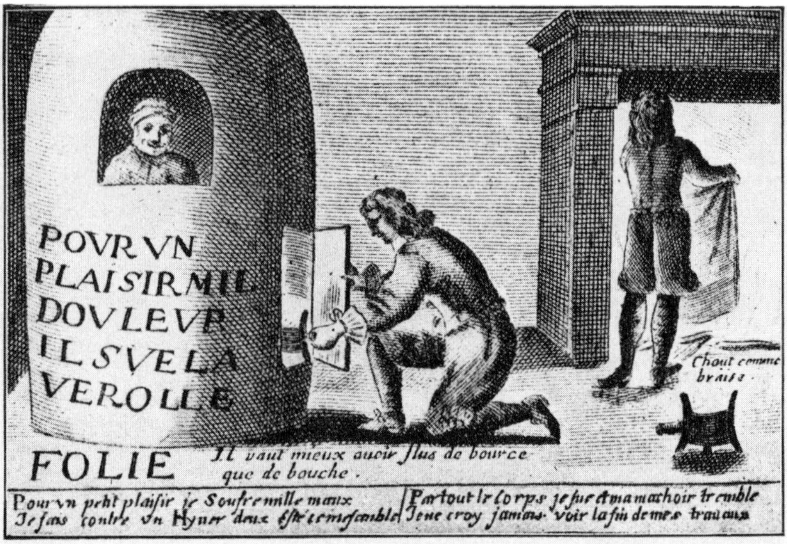

Figure 46
"For One Pleasure A Thousand Pains." Fumigation or sweating treatment for syphilis. From the collection of engravings by Jacques Laniet, Paris 1659–63 (Jeanselme 1931:195).

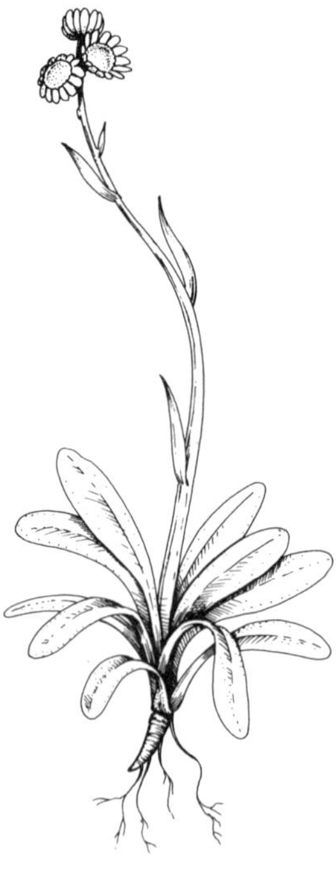

Figure 47
Senecio vulgaris (Figueroa Marroquín 1957:169).

Las Casas said that doctors and diviners were called upon for advice when a couple who wanted children could not have any. Lots were cast, and sometimes the prospective parents were told that they could not have children because they had committed a sin and therefore the gods would not send any. If they wanted children, they had to confess and perform penance (1967:2:226). Childless couples also resorted to herbs. A species of greenbrier (*Smilax cordifolia* Humb. & Bonpl.) was used in the seventeenth century in Guatemala to make sterile women fertile (Ximénez 1967b:247).

Herbal remedies were also employed to aid birth. In some areas the mother drank water mixed with pepper (*Capsicum* spp.). This acted as a cathartic and was said to purge recently delivered mothers (Fuentes y Guzmán 1972:3:32). Hernández said that chili acted as a purge. The powdered leaves were taken with atolli (1959:2:134).

In recent times the entire Cihuapahtli (*Montanoa tomentosa* Cerv.) plant has been used to make a tea to promote uterine contractions and facilitate birth (Mellen 1974:149). This remedy was also mentioned by Fuentes y Guzmán as being good for women's ailments (1969:1:241). Cihuapahtli was also mentioned in the *Cruz-Badianus Herbal:*

> If a woman has difficulty in labor, in order to deliver and bring forth the fetus with little effort, she should drink a medicine of the bark of the *quauhalahuac* tree and the herb *cihuapahtli* crushed in water, the small stone *eztetl,* and the tail of the small animal named *tlaquatzin* (Emmart 1940:190, 316).

Hernández said that *cihuapahtli mayor* cured women's illnesses and was beneficial to the uterus. The juice of *cihuapahtli hemionitico,* another species, was said to aid women giving birth. Hernández mentioned several other species of the plant which were also said to be good for women's illnesses (1959:2:293–98). In the *Florentine Codex* the cooked foliage was said to be drunk by a woman who was about to give birth. After the liquid was taken, the baby was born (Sahagún 1963:11:179–80). It is clear from the number of references to this plant in Guatemalan and Mexican sources that it was commonly known and used in aboriginal and colonial times to aid delivery.

Recently, in Chinautla, the midwife gave the mother a tea of eryngo (*Eryngium carlinae* Delar.) as a constituent to alleviate the pain of delivery (Reina 1966:241). Fuentes y Guzmán mentioned this plant as being used for medicinal purposes, but he did not say that it was used to aid birth (1972:2:116). In the Jacalteca area a small branch of fennel (*Foeniculum vulgare* Mill.) was boiled and the liquid taken before birth (Rodríguez Rouanet 1971:208). In colonial Yucatán a decoction of fennel leaves was used to increase milk and purge women after birth (Ossado 1944:537). During the seventeenth century fennel was used as an eyewash (Fuentes y Guzmán 1969:1:244), but as it was an introduced plant, it was not part of aboriginal treatment.

Many galactagogues were mentioned in the contemporary sources. Most of these plants were not discussed by colonial authors. In Jacaltenango, however, a dough of maize (*Zea mays* L.) was mixed with toasted cacao (*Theobroma cacao* L.) and ground up. The mother lacking milk took this hot or cold and sweetened (Rodríguez Rouanet 1971:120). Maize had many uses in the late seventeenth century (Fuentes y Guzmán 1969:1:227–28) as did cacao (Fuentes y Guzmán 1972:2:64–65; Gage 1969:152, 157).

The following remedies were other galactagogues used in modern times: a liquid made from the sweet potato (*Ipomoea batatas* Lam.) (Rodríguez Rouanet 1971:119); a tea made from a type of spurge (*Euphorbia lancifolia* Schlect.), a tea made from the breadnut tree (*Brosimum alicastrum* Sw.) (Mellen 1974:125), and the oil from the seeds of a type of dill (*Anethum foeniculatum* L.) taken in drops (Aguilar Girón 1966:354; Ossado 1944:536; Villacorta Calderón 1926:75). The heated leaves of the Barbados nut (*Jatropha curcas* L.) were placed on the breast of nursing mothers to increase milk flow (Morton 1981:449).

Other plants have been used to induce abortion. In Cobán the leaves of Mexican gianthyssop (*Agastache mexicana* Benth.) were cooked with other plants and the liquid drunk several times to promote abortion (Rodríguez Rouanet 1971:259). In Chajul a half pound of annatto (*Bixa orellana* L.) was cooked in five glasses of water. The brew was taken three times daily for five days for the same purpose (1971:261). Annatto seeds were taken in the Chortí area to avoid and relieve hemorrhages at birth (Wisdom 1940:289). In San Martín Sacatepéquez some branches of the southern maidenhair fern (*Adiantum capillus-veneris* L.) were cooked, and the drink was taken at breakfast for nine days for abortion. Afterwards a purge consisting of two ounces of English salt was administered (Rodríguez Rouanet 1971:260).

Several emmenagogues were mentioned by Ximénez and Fuentes y Guzmán. A species of greenbrier (*Smilax cordifolia* Humb. & Bonpl.) (Ximénez 1967b:247), a hot decoction of the leaves and stems of the Old World white horehound (*Marrubium vulgare* L.) (Fuentes y Guzmán 1969:1:241), the juice of the flowers or the flowers themselves of the

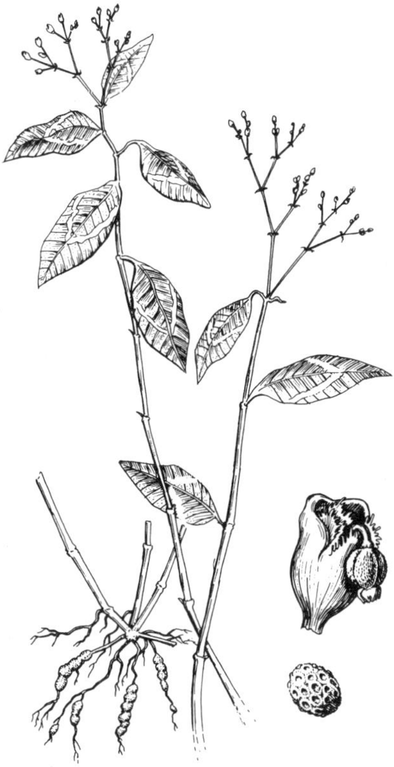

Figure 48
Euphorbia lancifolia (Rosengarten 1982:94).

Aztec marigold (*Tagetes erecta* L.) ground up and dissolved in water or wine (1969:1:246; Hernández 1959:2:220), and tlamiztatole, a beverage made by boiling maize (*Zea mays* L.) and adding pepper (*Capsicum* spp.) mixed with American wormseed (*Chenopodium ambrosioides* L.) (1969:1:228), were all considered good for menstrual problems. Among the Chortí the latter plant was taken for three days after delivery (Wisdom 1940:290). Hernández said that tlatonilatolli provoked urine and menstruation and heated and fortified the entire body (1959:2:291). In Mexico American wormseed was part of a mixture used to treat menstruation (López Austin 1972:139). Cihuapahtli (*Montanoa tomentosa* Cerv.) was another important emmenagogue, and a decoction of this plant was believed to clear an obstructed womb (Fuentes y Guzmán 1969:1:241; Hernández 1959:2:293).

Many remedies have been used in contemporary times for treating menstrual difficulties. Eryngo (*Eryngium carlinae* Delar.) was used in Verapaz to regulate menstruation (Dieseldorff 1940:192). It was also used in Chuchexic (Cosminsky 1972:370). This was one of the general medicinal plants contained in Fuentes y Guzmán's work (1972:2:116). It is considered to be a strong emmenagogue and may cause abortion (Aguilar Girón 1966:350).

The American storax (*Liquidambar styraciflua* L.) has been used in Santa Cruz Verapaz for menstrual pain (Rodríguez Rouanet 1969:81). Hernández said it alleviated infections of the uterus (1959:2:112), and Farfán also mentioned that it was good for causing menstrual blood to flow (1944:77). The leaves of wormwood (*Artemisia absinthium* L.) were cooked, and the liquid drunk for menstrual disorders (Rodríguez Rouanet 1971:252; Villacorta Calderón 1926:74). The husk of the coconut (*Cocos nucifera* L.) was used for the same thing. If the blood continued to flow, the husk was cooked in four glasses of water. The liquid was sweetened and drunk, four glasses a day for two days (Rodríguez Rouanet 1971:252). The coralbean tree (*Erythrina corallodendron* L.), which has sedative properties, has also been used in recent times as an emmenagogue (Wauchope 1948:50). The garden polypody (*Phlebodium aureum* John Smith), the southern maidenhair fern (*Adiantum capillus-veneris* L.), the resurrection selaginella (*Selaginella lepidophylla* Spring), tridax (*Tridax procumbens* L.), and rue (*Ruta graveolens* L.) (Villacorta Calderón 1926:74–76, 78) were other emmenagogues. Rue was also used in colonial Yucatán as an emmenagogue (Ossado 1944:546). Rue was used as a body wash to relieve labor and delivery pains as well as to stop post-delivery hemorrhages in the Chorti area (Wisdom 1940:288–89). The garlic guineahen weed (*Petiveria alliacea* L.) was used in Chuchexic for menstrual pains (Cosminsky 1972:367). It was also used by the Chortí as an emmenagogue (Wisdom 1940:287).

PART II

Spanish Influence on Indian Health and Medicine

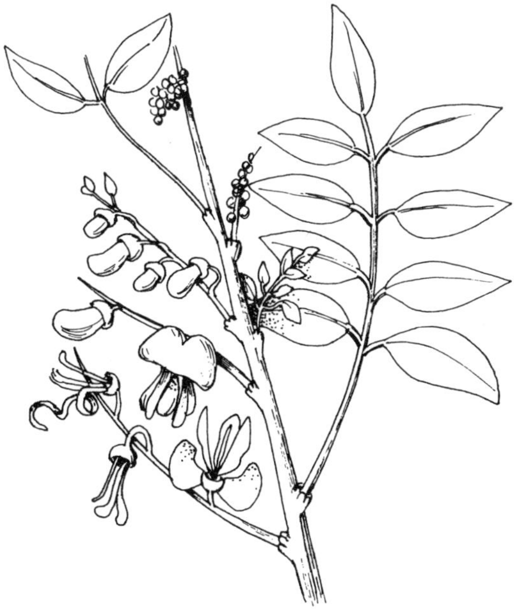

CHAPTER FIVE

The Introduction of Old World Diseases

Epidemics in the Sixteenth Century

Some Old World medical beliefs and practices were adopted by the native population of Guatemala after the Conquest, and the Spaniards made use of Indian knowledge. They used Indian doctors and exported some plant remedies to Europe. The major impact of the arrival of the Europeans in the New World, however, was the introduction of catastrophic epidemic diseases. The Europeans also contracted diseases endemic to the Americas, but the toll was far less severe than that suffered by the Indians.

Many writers have attempted to identify the epidemic diseases brought over by the conquerors and others (see for example, Cook 1946; Figueroa Marroquín 1957; MacLeod 1973; Schendel 1968). It is difficult to identify each outbreak with certainty because diseases were sometimes misdiagnosed, erroneously named, or were a combination of maladies (Crosby 1972:42–43).

For example, the Spanish word *viruelas* appears in many sixteenth century chronicles and is almost invariably translated as smallpox. Viruelas, however, refers specifically to the pimpled, pustuled appearance, which is the most obvious symptom of smallpox, and not to the disease. Sixteenth and seventeenth century Europeans may have used the word to refer to measles, chicken pox, or even typhus. Usually, what they called viruelas was smallpox (Crosby 1967:43). *Tabardillo* or *tabardete* (Spanish) are other words that appear in the colonial sources and are traditional Castilian terms for exanthematic typhus (Guerra 1966a:331). They came to be used to describe epidemic diseases characterized by fever.

It is also difficult to determine the mortality of various outbreaks. People were not statistically-minded during the colonial period, so their estimates of the numbers of people who died of epidemic diseases may be a more accurate measure of their emotions than of the number who really died (Crosby 1972:43). There is no doubt, however, that the overall mortality was very high. Murdo MacLeod listed all of the pandemics and local outbreaks of disease in Guatemala from 1519 to 1746 (1973:98–100). Christopher Lutz listed epidemic diseases in the capital, Santiago de Guatemala, and the surrounding region from 1519 to 1769 (1976:743–52).

Smallpox

Pedro de Alvarado entered Guatemala in 1523, but disease had preceded him, probably by means of Indian ambassadors from Mexico (MacLeod 1973:40). From 1519 to 1520 a virulent epidemic, which may have been measles (*sarampión,* Spanish) or smallpox (viruelas, *gran lepra* in Spanish) accompanied by pulmonary or pneumonic plague or typhus, spread to Guatemala from Cuba and Mexico (1973:98).

Smallpox is highly communicable in a non-vaccinated population with the mortality rate being around 30%. If it, or measles, occurred with plague or typhus, which seems to have been the case, this would explain the high mortality rate of the initial epidemic in Guatemala, which has been estimated at around one-third of the population (MacLeod 1973:98).

Smallpox is an acute infectious disease characterized by fever and the appearance on the surface of the body of an eruption which, after passing through various stages, dries up, leaving more or less distinct scars. It is one of the most contagious of all diseases and is spread by contact with infected persons or their surroundings (Thomson 1976:778). Smallpox has two main types, *variola major* and *variola minor,* with the former being the most severe. The virus is most often transmitted through the air in droplets or dust and enters the victim through the respiratory tract. Humans are the only source of the virus, and the period of infectiousness, beginning around the tenth day of the incubation stage, can last up to two weeks from the first appearance of the symptoms (Joralemon 1982:118–19).

High mortality can increase in areas of poor hygiene and poverty as a result of concomitant infection, particularly of the respiratory tract. Malignant smallpox is a serious form of the disease where the patient is from the onset overwhelmed with the prostration and quickly succumbs, the rash scarcely appearing at all (Thomson 1976:780). Perhaps the early Guatemalan epidemic was malignant smallpox.

Plague

Plague is characterized by fever, swelling of the lymphatic glands, a rapid course, and a very high mortality. It is caused by the bacillus *Yersinia pestis*. It occurs first as an epizöötic in rats, and the infection is spread to humans by the rat flea. After infection, an incubation period which varies from two to six days for bubonic and three to four days for pneumonic, elapses, and then the disease begins suddenly with fever, headache, great lassitude, and aching of the limbs. Fever, thirst, prostration, and weakness are characteristic. Swollen glands (buboes) occur in over two-thirds of the cases in the groin or armpit.

There is a rapidly fatal form, associated with great weakness, in which the bacteria enter the blood, and the person dies on the second or third day, or sometimes in a few hours (*septicaemic plague*). In other cases the lungs are particularly affected, and pneumonia develops with death on the fourth or fifth day. With this form the disease is transmitted directly from human to human by coughed-up sputum. This is said to be the most infectious and most fatal form of the disease and is called *pneumonic plague* (Thomson 1976:674–75; Ackerknecht 1972:9).

There is an ethnically-defined illness which was sometimes confused with the plague in colonial times. Snake (cumatz) illness seems to have had some symptoms in common with *k'ucumatz,* the Quiché name for pneumonic plague. Fuentes y Guzmán (1972:3:274) and Vázquez de Herrera (1944:4:309) both mentioned the snake illness. In one passage Fuentes y Guzmán stated that those who were attacked with it twisted and turned as a snake does and cried out in their pain cumatz! cumatz!, snake! snake! They did not die from the illness, nor did it last many days. In another passage Fuentes y Guzmán said that the malady came from eating children. He also said that it was thought to be caused by cold, and the snake was associated with water and cold. The cure was prolonged exposure to fire. The Indians were told by a Spanish priest that if they continued to eat children, they would be changed into snakes which would tear up their insides. Not long after the priest said this, an Indian woman, according to Fuentes y Guzmán, ate a child. That evening she began to feel sharp pains in her abdomen which twisted and turned like a snake. Her muscles, abdomen, stomach, and arms were affected by waves of pain. She suffered for three days with pains similar to those of labor, and began to expel deformed, growing snakes through her openings and died. Other Indian women and their husbands, who had aided them in eating children, suffered similar attacks but did not expel snakes (1969:1:390–91).

Vázquez de Herrera also described an epidemic called cumatz which occurred in Guatemala in 1650. He described it as a vehement attack in the stomach which spread throughout the body like a fever, affecting both the muscles and the nervous system, causing great pain. He also said that many of the victims had very high fevers and that the illness was usually fatal (1944:4:309). This probably referred to the plague which seems to have had some characteristics in common with the non-epidemic form of snake illness.

In the *Ritual of the Bacabs* "snake in the abdomen of a man" and "snake-pulsation in the abdomen of a man" were included as illnesses. In one type the victim was said "not [to] sleep, he does not curl up . . . because of it." The victim also had flatulence, fainted, sweated, and had morbid yawning. He hiccoughed and sighed. His breath was short. Tobacco (*Nicotiana* spp.) was mentioned as a cure in an incantation for snake in the abdomen (1965:40–45). Therefore, it is likely that cumatz is of pre-Columbian origin.

Tedlock described snake illness as it appeared recently in Momostenango:

> In the snake illness, there are sudden and extremely painful cramps in one or more of the following areas of the body: arms, legs, torso, wrists, elbows, ankles, knees, and neck. The muscles are taut and knotted, while the joints act as if they were dislocated. The person cannot turn, move, or walk about easily . . . Episodes of seizure by the snake illness are of relatively brief duration, lasting from a few minutes to a couple of days, but they are recurrent.

According to Tedlock, snake illness is due to a temporary, recurrent, stereotypic, unsought possession or hysterical psychosis, and this type of illness is one of several considered to be a call to become a diviner in Momostenango (1982:54–57). However, in the case reported by Fuentes y Guzmán (1969:1:390–91) the woman may also have had some type of parasites.

Typhus

Typhus is caused by *Rickettsia prowazeki* and is transmitted from lice to humans. The temperature of the victim rises suddenly on the third day, and the face and eyes become congested. The headache becomes more intense, and the patient becomes drowsy or delirious.

The characteristic rash which appears on the abdomen and spreads over the body, except for the face, may also appear at this point although it usually appears on the fifth or sixth day of the disease. Death from heart failure occurs on the fourteenth day, or the temperature falls, and the patient recovers (Thomson 1976:873).

Francisco Bravo, a physician practicing in Mexico during the sixteenth century, described typhus:

> The manner and form of invasion is this. A rather intense fever attacks those who are affected by the disease and persists in the same tenor without intermission for several days. With this are great distention of veins; severe aches and pains all over the body, especially in the head; . . . comotose symptoms and delirium; great illness of the face; thick reddish urine; large, vehement, fast, and frequent pulse; oppression of the heart; insatiable thirst; excessive dryness, roughness and blackness of the tongue from combustion of the humors; heaviness of the temples; and most intense heat of the entire body . . . In the skin of the whole body pustules break out which resemble mosquito bites, somewhat red or livid or black, concomitant with great intensity and ferocity of the symptoms (Jarcho 1957:427–28).

Another form of typhus is transmitted from rat to humans by fleas, and the agent is *Rickettsia mooseri.* It is usually milder than the other forms and has a lower mortality rate (Thomson 1976:873).

Measles

Measles is an acute infectious disease occurring today mostly in children. Among communities where measles is not prevalent, the old suffer equally with the young. There are few diseases so infectious as measles, and its rapid spread in epidemics is no doubt due to the fact that infection is most potent in the earlier stages. From ten to fourteen days after infection symptoms appear. There is sudden onset of acute catarrh of the mucous membranes. Sneezing, sometimes bleeding from the nose, red and watery eyes, cough, hoarseness, and occasionally diarrhea occur. Fever, rapid pulse, headache, thirst, and restlessness are other symptoms. Around the fourth day eruptions appear on the skin. Small spots of dusky red or crimson color are characteristic. The face becomes swollen and bloated. The rash lasts around a week. Measles may occur in a very severe or malignant form where the symptoms throughout are of urgent character, the rash feebly developed and of dark-purple hue, and there is great prostration of strength, accompanied by intense catarrh (Thomson 1976:539–41).

The epidemic of 1519–20 was called *chaac* by the Cakchiquels (Martínez Durán 1964:124) and was described in the *Annals of the Cakchiquels:*

> It happened that during the twenty-fifth year the plague began, . . . First they became ill of a cough, they suffered from nosebleeds and illness of the bladder. It was truly terrible, the number of dead there were in that period (1967:115–16).

Villacorta Cifuentes reviewed all of the information on smallpox and measles and made a good case that this epidemic was measles. He thinks that the symptoms described in the *Annals* passage quoted above and in another entry for a similar outbreak which occurred in 1560 are more characteristic of measles than smallpox (1976:50–57; *Annals* 1976:143). (See below for the passage referring to 1560.) In the sixteenth century smallpox and measles were not clinically differentiated, and the cough mentioned in the *Annals* passages for the years 1519–20 and 1560 would seem to support the measles hypothesis. Coughing is part of measles syndrome as are nosebleeds but neither routinely occur with smallpox (Villacorta Cifuentes 1976:53–54).

The Effect of the Epidemics

The first of series of sweeping epidemics struck in 1519–20 and Indian medicine was totally ineffective in dealing with it. From 1520 until the end of the eighteenth century, epidemics periodically ravaged native life. Measles (sarampión or *pequeña lepra* in Spanish), smallpox, fever (tabardillo), typhus, and pneumonic plague (*peste,* Spanish or k'ucumatz) in Guatemala (MacLeod 1973:19) led to a tremendous decline in the highland population while malaria and yellow fever decimated the tropical areas. Initially, many Indians believed that baptism was responsible for spreading the epidemics, and they brought the sons of slaves to the priests rather than their own children (Fuentes y Guzmán 1972:3:281).

From 1532 to 1534, a measles epidemic swept over Mesoamerica (MacLeod 1973:98). From 1545 to 1548, pneumonic plague struck in Guatemala, and several towns disappeared (1973:98). Many Indians also perished of an epidemic disease (probably measles) in 1560. The *Annals* said:

> In the sixth month after the arrival of the Lord President in Panagán, the plague which had lashed the people long ago began here. Little by little it arrived here. In truth a fearful death fell on our heads by the will of our powerful God. Many families [succumbed] to the plague. Now the people were overcome by intense cold and fever, blood came out of their noses, then came a cough growing worse and worse, the neck was twisted, and small and large sores broke out on them (1967:143).

In February of 1561, it was reported that the pestilence was widespread, and that Spanish officials were unable to collect tribute payments from the Indians since the healthy were so busy caring for the sick that they were unable to pay (Lutz 1976:743). In 1564, "Many people died of smallpox, which was then prevalent" (*Annals* 1967:145). In 1574, there was a pestilence in San Agustín, which was near Cobán. Four hundred people died within three months, and everyone in the town was ill. A Doctor Sedeño, who was in the town to count the people for tribute purposes, observed the lack of food and that there were not even forty healthy Indians in the entire town and that eight to ten Indians were being buried every day (Viana *et al.* 1955:25).

From 1576 to 1577, pneumonic plague and smallpox reoccurred (MacLeod 1973:98; Lutz 1976:744). In 1585 a great epidemic broke out in Quetzaltenango. The sum of twenty-one *pesos* (Spanish) was paid to the *corregidor* (Spanish) of the town and to the barber by order of the audiencia in Guatemala for medicines. The barber was sent to help cure the Indians (Lutz 1976:745).

In 1588, an epidemic of smallpox occurred among the children, but no adults died of the disease (*Annals* 1967:156). Perhaps this was chicken pox (*varicella*). By this time adults may have built up immunity to the disease. In 1590, another epidemic occurred "of coughs, chills, and fever from which the people died" (1967:158). From 1592 to 1593 there was a great pestilence in all of Guatemala (Lutz 1976:745).

Such virulent and widesweeping epidemics had either not been known in pre-Conquest times or were comparatively rare. Conquest and disease produced demoralization and physical debility and led to the profound spiritual weakening of Indian culture. Beginning with the epidemic of 1520, the Cakchiquel, for example, lost their ruler, his eldest son, and many other nobles (*Annals* 1967:115–16). This affected the succession to leadership, and most families, noble and commoner, lost some members during this period.

Remesal said that in 1530, Indians who died in the capital city of Santiago (Ciudad Vieja) were not being buried, and the dogs and birds were devouring their bodies (1932:1:53–54). The Cakchiquels had said the same thing had happened during the epidemic of 1519–20 (*Annals* 1967:116). In 1530, the town council of Santiago ordered that Christian Indians were to be buried in holy ground and non-Christians in the country so that their corpses would not be eaten by dogs (Fuentes y Guzmán 1969:1:199). These orders indicate that many deaths were occurring among the Indians during that time period. By the end of the sixteenth century, the population had dropped tremendously in surviving towns (see for example, MacLeod 1973:71, 131).

The Spaniards were powerless to arrest the progress of the epidemics. European medicine was not effective against these diseases, besides there were no European-trained doctors in Guatemala anyway until the late sixteenth century. Alvarado did not have an army surgeon when he entered the country but employed the services of a barber named Maese Francisco and some Indians who bled the conquerors (Fuentes y Guzmán 1972:3:282). Barbers performed this operation which was considered to be too menial a task for a doctor (Bettman 1962:74).

The conquerors also relied upon Indian doctors. When Alvarado was wounded in the leg during fighting, he said that he was forced to spend five days in an Indian town where the wound was treated (1954:42–43). Despite the care he received, his leg was shortened due to this wound, leaving him with a limp for the rest of life (Fuentes y Guzmán 1969:1:85). During the Conquest period, besides battle wounds, both Indians and Spaniards suffered from dysentery (Fuentes y Guzmán 1972:3:18), and both groups may have taken native herbal cures for it.

Fuentes y Guzmán said that the only medicine the Indians had for curing k'ucumatz was sleeping on a mat close to the hearth (1972:3:274). By the seventeenth century, it was no doubt generally known that ancient remedies had no effect on the plague, but some of the cures for fever mentioned in colonial sources may have been used to alleviate the symptoms of the disease. However, the Indians of San Antonio Aguas Calientes continued to bathe in the sulphur springs in their town to cure k'ucumatz (1972:3:274).

Estrada said that the Indians had many superstitions concerning illness and thought that whether a person died or not after contracting a disease had nothing to do with the treatment provided. When a person became ill, he was fed, and ate it or not and just died (1955:74). The fatalistic attitude of the Indians was probably based in the belief that catastrophic illnesses were a punishment sent by God. However, it is evident from other colonial sources that the Indians did continue to use ancient remedies to treat endemic illnesses.

The Spanish took many highland Indians to the coastal areas to build

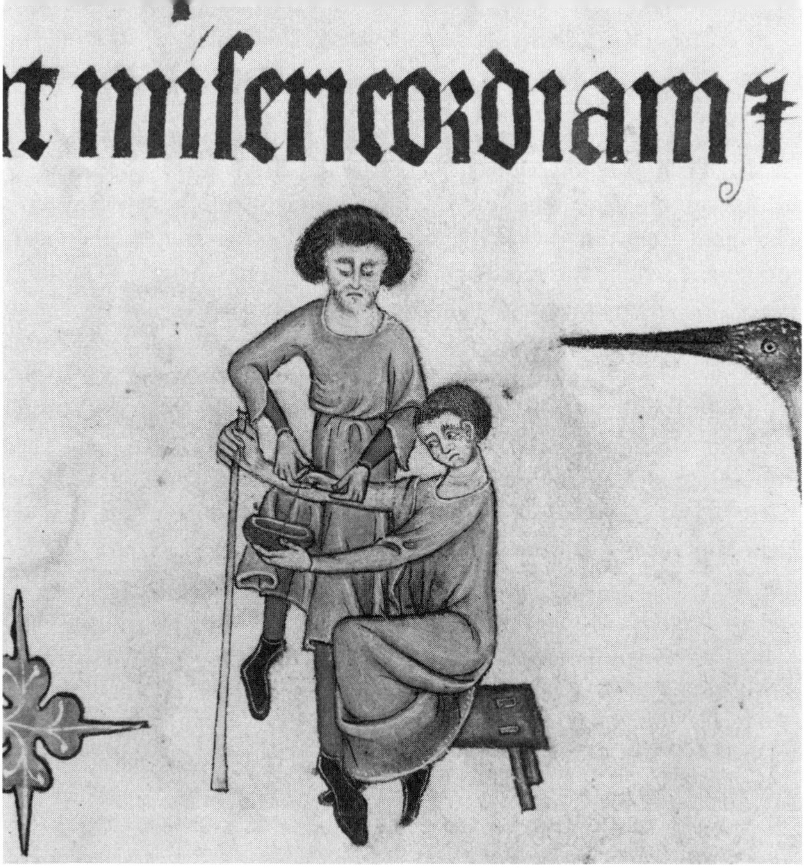

Figure 49
Barber Bleeding A Man. A barber-surgeon is shown bleeding a patient who steadies his arm with a "barber pole." This illustration is from the Luttrell Psalter (1340). The British Library, London. Add. Ms. 42130 f. 6.

ships and to work on cacao and indigo plantations (Fuentes y Guzmán 1972:3:293; MacLeod 1973:77, 185). Some of these Indians became sick and either died (Garcés 1973:384) or went home with tropical epidemic ailments. Diseases endemic to coastal areas were also spread in this way to the highlands.

Later Epidemics

Epidemics occurred every few years in Guatemala all throughout the sixteenth to eighteenth centuries (MacLeod 1973:98–100). In 1601, "a deadly epidemic began, attacking the throat of the women and men, who died after two days" (*Annals* 1967:159). Perhaps this was an outbreak of mumps. Mumps is due to infection with a virus and is highly infectious from person to person. It is predominantly a disease of childhood and early adult life, but it can occur at any age. The main symptom is swelling of glands, but fatigue, slight fever, and sore throat may precede the swelling by a day or two (Thomson 1976:574). The epidemic struck many Indian towns. There were so many people sick in Cobán that the priest in the monastery of Santo Domingo asked that the people be released from paying tribute (*AGC* A3.16:2801–40,493). From 1607 to 1608 a great epidemic which killed its victims in three days caused high mortality. In 1623 another epidemic claimed the lives of many children and adolescents (Lutz 1976:745). Gage described an epidemic which occurred from 1631 to 1632 and affected a wide area. He said:

> This fever in the very inward parts and bowels scarce continued to the seventh day but commonly took its victims away from the world to the grave the third or fifth day . . . It rotted their very mouths and tongues, and made them black as a coal before they died. Very few Spaniards were infected with this contagion (1969:263).

Ximénez said that it was peste and that many people died in the capital and provinces (1930:2:207). He called it tabardillo, and MacLeod identified it as typhus (1973:98).

Fuentes y Guzmán described an epidemic that he witnessed in 1647. It began first with a cold and then developed into "pains in the heart." Death resulted after three days. After examining the bodies, red worms were discoverd, which, biting the heart, caused death. The worms could only be killed by lemon juice. This remedy was used by the sick in their food and drink, and all were cured (1969:1:173).

In 1650 another pneumonic plague (k'ucumatz) epidemic occurred, and there were many deaths (MacLeod 1973:99). Vázquez de Herrera said that this epidemic took a terrible toll in and about the capital, because the Indians continued to follow ancient customs and treated the disease by bathing in hot, sulphurous baths (1944:4:309). They probably contracted pneumonia and died quickly. From 1665 to 1666 peste struck again in the highlands and the capital, resulting in many deaths (Lutz 1976:747). In 1680, Vázquez de Herrera said that there was an epidemic of smallpox (1944:4:313).

In 1686 Fuentes y Guzmán saw another epidemic which he referred to as dolor de costado. He said that many people died, mainly from lack of care and medicine (1969:1:173). According to MacLeod, this was typhus and/or pneumonic plague (1973:98). The disease killed more than one-tenth of the population of the capital (Vásquez de Herrera 1944:4:388). The President of the audiencia reported that the Royal Hospital of Santiago had only twenty-four beds but needed two hundred to care for the sick of all classes. This epidemic was very "violent," and those that suffered the most were "poor Spaniards, commoners, mestizos, mulattoes, and innumerable Indians" (Lutz 1976:747). Some people died suddenly while others expired with acute pains of the head, chest, and bowels. No remedy was found to check the progress of the epidemic although many of the diseased dead were opened to discover the cause of the disorder (Juarros 1937:162–63).

From 1693 to 1694 smallpox (viruelas, sarampión, tabardillo) devastated Santiago and Central America in general. The outbreak was very severe, and Fuentes y Guzmán contracted the disease. Once again, the poor suffered the most and died due to lack of food and medicine. A regidor (alderman) of Santiago reported that "every day many were buried in public, not counting those that are found thrown in the doors of churches, both infants and adults" (Lutz 1976:748; MacLeod 1973:98). Besides the epidemics described above, there were many others which affected only local areas (Lutz 1976:743–52; MacLeod 1973:99).

Herbal Remedies for Epidemic Diseases

There is practically no information in the Guatemalan colonial sources on herbal remedies used to treat epidemic diseases. Perhaps it was soon known that herbal remedies had no effect. It is also possible that some plants used to alleviate respiratory ailments and fever were given to a sick person to reduce their suffering even if it were understood that they would not recover. The contemporary literature mentions some plant cures in use today for epidemic-type diseases, but some of the worst diseases of colonial times, such as pneumonic plague and typhus, have not been problems in modern times.

Some remedies for measles have been given in recent times. In Camotán measles were treated with a drink and bath made from the boiled bark of the gumbolimbo tree (*Bursera simaruba* Sarg.) (Rodríguez Rouanet 1969:85). In Verapaz anil indigo (*Indigo fera suffruticosa* Mill.) was used against bacteria and measles. It was taken as a drink and was also used as a bath (Dieseldorff 1940:197). The Barbados nut (*Jatropha curcas* L.) has also been used today in Guatemala to treat measles. Heated plasters were applied to the soles of the feet with some mustard paste for fever accompanying the illness. Since the body is hot but the feet are cold, it was believed that the heat was drawn to them, and that the fever left through the soles (Simeon 1977:24–25). American wormseed (*Chenopodium ambrosioides* L.) and barley (*Hordeum vulgare* L.) were used to treat measles in Chuchexic (Cosminsky 1972:368). The Old World tamarind (*Tamarindus indica* L.) and the goldenshower senna (*Cassia fistula* L.) were other remedies for measles (Rodríguez Rouanet 1971:230, 233). In Colotenango, a drink of maize (*Zea mays* L.) with sugar was given. Then a separate drink of barley (*Hordeum vulgare* L.) water and linseed was used for measles (Valladares 1957:120). Oakes said that during a measles epidemic in Todos Santos the Indians put the sick children into the sweatbath, and most of them died of pneumonia as a result (1969:83–84).

In Verapaz vervain (*Verbena litoralis* HBK.) was used for smallpox (Dieseldorff 1940:196). Water of the goldenshower senna (*Cassia fistula* L.) was taken in Magdalena Milpas Altas for smallpox (Bremme de Santos 1963:557). Barley (*Hordeum vulgare* L.) was used for it in Chuchexic (Cosminsky 1972:368).

The sweatbath was used in Chichicastenango for smallpox (*loq'bal* in Quiché):

> When the eruption appears, if the spots are bright red, it is a good sign, but if they are somewhat black, it is a sign that the patient will die. When one sees a black eruption one goes at once to prepare the sweatbath. If the person is grown, he goes into the sweatbath to warm himself; if it is a child they put him in little by little, to warm his body so that the eruption will come out strong.

In Chichicastenango measles were treated in the same manner as smallpox (Bunzel 1967:144).

In Jocotán and Chiquimula the crossleaf calabash tree (*Crescentia alata* HBK.) was used for influenza. The water obtained from the fruit was drunk with a shoot of bulbstem yucca (*Yucca elephantipes* Reg.) (Rodríguez Rouanet 1969:83). Bathing in water containing the Old World rosemary plant (*Rosmarinus officinalis* L.) or eucalyptus (*Eucalyptus globulus* Labill.) was another treatment for influenza (Simeon 1977:22). Perhaps these influenza remedies were used formerly for plague.

Although epidemic diseases were the most detrimental of the post-Conquest introduced diseases, there were other diseases which were confined to specific areas or affected Indian health to a lesser degree.

Erysipelas

Erysipelas is caused by a streptococcal infection of the skin (*Streptococcus pyogenes*) or the reticular lymphatics of the mucous membranes. It begins suddenly and is characterized by chills, fever, local erythema, and a burning sensation over the slightly elevated lesions. *Barefoot Doctor's Manual* 1974:436). It is highly infectious, and the area of redness spreads. There is usually considerable pain with heat and tingling in the affected part. An attack usually last a week to ten days (Thomson 1976:313–14).

Only one plant is mentioned in the Guatemalan colonial literature as being a treatment for erysipelas, and this is the black nightshade (*Solanum nigrum* L.) (Fuentes y Guzmán 1969:1:243). This plant has been used in San Raimundo and San Pedro Ayampuc in contemporary times as a remedy for erysipelas (Villacorta Calderón 1926:77). Hernández mentioned that the leaves of the tamarind (*Tamarindus indica* L.) were applied to affected areas in Mexico and worked well (1959:3:173).

Modern remedies have also included the Jamaica bitterbush (*Picramnia antidesma* Sw.) (Aguilar Girón 1966:364) and the leaves of the Mexican cedar (*Cedrela mexicana* M. Roem). The leaves of the latter were cooked and one-half a glass was drunk (Rodríguez Rouanet 1971:113). Eryngo (*Eryngium carlinae* Delar.) was another herbal treatment (Villacorta Calderón 1926:75).

Leprosy

Leprosy is a chronic disease which affects the skin in particular but also the mucous membranes and nerves. The causative organism is the *Myobacterium leprae* which is transmitted by contact with open cases of leprosy. The infection usually takes place through the skin and then spreads along the nerves. There are two types of leprosy: tuberculoid and lepromatous. The former runs a relatively benign course and is often self-healing; the latter is steadily progressive.

In the lepromatous form skin manifestations range from areas of whitening of the skin to massive nodules. Nerve manifestations range from localized swellings of the nerve to extensive areas of anaesthesia in the skin. The ultimate destruction of the nerves leads to deformities. The eyes may also be affected, leading to blindness (Thomson 1976:501–502).

Leprosy is probably an Old World disease, and it was endemic in Extremadura, the homeland of many of the conquistadors. In aboriginal Mesoamerica, however, there were skin diseases which were similar in appearance to leprosy.

In 1638 the Hospital of San Lázaro was founded and located west of the capital. It was designed for those who had leprosy and elephantiasis so the disease was prevalent enough by then to require a hospital for lepers (Asturias 1958:68). Many lepers were said to be in the capital and in the countryside (*AGC* Al.7:2053–14299). The piedmont town of San Juan de Los Leprosos got its name due to the many lepers residing there (Fuentes y Guzmán 1972:2:38–39).

There are no specific remedies mentioned in the Guatemalan colonial sources for leprosy, but those employed for skin disorders may have been used. In recent times oil from the seeds of annatto (*Bixa orellana* L.) has been put on affected parts of the body (Rodríguez Rouanet 1971:167). Hernández said that the same remedy was used for mange and sores in Mexico (1959:2:28). The Barbados nut (*Jatropha curcas* L.) has also been used to alleviate leprosy in recent times in San Raimundo (Villacorta Calderón 1926:78).

Malaria

There is some controversy as to whether malaria was present in the New World prior to contact. The carriers of malaria, mosquitos belonging to the subfamily *Anophelinae,* were probably present in the New World before the Conquest. Nevertheless, it is possible that the plasmodia parasites responsible for the disease were not present prior to the arrival of infected persons from Europe, or more likely, Africa (Joralemon 1982:111). The vagaries of host and geographical distribution of the American primate plasmodia support the conclusion that these parasites have not been established in the New World for a very long period of time. Mammalian malaria was probably absent from the Americas prior to European contact (Dunn 1965:389–90).

There is no information about malaria being more deadly to Indians than Europeans. This may be used as an argument that malaria must have been present in pre-Columbian America and that Indians had a degree of immunity to it. If malaria did exist in the New World before Columbus, it must have had a patchy distribution.

Although there is no mention of legerbark cinchona (*Cinchona ledgeriana* Moens & Trimen) in the available written records of the Aztecs, Mayas or of early Spanish chroniclers, the Indians of Ecuador seem to have known that the bark was good for malaria because they cured the ailing corregidor of Quito with it. This was sometime between 1630 and 1640, and the Spaniards did not seem to know of its properties before that time (Villacorta Cifuentes 1976:74). Perhaps some form of malaria was known to Indians of certain areas in pre-Hispanic times, and some of these Indians may have made use of the ledgerbark cinchona.

Malaria consists of a series of febrile attacks and chills at first and later assumes a chronic form with a tendency towards frequent relapses. The parasites are protozoa, belonging to the genus *Plasmodium.* The specific names for benign tertian, quartan, and malignant malaria are, respectively, *P. vivax, P. malariae,* and *P. falciparum* (Thomson 1976:530–32). Humans are infected by the parasites injected by the bite of infected mosquitoes.

P. vivax has a low mortality rate in untreated adults. The infection is characterized by relapses that occur over a period of at least two years after primary infection. Relapses also occur with *P. malariae* but are much rarer than after infection with *P. vivax. P. falciparum* often produces a fulminating infection in the nonimmune patient. If untreated, the infection may progress rapidly to a fatal termination. If treated early, the infection usually responds to antimalarial drugs. If treatment is inadequate, reoccurrence is possible due to parasites persisting in the blood (Goodman and Gilman 1970:1095).

Fuentes y Guzmán said that from 1682 to 1689 the people of San Juan Amatitlán suffered from an epidemic [very probably malaria] characterized by fever and chills which coincided with the victims' return from the south coast, a tropical area (1969:1:247). Malaria was probably quite common in tropical areas by the late seventeenth century.

Colonial sources do not specifically mention cures for malaria, but fever remedies were probably used. There are some herbal remedies which have been used in modern times specifically for malaria, and these may have been used in earlier times as well. For example, teas made from the fruit of the *soncoya* (Spanish) (*Annona purpurea* Moc. & Sessé) and the ledgerbark cinchona (*Cinchona ledgeriana* Moens & Trimen) were used for malaria (Mellen 1974:135). Hernández mentioned a plant which may have been a species of cinchona and said it cut fevers short (1959:2:190). The bark of the billywebb sweetia (*Sweetia panamensis* Benth.) was another malaria remedy (Mellen 1974:135; Villacorta Calderón 1926:75). The bitter leaf decoction of the Mexican sunflower (*Tithonia diversifolia* Gray) and the bark decoction of a type of bitterwood (*Trichilia havanensis* Jacq.) were used for malaria (Morton 1981:407, 973). Humboldt's willow (*Salix chilensis* Mol.) (Wauchope 1948:50), jimson weed (*Datura stramonium* L.), cihuapahtli (*Montanoa tomentosa* Cerv.) (Hernández 1959:3:67; Villacorta Calderón 1926:79, 80), and vervain (*Verbena litoralis* HBK.) were other malaria remedies (Cosminsky 1972:367). The root decoction of greenbrier (*Smilax spinosa* Mill.) has also been taken in Guatemala to prevent malaria (Morton 1981:85).

Onchocerciasis

Many Indians of the tropical and piedmont areas suffered from blindness. Vázquez de Herrera described the situation in those areas. He said that in some towns most of the inhabitants were blind. This situation characterized Magdalena in Siquinalá and the town of San Juan de los Leprosos. Three towns adjacent to San Bartolomé were "well populated with blind Indians," and Vázquez de Herrera referred to that blindness as "a plague which has spread like contagion in some towns of the coast" (1944:4:55–56; 350). Fuentes y Guzmán said that most of the Indians of Malacetpeque were blind due to very large cataracts (nubes) (1972:50), but it is not clear if this referred to onchocerciasis.

In some instances blindness may have been due to leprosy, but in others it was probably due to onchocerciasis (*enfermedad de Robles,* Spanish), a disease believed to have been introduced into the New World from Africa (Schendel 1968:218). Onchocerciasis is caused by *Onchocera volvulus,* a filarial worm transmitted by gnats of the genus *Simulium.* Nodules form on various parts of the body, and the vision may be eventually affected if the worm invades the optic nerve (Thomson 1976:652).

Villacorta Cifuentes made a case for the presence of onchocerciasis prior to the arrival of the Europeans. Medical studies were carried out by the Center of Medical Investigations of Kumba, Africa on the relationships within the *O. volvulus-Simulium* complex. Two types of *O. volvulus* were identified in West Africa. To study the potential of ingestion and development of both types two infected volunteers were taken to Guatemala. The growth of the Africa parasite was slower in Guatemala than in Africa, and the attraction exercised by the *Simalium* gnats over the microfilariae of the Guatemalan type did not exist on the microfilariae of the African type. These diffferences were very marked and may indicate that there is a native form of onchocerciasis, and that the disease was not imported to the New World by African slaves.

Some archaeological evidence has also suggested the pre-Columbian existence of this disease. A few skulls have been found with holes that may have been caused by onchocerciasis. One came from Zaculeu, which is in the onchocerciasis zone today. A modern skull of a woman who had died of onchocerciasis was exhumed and showed a hole which was similar to those of the ancient skulls (Villacorta Cifuentes 1976:76–83). People who had onchocerciasis were also found in highland towns during the colonial period. It is possible that there was a native form of the disease, and that an Old World variety (or varieties) was brought over by African slaves. No specific cures are given for onchocerciasis, but treatments used for other eye disorders were probably used.

CHAPTER SIX

European Medicine in Colonial Guatemala

The Church and Medical Care

The Spaniards were interested in native herbology and viewed it as part of the domain of medicine. They separated herbal knowledge from accompanying religious rituals which they considered as paganism (Cosminsky 1983:160). Priests played a major role in attempting to stamp out paganism wherever they found it. They were not entirely successful, as can be seen by the survival of many aboriginal religious and medical rituals in the Guatemala highlands down until modern times.

The church also played a part in the introduction of European medical thinking into colonial society. Guerra has indicated that the Catholic church may be singled out as the most important cultural factor in the evolution of Spanish American medicine in post-Conquest times (1969:179). The priests were also nurses, and each monastery had an infirmary (Vázquez de Herrera 1940:3:19).

In 1530, Jorge de Alvarado, the brother of the conqueror, indicated a place in the new capital (Ciudad Vieja) where a hospital was to be constructed for treating the poor and travelers (*Libro Viejo* 1934:29; Remesal 1932:1:52). It was completed a few years later and was named Hospital de la Misericordia (Martínez Durán 1964:127). The hospital served mainly to house the sick, orphans, and old men (Asturias 1958:65). As there were no European doctors in Guatemala during the first years after the Conquest, the Hospital de la Misericordia was staffed by the priests (Martínez Durán 1964:128, 144).

In 1541, Fray Matías de Paz, a Dominican, also had a house with a straw roof in the newly founded capital. This represented the humble beginning of the Hospital de San Alejo, the first to be dedicated to the treatment of sick Indians. The hospital eventually came to be located near the Dominican Monastery. Fray Matías sought out the ill and, when necessary, carried them to the hospital himself (Remesal 1932:2:341; Vázquez de Herrera 1944:4:380).

In the mid-sixteenth century Bishop Francisco Marroquín founded a hospital called Hospital de Santiago for Spaniards. In 1559, it was joined to San Alejo, and the name was changed to Hospital Real de Santiago. It turned out that both the Indians and the clergy were dissatisfied with this merger, and in 1569 (or 1578, according to Remesal), the two hospitals once again became separate, remaining so until the late seventeenth century (Asturias 1958:67; Villacorta Calderón 1942:225).

Remesal said that there was a doctor of sorts treating the citizens of the capital by 1541. This was the notorious Doctor N. who was not professionally trained, and according to people who knew of his work, he killed more people than he cured. The situation became so bad that the town officials ordered that if a person called Dr. N. to treat someone who was ill, and the patient died or got worse, then the one who called him would have to take the blame (Remesal 1932:1:255). The first real doctor, Juan de los Ríos, arrived in Guatemala in 1543, eliminating the need for Dr. N. (Martínez Durán 1964:144). By the end of the sixteenth century, there were several trained doctors and surgeons in the capital, but doctors could not receive medical degrees in Guatemala until after the University of San Carlos was founded in 1676 (1964:144–45, 206). All of this did not affect the Indians in any case. They had to rely on their own curers or the priests.

During the seventeenth century, other hospitals, such as the Hospital de San Pedro and the Hospital de San Juan de Dios, were founded. The latter was the most elaborate and had five rooms dedicated to treating men. These rooms were for medicine, surgery, venereal diseases, contagious diseases, and the treatment of wounded criminals. The last room had iron bars. There were also two rooms for women, one being for medicine and the other for surgery. This hospital primarily treated Spaniards (Asturias 1958:68, 82). Indians were brought in from the provinces to work there and in the other hospitals of the capital, but they had only San Alejo for treatment (*AGC* Al.7 2053–14299).

By the mid-seventeenth century, San Alejo was in a ruinous state. It was responsible for seventy-two Indian towns; yet it had only twenty-four beds. It is easy to see why Indians continued to rely on traditional medicine. San Alejo received only 1,300 pesos to cover expenses, which was barely enough to keep it functioning (*AGC* Al.7 2053–14299, Al.7 2049–14238). In fact, some of this money came from houses owned and rented out by the hospital. Fuentes y Guzmán said that the Indian hospital was poor, and that the Indians died more from need than from their illnesses (1969:1:170).

Although there seems to have been more doctors in the capital during the late sixteenth and early seventeenth centuries, by the eighteenth century, hospitals in the capitals had become little more than infirmaries due to a chronic shortage of funds and competent personnel (Martínez Durán 1964:145–47, 299). By 1723, there was only one doctor in Santiago (Salazar 1951:84).

If the situation had deteriorated in the capital, it is not difficult to imagine the plight of the provinces. People residing there relied mainly on priests or native curers. Sixteenth-century European medicine also stressed herbal remedies (Cook 1946:325), and it was probably during this time that Indians began incorporating Old World medicines into their body of herbal treatments.

After the mid-sixteenth century, some provincial towns had churches with resident priests. The Indians were treated by these men and no longer had to rely only on traveling friars. For example, Fray Gonzalo Méndez, a Franciscan, treated the Tzutujil in Santiago Atitlán. Some of the Indians also learned to assist the priests (Vázquez de Herrera 1938:2:30). The churches, however, were not hospitals with trained medical personnel but were religious establishments. Spanish medicine diffused out from the capital slowly. Quetzaltenango, the second largest city in Guatemala, did not have a hospital until the nineteenth century when the Hospital de Occidente was constructed (Aguirre 1972:244). It is therefore not surprising that much of the native medical system survived until the modern period.

The Accommodation of Catholicism and Indian Medical Beliefs

After the establishment of the system of religious brotherhoods (cofradías), probably in the late sixteenth century, the brothers (*cofrades*) assisted the local priests in visiting sick people and administering the sacraments. If a member became ill, the cofradía saw to it that he was cared for (Fuentes y Guzmán 1969:1:362; Vázquez de Herrera 1944:4:36). Through the cooperation between the priests and Indian cofradía members, medical knowledge was exchanged.

Native treatment specialists probably began to exercise their curing role through the cofradía structure as they often do today in the highlands. This may have been especially true after the mid-seventeenth century, when there were fewer priests living in the more remote Indian areas, and there was a resurgence of ancient customs.

Of course, the priests were not always accepting of native medical practices. As mentioned previously, they tried to prevent the Indians from bathing so often, and their idea that this was harmful must have been confirmed as they witnessed the deaths of many sick people who emerged from the waters of sweatbaths. The priests also discouraged circumcision (Schendel 1968:87), which probably led to an increase of penile cancer. The church practice which most seriously affected native health was congregating Indians into focal towns. This facilitated the spread of epidemics and increased mortality.

The values and practices which are the most easily transferable are those which are most consonant with the ideology and behavioral standards of the host culture. New roles for which "analogue roles" exist in the host culture will be most easily accepted (Landy 1978:237). Many aboriginal beliefs about illness causation were compatible with Catholic beliefs. For example, the pre-Columbian idea that many illnesses were sent by the gods as a punishment for sin or ritual error continued on after the Conquest with Catholic religious figures replacing the ancient gods. Saints were patrons of various illnesses, and illness frequently took on moral tones. Medical books included many prayers (*novenas,* Spanish) and religious tracts for preventing and curing illness (Guerra 1969:183). Sorcery as an explanation for illness existed in the New and Old Worlds, and this belief has also survived into modern times.

There are several examples in the colonial writings which illustrate how Catholicism began to influence native attitudes regarding illness. Vázquez de Herrera reported a case of an Indian who was dying. This man had a vision of a "resplendent personage" who comforted him and asked him why the Indians did not celebrate the fiesta of San Pascual Bailón. The sick man replied that he was not familiar with that particular saint. The personage promised that the saint would be the protector of the Indians if the fiesta were celebrated and the cult initiated. It also promised to give the Indians a sign and to free them from the ravages of the current epidemic. The sick man was told that he would die in nine days. After that, the epidemic would stop, and there would be no more deaths. The Indian summoned the cofrades and related the details of the vision to them. They initiated the cult, the sick man died in nine days, and the epidemic ceased. Afterwards, other towns took up the cult (1944:4:309–10).

There are other examples in the colonial literature of sick people reportedly having been cured by saints. In the piedmont town of San Francisco, the Indian cook in the monastery became ill and was reportedly cured by San Diego el molonel around 1650 to 1660 (Vázquez de Herrera 1944:4:310). In 1686 an Indian in San Pablo Jocopilas, sick with an illness similar to elephantiasis, had a vision that a light fell upon his leg and cured him (1944:4:315–16). No doubt these types of religiously inspired visions were characteristic of pre-Hispanic times, too.

Some pre-Columbian pilgrimage centers, such as that at Esquipulas, took on Catholic characteristics and became famous for curing illness. Black idols existed in ancient times and were also found during the colonial period (Borhegyi 1959:45–46; Gage 1969:281). The most important Maya merchant god Ek Chuah (*ek* means black in Yucatec) was depicted as black in the codices and vase paintings, except for a red area around the lips and chin. Merchants prayed to Ek Chuah for a safe return home. Ikal Ahau, or Black Lord, was a death god among the Tzotzil (Thompson 1972b:306–307, 323). Some of these black gods may have acted as protectors, and the black Christ of Esquipulas may have replaced one of these protector idols.

By the early seventeenth century, people began to claim that the Black Christ cured them of various illnesses. In 1621 an Indian named Juan Andrés was cured of sores on his legs, and in 1680 a blind Indian was cured. A completely paralyzed person was restored to health. People also came to the shrine because of the curative powers of the sulfurous springs of the Río de los Milagros which ran nearby.

The image of the Black Christ was officially recognized as having curative powers in 1737 when the Archbishop of Guatemala was healed of a contagious illness after visiting the shrine (Borhegyi 1959:46). In the case of the Black Christ, both Spaniards and Indians recognized the powers of a religious figure that had strong pre-Columbian antecedents.

Reina described the rituals performed by a sick person at the shrine of the Black Christ in recent times:

> If part of the body is ill, a person is encouraged to take a replica of that part made in wax and leave it with the Christ. A young informant had a pain in his chest for several months and went to Esquipulas to request total recovery. He said, "I had faith that the Christ could cure me . . . I left the upper part of a body made of wax, and then I went to the nearby river and bathed myself. The pain has never returned" (1966:176–77).

The Influence of European Medical Beliefs on Indian Medicine

Although the practice of Spanish medicine by trained medical personnel was confined mainly to the capital in colonial times, some European medical beliefs did reach the Indian areas and were incorporated into the native medical system.

A discussion of the European medical system and humoral theory is necessary to an understanding of Indian medicine as it has been practiced since the early sixteenth century. The fifteenth to the seventeenth centuries was a period of great medical advance in Spain. However, little of this knowledge made its way to Guatemala, and by the time Spanish medicine did begin to influence the country in the eighteenth century, it had greatly declined in quality (Martínez Durán 1964:139).

In sixteenth century Europe, the university-trained doctor stood at the top of the medical hierarchy. The surgeon, who sutured holes in the intestines, removed tumors, repaired rectal fistulas, and performed plastic surgery on the lips and nose, was below him. The barber-surgeon treated external ulcers, fractures, pulled teeth, and performed bleeding and cupping (Lyons and Petrucelli 1978:454, 456). Cupping was often perfomed in bath houses. There was also the apothecary who dabbled in medicine but was supposed to obey the university-trained doctor (Bettmann 1962:108).

Although the university-trained doctor was the most respected medical practitioner, great progress was made in surgery in Europe during the sixteenth century, which correspondingly raised the prestige of the surgeon. During the latter half of the sixteenth century, the apothecary also rose in status and was often ahead of the university-trained physician in equipment and scientific knowledge. New drugs were arriving from the West and the Far East which were prepared in the apothecary's shop (1962:126–28). There was a heavy reliance on herbal medicine in Europe, but it was not until the seventeenth century that European medicine became scientifically oriented.

Humoral Theory

Spanish medicine at the time of the Conquest was based on classical Greek and Roman tradition as modified during transmission by way of the Arab world. The Hippocratic doctrine of the four humors (blood, phlegm, black bile (melancholy), and yellow bile (choler)) formed the basis of European medical theory (Foster 1953:201–202). This theory stated that there were four primary and opposing qualities:

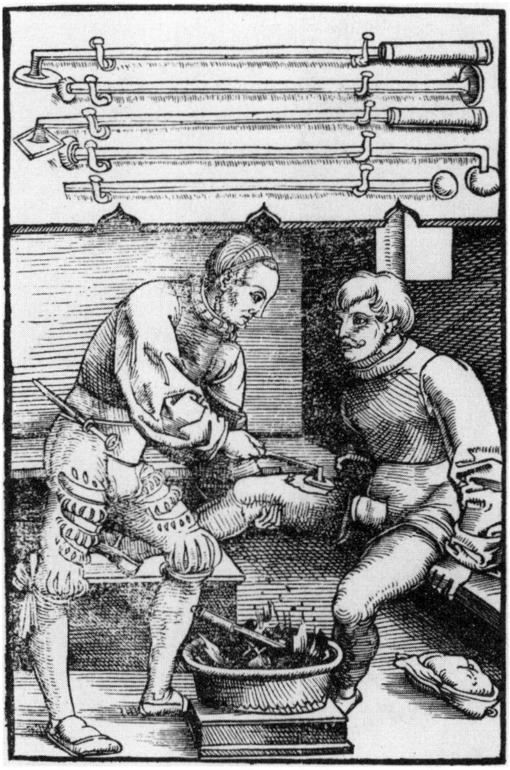

Figure 50
Cauterization. Woodcut by Johannes Wechtlin showing a selection of cauterizing irons at top and a patient having his thigh cauterized after injury (Gersdorff 1967:70).

hot/cold and wet/dry (Logan 1973b:387). All substances possessed two of the four qualities: humid (water) or dry (earth) and cold (air) or hot (fire). All matter was considered to be composed of varying proportions of water, earth, air and fire (Neuenswander and Souder 1980:142). Blood was thought to be hot and wet, yellow bile hot and dry, phlegm cold and wet, and black bile cold and dry (Foster 1953:202). Illness was primarily attributed to phlegm and disequilibrium of the humors, development of tumors and growths (*carnosidades,* Spanish), inflammations and retentions, or to temperament (Chinchilla Aguilar 1963:44). The seasons were also taken into account as they were associated with the humors (Andrews and Hassig 1984:32).

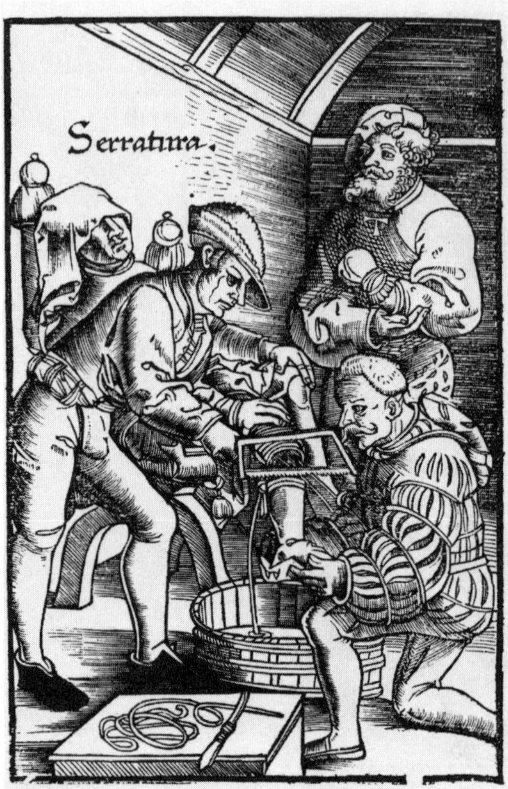

Figure 51
Amputation. The surgeon sawed between the bandages, wound around the leg, and then covered the stump with the bladder of a bull or hog (Gersdorff 1967:30).

Much of Spanish medical theory during the sixteenth century was based on the concept that people, illnesses, medicines, and most natural objects had complexions. The complexion was defined according to its specific properties of hot/cold and wet/dry. When determining the complexion of an illness or its cause, the physician would also attempt to understand the natural complexion of the patient. Harmony could then be resored by diet, internal medicines, purging, vomiting, bleeding, and cupping (Foster 1953:203).

In the Hippocratic system hot and cold do not refer to temperature but to the effects an item has on the body. Curing illness was a matter of correcting imbalances in the humors by adding or subtracting heat, cold, dryness, or wetness. For example, today in Latin America overconsumption of cold foods is thought to cause chills and coughs. Hot and cold illnesses can be cured by eating foods of the opposite quality (Logan 1978:183). Rather than combating hot and cold illnesses by consuming foods with the opposite elements, in some areas what is actually done is to avoid "shocks" between the two extremes (Neuenswander and Souder 1980:151). Extremely hot and cold foods are not eaten together.

Binary opposition assumed great importance in sixteenth century Spanish medicine. It was also important among the native Mesoamericans. Aboriginal cosmology and medicine had a component that closely paralleled, and therefore greatly facilitated, the adoption of Spanish humoral medicine. Dualism was a primary feature of the pre-Columbian world view, and equilibrium was considered important in maintaining health (Logan 1977:97; López Austin 1980:1:300–303).

The dualistic world view in pre-Columbian times was applied to the entire cosmos, and even today the hot/cold classification is applied widely. In contrast, the Hippocratic Theory was used in Europe only in relation to illness, medicine, and health (1980:1:306–307). Hot and cold medicines were mentioned in the *Cruz-Badianus Herbal,* the *Florentine Codex,* and by Hernández who reported that hot and cold were native classifications. However, all three sources may have had some European organizational and conceptual influence. Some native therapeutic treatments did employ hot/cold concepts to restore body equilibrium. Some, such as bathing in hot or cold water, were considered scandalous by the Europeans (1980:1:309) who viewed any type of bathing as an abomination (Vogel 1973:47); therefore, it is not likely they were of European origin.

The humoral theory coincided very well with pre-Columbian views on equilibrium and disequilibrium. Certain stresses or behaviors, such as sexual transgressions, could produce an abnormal distribution of hot and cold within the body according to Aztec medical theory. Many medicines were used to regulate the relationship between cold and hot and keep it evenly distributed (1980:1:301–302). The Aztecs also believed that in excess the four types of phlegm: white, yellow, green, and purulent were responsible for many alterations of the body (1980:1:192).

Although it has been pointed out that the hot/cold classification was pre-Conquest (1980:1:306–18), there is less evidence for the aboriginal existence of the wet/dry category. It was found to exist in Joyabaj, but it only applied to illness (Neuenswander and Souder 1980:144). The existence of the wet/dry classification may be explained as a post-

Conquest introduction which would indicate why it is not so widespread in the Guatemala highlands today. It could also have been aboriginal but of lesser importance in those times than the hot/cold dichotomy.

The Spanish priests superimposed the European hot/cold concept over the pre-Hispanic Maya system, keeping the same terminology, and extended it to illness. Perhaps the wet/dry distinction was applied to illness but not to therapy in aboriginal times. It may have continued to operate in that area among some groups (Neuenswander and Souder 1980:163). The humid/dry qualities came to be used to categorize illnesses in agreement with the etiology and prognosis. "Good" was synonymous with the "humid" and the "bad" with the "dry." Humid illnessees were considered benign and were treated with simple remedies. Dry illnesses were seen as being supernatural and malign, and required religiously oriented curing ceremonies (1980:145, 157). The wet/dry classification and the intensity grading scale still exist in several other areas besides Joyabaj today which would tend to support the pre-Hispanic existence of these aspects (Logan 1977:94; Madsen 1955:125; Wisdom 1940:323–24).

The hot/cold classification is an important principle of the native medical system existing today in the Guatemala highlands. Hotness and coldness are still considered to be innate qualities possessed by the substance in question although physical temperature sometimes plays a role. Whether the substance is hot or cold is determined primarily by its effect of sensation upon the temperature of the body or on an illness. Color and sex, cooking or type of preparation, and exposure to the sun (hot) and water (cold) also determines the quality in some areas. For example, the sun is hot so things exposed to the sun become hotter. The body is affected by the quality of an item and the physical temperature of the environment. Overexposure to one class or to opposite extremes disturbs the body equilibrium and may cause illness (Cosminsky 1972:97–98; 1977a:203).

A third category, fresh or cool, exists in some highland towns. Items in this category are considered to be good and are often equated with nourishing foods (*alimentos,* Spanish) (Cosminsky 1975:183–84). Today all foods, beverages, herbs, and medicines are classified as hot or cold (see Logan 1973b:392–93 for some of these classifications).

Generally, in modern times, a healthy body is viewed as being in a balanced state of hotness and coldness. In Santiago Atitlán, however, it was believed that the natural state of the body was warm or a little hot. Deviations from this to any degree could result in illness (Douglas 1969:270; see also Neuenswander and Souder 1980:162). It was also believed in Santa Lucía Utatlán that it was less dangerous to eat relatively hot foods when one is cold than to eat cold foods when one is hot (Cosminsky 1977a:204). This probably stemmed from the belief in classical humoral theory that a healthy body should be preponderantly hot (Foster 1953:205). Fresh or cool (*fresco,* Spanish) substances, rather than cold ones, were those regarded as the best to treat hot illnesses (Cosminsky 1977a:204). The fresco category, however, is probably the result of acculturation to modern Western medical concepts and nutritional knowledge (Cosminsky 1975:188).

Although the humoral theory of medicine is still important in the traditional medical systems of Middle America today, it has long since lost influence in Europe. In 1761, Giovanni Battista Morgagni destroyed this ancient theory of illness through the publication of his work titled *De Sedibus et Causis Morborum (On the Sites and Causes of Diseases*). He proved that pathologic anatomical changes in the internal organs were responsible for the clinical symptoms of disease (Lyons and Petrucelli 1978:477, 481).

Some herbal medicines were used in colonial Guatemala to restore the equilibrium among the humors and promote health. In the sixteenth century spices were important drugs and were thought to influence the bodily humors. In fact, they ranked second only to cathartics as the most popular remedies (Guerra 1966b:29–30). The need to maintain a clean stomach or, if necessary, to "clean it" with purges was basic to classic Spanish thought (Foster 1953:206).

Fuentes y Guzmán said that cihuapahtli (*Montanoa tomentosa* Cerv.) destroyed and reduced phlegm and coldness contained in the stomach (1969:1:241). The Aztec marigold (*Tagetes erecta* L.) was thought to heal illnesses coming from cold causes and, when taken as an emetic, it was said to evacuate the humor through cold and sweat (1969:1:246; Hernández 1959:2:220). The castor plant (*Ricinus communis* L.) was used for any cold related illnesses (Fuentes y Guzmán 1972:3:35).

Chilatole (from Nahua *chilatolli*), a beverage made from maize (*Zea mays* L.) and pepper (*Capsicum* spp.), was believed to expel and destroy the pituitary humor (1969:1:227). The pineapple (*Ananas comosus* Merr.) was thought to dissolve the phlegm that blocked the bladder (1972:3:29). Colored sapotas, such as the green sapota (*Pouteria viridis* Pitt.), were considered to be very good for the health; the seeds were used in cacao (*Theobroma cacao* L.) to destroy phlegm and other viscous humors (Fuentes y Guzmán 1972:2:116). According to Ximénez, any sick person could by eating any type of sapota be helped (1967b:262–63).

The spearleaf saltbush (*Atriplex hastata* L.) was said to purge the choleric humor (1972:3:306). Club moss (*Lycopodium dichotomun* Jacq.) was said to evacuate all of the humors (1972:2:42–43).

Pasmo, from pasmada meaning chilled or numbed in Spanish, was a cold-caused illness frequently mentioned by colonial Spanish writers. It was characterized by such symptoms as loss of appetite, being physically run-down and cold, and having pain in the bones. It was believed to be an attack of cold on a person who was overheated (Adams and Rubel 1967:343; Alonso Pedraz 1958:3167). Fever and pasmo could be brought on by being drenched in a heavy rain, or by sweating a lot from working or walking and then catching cold. If not treated immediately, the victim became feverish and got the illness (Estrada 1955:75). Recently, it has also been thought that the illness could result from eating foods which are too hot or too cold (Adams 1957:363), or by using hot and cold in sequence too quickly (Winter 1972:143).

Fuentes y Guzmán said that the shoots of the avocado (*Persea americana* Mill.) were cooked and the hot liquid administered to any person who had fallen down and received a shock. It preserved the person against pasmo and cold. He said that there was no rustic nor untutored man who did not know about the virtues of the avocado and who did not use it frequently (1969:1:239). The century plant (*Agave americana* L.) preserved those with wounds from pasmo (1969:1:218). Curarina (*Cissampelos pareira* L.) remedied those touched by air (aire), colds, fevers, pasmo, and other illnesses (1969:1:229). Cambray (*Cosmos sulphureus* Cav.) (1972:2:116) and cudweed (*Gnaphalium attenuatum* DC.) (1969:1:242) were other herbal medicines taken for pasmo according to the chronicler.

The tamarind (*Tamarindus indica* L.) was used for illnesses thought to be caused by heat (Ximénez 1967b:249; Hernández 1959:3:173). In recent times the tamarind has been used to treat several ailments (Rodríguez Rouanet 1971:314–15). Fuentes y Guzmán also mentioned the sweatbath as a "hot" cure used to treat fevers (1972:3:91). Today in Colotenango the sweatbath and massage are still used for illnesses where it is desired to eliminate aire (air) or *frío* (Spanish; cold) (Valladares 1957:125).

PART III

Analysis of Medicinal Plants

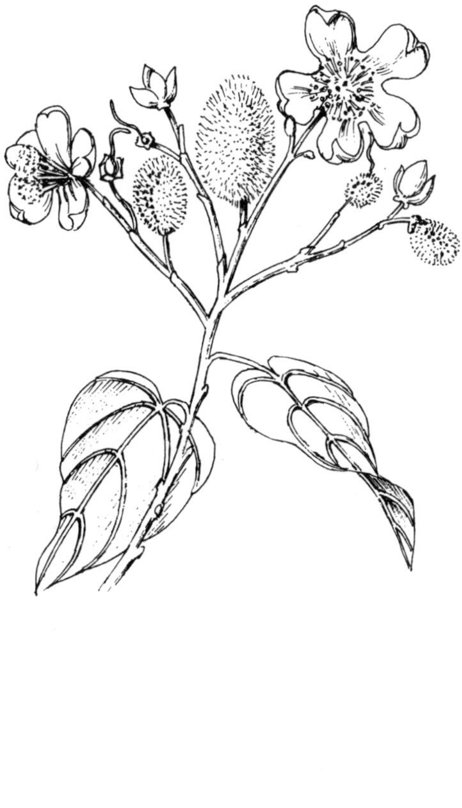

CHAPTER SEVEN

Plant Analysis

In this section plants used in the first two parts of this work are analyzed to discover their active constituents and to see if they are effective in stated applications. The origin, common name, uses, constituents, activity, and, in a few cases, method of collection, are given when known. The treatment is uneven due to the fact that many plants have not yet been properly studied.

Crude drugs used by native curers were vegetable or animal products which consisted of natural substances that had undergone only collection and drying (Tyler et al. 1981:4). The medicinal value of the plants discussed above is due to the presence in the plant tissue of a chemical substance, an active principle, which produces a physiological effect (Thomson 1978:11). Many of the herbal medicines in use today and in the past have had little pharmacologic testing. Even when the chemicals are known, there are often only minimal tests which give information on their activity and effectiveness. Just because an herb has been used for hundreds of years does not mean that it has any pharmacologic value. Conversely, just because no pharmacologic activity can be found does not necessarily mean that it is useless (Spoerke 1980:7–8).

Medicinal plants are defined as those which contain one or more active constituents capable of preventing or curing a disease. Some plants are composed of a range of effective compounds and can produce very different effects according to the way the drug is treated. In other plants the medicinal action may be due to one component or to the combined effect of two (or more) components (Schauenberg and Paris 1977:10). The plants contained in this work will be discussed below in alphabetical order according to the Latin binomial nomenclature.

Acacia hindsii Benth.

Origin: New World
Common Names: acacia (Eng.**); *cornizuelo* (Sp.**); *ixcanal* (Nah.**)
Uses: pain of spider bites

Acrocomia vinifera Oerstd.

Origin: New World
Common Names: palm (Eng.); *coyolli* (Nah.); *mop* (Q.*)
Uses: diuretic; elephantiasis
Collection: The sap is collected from gashes made in the crown of felled palms (Morton 1981:52).

Adiantum capillus-veneris L.

Origin: Old and New Worlds
Common Names: southern maidenhair fern (Eng.); *avenca* (Sp.); *cabello de Venus* (Sp.); *culantrillo* (Sp.); *chib* (Q.)
Uses: abortion; emmenagogue; medicinal; toothache
Constituents: The southern maidenhair fern contains mucilage, tannins, gallic acid, sugars, bitter principles, capillarine, and minute quantities of essential oil (Stuart 1979:144).
Activity: The plant is pectoral, bechic, and is also a weak diuretic, and expectorant. The southern maidenhair fern has been primarily used in chest complaints such as respiratory catarrh, and coughs. It has been a constitutent in cough medicines (Stuart 1979:144; Wren 1973:194).

As the plant is a mild emmenagogue (Stuart 1979:144), it may stimulate menstruation, but it would probably not cause abortion in most pregnant women. Due to its mucilage and tannin content, the southern maidenhair fern would soothe a toothache and serve as a mild antiseptic but stronger remedies would be more effective.

Fuentes y Guzmán mentioned this plant as a medicinal and said it was one whose virtues were well known (1969:1:243–44) so perhaps it was used as a cold remedy in earlier times.

---

*Origins are taken from Morton (1981).
**Eng. = English; Sp. = Spanish; Nah. = Nahua; Q. = Quiché

Agastache mexicana Benth.

Origin: New World
Common Names: Mexican gianthyssop (Eng.); *toronjil* (Sp.)
Uses: abortifacient; medicinal; menstrual disorders; stomachache

Agave americana L.

Origin: New World
Common Names: century plant (Eng.); *maguey* (Sp.); *metl* (Nah.); *qui* (Q.)
Uses: antispasmodic; cathartic; coughs; diuretic; expectorant; fevers; kidney inflammation and pain; pasmo; rheumatism; sores; urinary pain; wounds
Constituents: The leaf contains acrid volatile oil, agave gum, phloinolic acid, oxalic acid and oxalates, saponside, cutin, hecogenin (a steroid sapogenin), a sapogenin, and a sugar (agavose) (Stuart 1979:146).
Activity: The leaf juice has soothing and demulcent properties and would thus form a protective coating over inflamed tissues of the stomach and intestinal tract. This would result in a quieting effect on the stomach, and reduce irritation in the intestine that might be caused by diarrhea or dysentery (Weiner 1980:34). These properties are also responsible for the plant's vulnerary properties, and it is effective for healing wounds and sores. The fresh or dried leaf, the juice, root, and gum are purgative, diuretic, insecticidal, and act as an emmenagogue (Stuart 1979:146).

Although its purgative and antidiarrhea effects seem inconsistent, different results may be obtained by varying dosages and using different parts of the plant. No information was found concerning any activity against coughs, fevers, rheumatism, kidney inflammation and pain, or urinary pain. Nor was any information found regarding the century plant's value as an expectorant.

Toxicity: Symptoms of poisoning include nausea, vomiting, diarrhea, visceral vasodilation, and hemorrhage. Dermatitis, liver damage, and photosensitization may also result (Spoerke 1980:19). (This action is due to the saponins and oxalates. Oxalic acid is a powerful corrosive agent.) In general, the symptoms of oxalate poisoning are those of the local irritant effects and hypocalcemia. Not all plants containing oxalate cause poisoning, and symptoms are probably related to quantity present (Goodman and Gilman 1970:828).

Ananas comosus Merr.

Origin: New World

Common Names: pineapple (Eng.); *piña* (Sp.); *matzahtli* (Nah.); *ch'ōp̄* (Q.)

Uses: diuretic

Constituents: Ripe pineapple contains calcium and thiamine but is low in iron, carotene, and phosphorus. Ascorbic acid varies from low to fair. Of the non-volatile acids, 87% is citric and 13% ℓ-malic. The fruit, juice, and entire plant contain the proteolytic enzyme bromelain (or bromelin).

Activity: Although the pineapple was only mentioned in the colonial Guatemalan sources as a diuretic, it has wider applications and may have been used for other ailments in those times as well.

Bromelain is usually combined with pancreatin, an animal enzyme, in the preparation of digestive aids (Morton 1977:40, 43). It also reduces edema and accelerates tissue repair. Its effectiveness is apparently owing to depolymerization and permeability modifications that it induces following oral administration. Bromelain is found in the juice of the fruit and the stem of the plant (Tyler et al. 1981:291).

As an anti-inflammatory agent, bromelain is given after dental, gynecologic, and general surgery. It is used in treating sprains, contusions, hematomas, abcesses, and ulcerations (Morton 1977:43). The juice of the unripe fruit is highly irritant and abortifacient (Morton 1981:62) and is also a diuretic.

Toxicity: Unripe pineapple is poisonous and causes violent purgation (1977:43).

Given its proven beneficial qualities, the lack of more widespread use of the pineapple according to the early Guatemalan sources may represent an error of omission.

Anethum foeniculatum L.

Origin: Old World
Common Names: dill (Eng.); *hinojo eneldo* (Sp.)
Uses: galactagogue; gastric and stimulant

Annona purpurea Moc. & Sessé

Origin: New World
Common Names: *soncoya* (Sp.); *anona morada* (Sp.)
Uses: malaria
Constituents: The plant contains the alkaloids glaziovine, *O*-methylatheroline, and oxopurpureine (Morton 1981:225).
Activity: Glaziovine is reported to have tranquilizing and antidepressant properties (Reynolds and Prasad 1982:1713). It may therefore have a calming effect on the chills associated with malaria.

Annona reticulata L.

Origin: New World
Common Names: custard apple (Eng.); *anona* (Sp.); *cuauhtzapotl* (Nah.)
Uses: diarrhea; dislocations; dysentery; fractures
Constituents: The leaves, bark, unripe fruit, and seeds contain much tannin. The bark contains the alkaloid anonaine.
Activity: The sap of the tree causes severe inflammation when it comes in contact with the eyes. The bark, seeds, leaves, and roots are more actively insecticidal than these parts of related species (Morton 1981:226). Tannin has an astringent effect and acts on the gastrointestinal tract, causing constipation. The plant would, therefore, aid in alleviating dysentery and diarrhea. Its astringent, antiseptic, and insecticidal properties would help in healing fractures, especially if the skin were punctured or abraded but the custard apple would probably not be useful in cases of dislocation.

Argemone mexicana L.

Origin: New World

Common Names: Mexican prickly poppy (Eng.); *cardo santo* (Sp.); *chicallotl* (Nah.)

Uses: cathartic; evil eye; eye disorders; kidney stones; tonic

Constituents: The toxic alkaloids sanguinarine, berberine, protopine, and others are found in the whole plant or seeds (Lewis 1977:31). The seeds contain a high content of oil, water, mineral salts, sugar, gum, casein, albumin (a protein), gluten, starch, and a woody principle. The active constituent is a volatile oil of the seed (Lozoya and Lozoya 1982:163, 165).

Activity: Protopine acts on the musculature of the uterus, and berberine has cholagogue and antibiotic properties.

Administered orally, the oil is a drastic purgative. The alkaloids modify cardiac function, stimulating the tone and force of contraction of the heart and prolonging the refractory period (Lozoya and Lozoya 1982:165, 167). Berberine is reported to have mild local anaesthetic effects on mucous membranes (Reynolds and Prasad 1982:317). The activity discussed above probably accounts for the plant's use as a tonic.

Fuentes y Guzmán said that the yellow liquid that exuded from the stem and leaves of the Mexican prickly poppy was used as an eyewash for cataracts even though it was caustic (1969:1:240). The antibiotic properties of berberine would help to alleviate eye inflammations and pain, but the seed oil should not be used because it causes glaucoma (Morton 1981:241). Because of its caustic nature, the Mexican prickly poppy may have had some effect on cataracts, but it must have been a dangerous remedy. No specific information was found as to the plants' ability to affect kidney stones. Perhaps its anaesthetic properties helped to alleviate the pain. Evil eye may result from a variety of causes, and it is possible that some of the symptoms were alleviated by using this plant.

Toxicity: The seeds, which are rich in sanguinarine, are highly toxic (Lozoya and Lozoya 1982:148–49). The alkaloids in the seeds have produced dilation of capillaries which can cause fluids to leak into the tissues. Symptoms in animals include nausea, vomiting, diarrhea, visual difficulties, swelling of the abdominal cavity, generalized edema, dizziness, fainting, coma, and cardiac toxicity.

Humans may develop similar symptoms by eating the seeds (Spoerke 1980:145–46). In India, the seed oil is a common adulterant of mustard and sesame seed oil and has been found to be the cause of epidemic edema and glaucoma (Morton 1981:241).

Aristolochia maxima L.

Origin: New World
Common Names: Dutchman's pipe (Eng.); *canastilla* (Sp.); *guaco* (Sp.); *tlacopahtli* (Nah.)
Uses: antidote; antispasmodic
Activity: Almost all species of *Aristolochia* are thought to be good against snake bite, but no experimental studies have been made to confirm this activity (Martínez 1944:234).

Artemisia absinthium L.

Origin: Old World
Common Names: absinthe (Eng.); wormwood (Eng.); *ajenjo* (Sp.)
Uses: cholagogue; fever; liver pain; menstrual disorders; stomachache; tonic
Constituents: Wormwood contains approximately 0.5% of a volatile oil with bitter substances such as absinthin, a diterpenic lactone that is an azulene (a blue liquid hydrocarbon) derivative. The volatile oil is composed of (+)-thujone (a ketone), thujyl alcohol, esters of thujyl alcohol, and other terpenoid compounds (Tyler et al. 1981:500). Wormwood is a glucoside and also contains resins, starch, and santonin, a lactone glycoside (Stuart 1979:158).
Activity: Wormwood has been used medicinally since the time of the Greeks and probably long before (Moerman 1982:201). In Europe, wormwood was formerly steeped in alcohol and used as an aperitive to promote digestion. The manufactured liquor came into disrepute with the discovery of its intoxicating potency and deleterious effects on mental faculties (Morton 1981:908). The bitter principle and volatile oil do stimulate secretions and promote appetite and account for the plant's reputation as a tonic. Worm-

wood has been used to aid digestion and alleviate abdominal colic (Stuart 1979:158). It is one of the best gastric tonics used for dyspepsia, stomach pains, and liver deficiencies (Schauenberg and Paris 1977:167). It stimulates the flow of bile from the liver (Weiner 1980:205).

The antihelmintic effect, from which the plant gets its English name, is due to santonin (Stuart 1979:158). Some researchers have not been able to find experimental evidence to corroborate the antihelmintic effects of wormwood, but water extracts given to animals by mouth have been shown to produce cathartic action. Despite this, the same researchers claim that it is an excellent worming agent (Weiner 1980:205). Although no mention was made in the Guatemalan sources of the plant's value as a vermifuge, it may have been used for that purpose since it has been used for worms in nearby areas (Morton 1981:908). *Artemisia vulgaris* L. may have been confused with wormwood as it was said to be used as a vermicide in contemporary times (Villacorta Calderón 1926:76).

Wormwood is also antipyretic and antiseptic (Stuart 1979:158). It is also an emmenagogue and a diuretic (Schauenberg and Paris 1977:167), and this would account for its use for menstrual problems. Prior to the introduction of quinine, it was highly regarded as a remedy for intermittent fevers (Weiner 1980:205).

Toxicity: The oil has been associated with acute and chronic toxicity, presumably largely because of its thujone content (Tyler et al. 1981:500). Habitual use of wormwood causes convulsions, restlessness, and vomiting. Overdose causes vertigo, cramps, intoxication, and delirium (Stuart 1979:158). Because the liquor affects the central nervous system, its prolonged use produces irreversible nervous degeneration. Serious psychic, motor, and sensory perturbations occur which may lead to the total degeneration of the victim (Schauenberg and Paris 1977:167).

Artemisia vulgaris L.

Origin: Old World
Common Names: mugwort (Eng.); *incienso* (Sp.)
Uses: cholagogue; fractures; rheumatism; sores; stomachache; vermicide

Constituents: Mugwort also contains thujone. Various polyacetylenes occur in the root and flowers (Morton 1981:909). It also contains volatile oil, resin, tannin, and absinthin, the bitter principle, which stimulates digestion (Stuart 1979:159).

Activity: In Europe mugwort has been used since ancient times for gynecological disorders, epilepsy, and other nervous problems (Morton 1981:910). Certain of its extracts injected into laboratory animals produce a sedative effect. Therefore, it is possible that this effect could be beneficial to a person experiencing an epileptic fit (Weiner 1980:135–36). The plant would also be good for rheumatism due to its calming effect.

Mugwort is an effective stomach remedy because it stimulates digestion. This may also account for its use as a cholagogue. Mugwort contains tannin which has a mild astringent and antiseptic effect which would aid in healing fractures and sores. Although Villacorta Calderón mentioned mugwort as a vermicide (1926:76), he probably confused the plant with wormwood.

Toxicity: Large prolonged dosage injures the nervous system (Stuart 1979:159).

Atriplex hastata L.

Origin: New World

Common Names: spearleaf saltbush (Eng.); *armuelle silvestre* (Sp.); *quilitl* (Nah.)

Uses: cathartic for the choleric humor; scars; sores

Bixa orellana L.

Origin: New World

Common Names: annatto (Eng.); *achiote* (Sp.); *achiotl* (Nah.)

Uses: abortifacient; after-birth hemorrhage; burns; diuretic; dysentery; evil eye; fever; heart stimulant; leprosy; mange; scars; skin eruptions; sores; urinary disorders

Constituents: Annatto is composed of 13.000% moisture, 7.972% ash, 8.547% glucose, 2.952% nitrogen, 18.450% albuminoids, 49.079% cellulose, and materials not assayed (Martínez 1944:25). The red pulp extracted for coloring purposes has been assayed for vitamin A activity. It contains 1,000 to 2,000 I.U. of vitamin A per gram of oily extract. The seed contains a toxic alkaloid. The leaf oil is rich in the rare tetracyclic sesquiterpene hydrocarbon ishwarane (Morton 1981:572).

Activity: It is not clear that annatto has any medicinal properties, other than containing vitamin A. Since vitamin A is beneficial for skin problems (Adams 1976:86–87), annatto would have been helpful in preventing skin eruptions and in treating other skin problems such as mange, sores, and scarring. This may also explain its use in cases of burns or leprosy. The reason that it was used to treat so many illnesses probably stems from the fact that it was mixed into the aboriginal cacao drink which was thought to be generally healthful. No information was found, however, as to whether annatto is effective for any of the other uses mentioned in the Guatemalan sources.

Collection: In the early seventeenth century, Vázquez de Espinosa described how annatto was collected and prepared:

> It produces a flower . . . which develops into a fruit composed of red granules . . . When these are ripe and the proper time has come, they pick them and squeeze and rub them under water until they come apart and lose their husks; then they boil this water in large kettles . . . As it boils, they skim off the greasy scum which comes to the top and put it in another vessel; then they strain it through cloths or strainers; cooling, it comes out like a dough; they make bars or cakes out of this, and cure and dry them in the sun (1968:238).

Boerhaavia erecta L.

Origin: New World

Common Names: erect spiderling (Eng.); hogweed (Eng.); *anisillo* (Sp.)

Uses: hemorrhoids

Constituents: All parts contain calcium oxalate (Morton 1981:191).

Bombax ellipticum HBK.

Origin: New World

Common Names: bombax (Eng.); *flor de doncella* (Sp.) *flor de señoritas* (Sp.); *xiloxochitl* (Nah.)

Uses: abdominal obstructions; clean kidneys; colds; coughs; diuretic; respiratory problems; sores

Borreira ocimodes D.C.

Origin: New and Old Worlds
Common Names: button plant (Eng.)
Uses: rheumatism
Activity: The dried plant has a distinct odor from coumarin (a lactone). A person making extracts of the plant by the vacuum method continuously for twenty-four hours became profoundly affected by the stupefying emanation (Morton 1981:853). This may account for its use in treating rheumatism.

Bourreria huanita Hemsl.

Origin: New World
Common Names: strongbark (Eng.); *izquixochitl* (Nah.)
Uses: blisters; irritation; rash

Bromelia karataas L.

Origin: New World
Common Names: bromelia (Eng.); wild pinguin (Eng.); *piñuela* (Sp.)
Uses: vermicide
Constituents: The chemical composition of 100 g of peeled, seeded, ripe fruit is: moisture, 87.4 g; ether extract, 0.32 g; crude fiber, 0.3 g; nitrogen, 0.238 g; ash, 0.87 g; calcium, 52.8 mg; phosphorus, 8.0 mg; iron, 0.69 mg; carotene 0.015 mg; thiamine, 0.067 mg; riboflavin, 0.026 mg; niacin, 0.370 mg; ascorbic acid, 38.0 to 56.3 mg (Morton 1981:63).

Brosimum alicastrum Sw.

Origin: New World
Common Names: breadnut (Eng.); *ramón* (Sp.); *tlatlacoyoctic* (Nah.)
Uses: galactagogue

Constituents: The seed contains an essential oil, fat, resin, wax, mucilage, starch, albumin, dextrin (a polysaccharide), glucose, and sugars.

Activity: The sap obtained by tapping the trunk or crushing the immature tree is sold as "vegetable milk" at high prices in Guatemalan pharmacies (Morton 1981:141). In recent times the breadnut has been used as a galactagogue (Mellen 1974:125). Its reputation as "vegetable milk" may be the reason for this use although some Mexican physicians verified that preparations made from the seeds were effective as a galactagogue (Martínez 1944:58).

Bursera simaruba Sarg.

Origin: New World
Common Names: *gumbolimbo* (Sp.); *palo jiote* (Sp.); *xiotl* (Nah.)
Uses: diarrhea; fever; measles; scars; venereal sores

Caesalpinia coriaria Willd.

Origin: New World
Common Names: dividivi (Eng.); *nacazcolotl* (Nah.); *zumaque* (?)
Uses: toothache
Constituents: The mature pods of this plant contain 30 to 50% tannin (Morton 1981:282).
Activity: The antiseptic and astringent properties of tannin in the dividivi may alleviate toothache.

Calophyllum brasiliense var. *rekoi* Standl.

Origin: New World
Common Names: beautyleaf (Eng.); *calaguala* (Sp.); *leche de María* (Sp.)
Uses: wounds

Campyloneurum phyllitidis Presl.

Origin: New World
Common Names: strap polypodium (Eng.); *lengua de ciervo* (Sp.); *lengua de vaca* (Sp.)
Uses: purify liver

Capsicum spp.

Origin: New World

Common Names: *Capsicum* spp.: pepper (Eng.); *Capsicum annuum* var. *minimum* Heiser: red pepper (Eng.); *chile largo* (Sp.); *chilli chiltecpin* (Nah.); *chilli huacqui* (Nah.); *īc; (Q.)*

Uses: antidote; cathartic; evil eye; expectorant; expel and destroy the pituitary humor; menstrual disorders

Constituents: Capsicum, or red pepper, is the dried, ripe fruit of the plant. Capsicum contains capsaicin (a phenolic amide) (about 0.02%), an extremely pungent principle, in the dissepiments of the fruit. Capsicum also contains about 1.5% of a volatile oil, a fixed oil, carotenoids, up to 0.2% of ascorbic acid (Tyler et al. 1981:155–56), and palmitic acid (Stuart 1979:166). It is a useful source of vitamin C.

Activity: Capsaicin has a very peppery taste and even in small quantities irritates the skin and mucosa and produces a burning sensation. This would cause it to be an expectorant. Its continued application causes dermatitis, with the eventual production of swellings and blisters (Schauenberg and Paris 1977:28–29). Handling the fruits may inflame the palms, and contact with the eyes causes intense irritation and tearing (Morton 1981:789).

Fuentes y Guzmán said that those who frequently ate red pepper were protected against poison (1972:3:32), and red pepper can soothe a bite due to its counter-irritant and pain-blocking properties. Capsicum blocks the movement of pain in some nerve fibers by causing the release of a pain-killing substance (*Los Angeles Times* 1983:29). It would, therefore, be useful for menstrual disorders. Hernández rightly noted, however, that if used in excess, it could cause inflammation (1959:2:138).

Taken internally, red pepper aids in atomic dyspepsia and flatulence (Trease and Evans 1983:376). In excess, however, capsaicin can cause gastroenteritis, and permanent lesions of the kidneys (Schauenberg and Paris 1977:28). Irritation of the gastrointestinal tract can produce diarrhea. Therefore, red pepper is an effective purge, although a harmful one if used excessively. Evil eye can have many different symptoms, and red pepper may have alleviated some of them. It was not effective when used according to humoral theory to expel and destroy the pituitary humor.

Toxicity: Indians in Yucatán sometimes employ the toxic root for deliberate poisoning (Morton 1981:789).

Carapa guianensis Aubl.

Origin: New World
Common Names: Guiana crabwood (Eng.); *andiroba* (Sp.)
Uses: mouth disorders
Constituents: The bark and seeds of this plant contain unnamed alkaloids and the bark contains 12% tannin. The seeds contain 7-deacetoxy-7-ketogedunin and the furanoid tetranortriterpene, andirobin (Morton 1981:401).
Activity: The tannin content of the Guiana crabwood bark would make it somewhat useful in treating mouth disorders.

Carica papaya L.

Origin: New World
Common Names: papaya (Sp.); *chichihualxochitl* (Nah.); *papaya* (Q.)
Uses: vermicide
Constituents: Papain (the dried and purified latex of the fruit) contains several enzymes: one or more proteolytic enzymes, among which is peptidase I which is capable of converting proteins into dipeptides and polypeptides (amides); a renninlike, coagulating enzyme that acts on the casein of milk; an amylolytic enzyme (which converts starch into soluble products); a clotting enzyme similar to pectase; and an enzyme that has a feeble activity on fats (Tyler et al. 1981:290–91). The seeds contain a glycoside, caricin, and myrosin (an enzyme) (Spoerke 1980:131).

The roots and leaves of papaya contain the bitter alkaloid carpaine which acts on the heart like digitalis but is destroyed by heat. Two new alkaloids, dehydrocarpaine I and II, have been found in the leaves in higher concentrations than carpaine. Dried papaya seeds yield 600 to 760 mg per 100 g BITC (the aglycone of glucotropaeolin benzyl isothiocyamate) (Morton 1981:596–97).
Activity: In veterinary practice, papain has been demonstrated to be a safe and effective anthelmintic, especially in treating weak or pregnant dogs (Morton 1977:229). It has been used as an ame-

bicide in Central America (Lewis 1977:292) and a vermifuge especially for tapeworm (Tyler 1981:165).

Papain is used as a digestant for proteins and to soothe digestive disturbances (Morton 1981:596–97; Tyler et al. 1981:291). No reference was found in the Guatemalan sources of papaya being used as a digestive aid, but it may have been used for this purpose.

Toxicity: Fresh latex is a severe gastric irritant if ingested and has been used in poisoning (Morton 1977:229).

Collection: Shallow cuts made on the surface of the fully grown but unripe fruit cause them to exude latex. After collection, the coagulated latex is shredded and dried to yield crude papain (Tyler et al. 1981:290).

Cassia fistula L.

Common Names: goldenshower senna (Eng.); *cañafistula* (Sp.); *cuauhayohuachtli* (Nah.)

Uses: cathartic; colds; coughs; fever; kidney and urinary disorders; measles; smallpox

Constituents: Goldenshower senna contains anthraquinones (glycosides) (Lewis 1977:282) and mucilage (Harris 1972:77). The pulp is lower in rhein (a yellow crystalline acid) and sennidin-like compounds (sennoside A and B) than related sources of senna (Morton 1981:292). It also contains about 50% sugars, coloring matter, and a trace of volatile oil.

The heartwood is reported to contain barbaloin (a glycoside) and rhein together with a leucoanthocyanidin (Trease and Evans 1983:394). The flowers contain rhein, kaempferol (a flavonol) and fistulin (a bianthraquinone glycoside) (Morton 1981:293).

Activity: The plant is a purgative with the action stemming from the anthraquinones which exert their action by increasing the tone of the smooth muscle in the wall of the large intestine (Tyler et al. 1981:58). Either the pulp or the dried fruit may be used as a laxative (Lewis 1977:282; Wren 1973:70).

Goldenshower senna was an important cathartic during the seventeenth century, and royal attempts to stimulate its cultivation in Guatemala show that it was considered to be of some consequence as an article of trade. Coastal Honduras and Verapaz were the main areas of production (MacLeod 1973:65–66). No information was found concerning the activity of the plant against the other uses mentioned.

Toxicity: Anthraquinones are toxic in overdose (Lewis 1977:42).

Cassia occidentalis L.

Origin: New and Old Worlds

Common Names: coffee senna (Eng.); *habilla* (Sp.); *ehecapahtli* (Nah.)

Uses: fevers; skin disorders

Constituents: The seeds of coffee senna contain chrysophanol (a phenol), physicion, emodin (a phenol), cassiolin, α_3-sitosterol, and three other 1,4,5-trihydroxyanthraquinone derivatives; islandicin; helminthosporin, and xanthorin. The dried, powdered roots yield physicion and phytosterols (Morton 1981:298).

Activity: In one pharmacologic assay, the leaves and stems showed hypotensive activity. In El Salvador and Guatemala, the roots are said to be antispasmodic. The decoction is taken in difficult cases of menstruation, hysteria, and rheumatism (Morton 1981:298). Therefore, the plant appears to have sedative properties. The antispasmodic properties of the roots may account for the plant's use as a febrifuge. It may have alleviated chills associated with fevers. The yellowish powder chrysarobin has also been used topically for psoriasis and other chronic skin diseases (Ortíz de Montellano 1975:219; Reynolds and Prasad 1982:492). The plant may therefore be effective for those types of disorders.

Toxicity: Coffee senna is fatally toxic to cattle. Rabbits and sheep have also been poisoned by the leaves and pods (Morton 1981:298).

Castilla elastica Sessé

Origin: New World

Common Names: Panama gum tree (Eng.); *hule* (Sp.)

Uses: eye disorders; medicinal; muscular cramps and pain

Ceanothus coeruleus Lag.

Origin: New World
Common Names: azure ceanothus (Eng.); *palito de hierro* (Sp.); *tlalixtli* (Nah.)
Uses: throat disorders

Cecropia peltata L.

Origin: New World
Common Names: shieldleaf pumpwood (Eng.); *guarumo* (Sp.)
Uses: cardiac tonic; diuretic; whooping cough

Cedrela mexicana M. J. Roem

Origin: New World
Common Names: Mexican cedar (Eng.); *cedro* (Sp.)
Uses: erysipelas; fever; mouth disorders; tonic

Cedrela salvadorensis Standl.

Origin: New World
Common Names: Salvador cedar (Eng.); *cedro macho* (Sp.)
Uses: vermicide

Chenopodium ambrosioides L.
Origin: New World
Common Names: American wormseed (Eng.); wormseed goosefoot (Eng.); *epazotl* (Nah.)
Uses: asthma; blood purifier; diuretic; measles; menstrual disorders; skin disorders; vermicide
Constituents: American wormseed contains 1 to 2 % of volatile oil and some saponins in the roots (Spoerke 1980:138–39) as well as 342.300 mg calcium, 8.630 mg iron, 3.578 mg carotene, 0.297 mg riboflavin, and 99.200 mg ascorbic acid per 100 mg edible portion. The plant also contains geraniol (an alcohol), cymene (a liquid aromatic hydrocarbon), terpinene, butryic acid, methl salicylate, magnesium sulphate, magnesium phosphate, chenopo-

dium sapogenin, a pentacyclic tripenoid, and urease (an enzyme). The older the plant, the greater the saponin content (Morton 1981:176–77).

The main constituents of the oil are 60 to 80% ascaridol, 20% ρ-cymene, α-limonene, and *d*-camphor. The volatile oil is distilled with steam from the fresh, aboveground parts of the flowering and fruiting plant (Claus et al. 1970:194–95).

Activity: Ascaridol, an unsaturated terpene peroxide, is the most active, if not the sole active agent in the plant (Spoerke 1980:139). The seed oil paralyzes intestinal worms, which must then be expelled with a purgative. It has been mixed with castor oil and marketed in Guatemala and El Salvador under the name "Tiro Seguro" (Sure Shot) (Morton 1981:176–77). The oil is an effective anthelmintic against roundworms and hookworms (Hatcher and Batton 1944:83). There is no agreement as to whether other terpenes present in the oil also possess vermifuge activity, but the potency of the total oil is superior to ascaridol administered in pure form.

American wormseed has also been used against intestinal amebae (Vogel 1973:326). The fungicidal action of another constituent, 2p-cimenol, has been demonstrated (Lozoya and Lozoya 1982:40). The oil decreases blood pressure, heart rate, and central nervous system activity. There is some decrease in gastric mobility leading to constipation. It is also an irritant (Spoerke 1980:139).

The plant is not effective against venereal disease ("blood purifier") but would be effective for skin problems due to the antiseptic and fungicidal properties of ascaridol. Wren claims that the plant is antispasmodic (1973:328), and this may be why it was used for asthma and menstrual disorders during the colonial period. As it is an irritant, it may also be effective as a diuretic. Although it is not effective against measles, its use for that disease may stem from its fungicidal properties which may cause it to be effective on some skin disorders. Perhaps it was believed that it would be effective on the red spots which characterize measles.

Toxicity: The therapeutic dose for worms is close to minimum toxic levels, and death may result (Lewis 1977:291). Mild reactions are headache, dizziness, and nausea. More pronounced symptoms include vomiting (sometimes bloody), deafness, tingling of the extremities, and depression. Acute poisoning brings on vomiting, convulsions, weakness, drowsiness, cardiac and respiratory disturbances, and may be fatal (Morton 1981:177–78).

Chiranthodendron pentadactylon Larr.

Origin: New World
Common Names: monkey hand tree (Eng.); *mano de mico* (Sp.); *macpalxochitl* (Nah.); *q'anaq'* (Q.)
Uses: hemorrhoids
Activity: In pharmacologic assay, the flower has shown anti-inflammatory and antiatherogenic activity (Morton 1981:549). Therefore, it would aid in reducing the inflammation of hemorrhoids.

Chulbalam

Origin: New World
Common Names: *chulbalam* (Q.)
Uses: diuretic

Cinchona ledgeriana Moens & Trimen

Origin: New World
Common Names: legerbark cinchona (Eng.); *quina* (Sp.); *chichiccuahuitl* (Nah.)
Uses: fever; malaria
Activity: The earliest record of the use of cinchona occurred in 1633, in a book written by an Augustinian monk named Calancha of Lima, Peru. By 1640, the drug was being employed against fevers in Europe (Gilman et al. 1980:1054). Malaria had baffled the medical profession for ages (Bettman 1962:159). *Cinchona ledgeriana* Moens & Trimen, probably the most valued of the cinchonas, was named in honor of Charles Ledger who obtained the seeds in Bolivia in 1865. The seeds were bought by the Dutch for their Javanese plantations (Trease and Evans 1983:614).

Constituents: The alkaloids contained in cinchona are mainly formed in the middle layers of the bark. There are some twenty-five related alkaloids, of which the most important are quinine, cinchonine, and cinchonidine, the average yield being 6 to 7%. Another constituent of cinchona is cinchotannic acid, from 2 to 4% (Tyler et al. 1981:217).

Activity: Quinidine has antimalarial, antipyretic, and oxytocic action. However, its actions on cardiac muscle are more intense than those of quinine (Gilman et al. 1980:768). It is also used for prevention of cardiac arrhythmias (Trease and Evans 1983:617). Today quinidine is the main cinchona alkaloid employed therapeutically, but quinine is still used for falciparum malaria (Tyler et al. 1981:217–18).

Toxicity: Contact dermatitis and/or asthma occasionally occur in factory workers where cinchona bark is ground (Morton 1977:349). Quinine has been implicated in visual and auditory defects, including those which are congenital (Lewis 1977:96). When taken orally, hearing and vision are particularly disturbed (Gilman et al. 1980:1056). Excessive doses can lead to a condition known as cinchonism or quinism, marked by buzzing in the ears, deafness, headache, vertigo, and nausea (Weiner 1980:66).

Cissampelos pareira L.

Origin: New and Old Worlds

Common Names: *alcotán* (Sp.); *curarina* (Sp.); *raíz de la estrella* (Sp.); *iztacoanenepilli* (Nah.); *alkotan* (Q.)

Uses: aire; antidote; colds; fever; pasmo; tonic

Constituents: The root contains 0.72% total alkaloids, including curine, hayatidine, hyatine, hyatinine, bebeerine, cissamine, isochondodendrine, menismine, pareirine, and cissampareine. The root also yields the alkaloids dehydrodicentrine, dicentrine, cyclenine, and insularine.

Activity: The bitter root decoction of curarina, 20 g boiled for fifteen minutes in one liter of water, or an infusion prepared by steeping the macerated root for several days, is widely acclaimed in tropical America as a remedy for the bite of snakes and other poisonous animals (Morton 1981:216–17). However, no data was found which could verify this activity. Martínez said that the plant was a bitter tonic (1944:154–55), and this is probably the reason for its use in cases of colds, aire, pasmo, and fevers.

Clusia rosea Jacq.

Origin: New World
Common Names: copey clusia (Eng.); balsam (Eng.); *manzanarrosa de ratón* (Sp.)
Uses: fractures; toothache
Constituents: The plant contains triterpenoids such as aplotaxene, friedelin, α-friedelinol, β-friedelinol; also present are oleanolic acid and sitosterol. The pigment in the latex has been identified as xanthochymol (Morton 1981:565–66).
Activity: The latex is dangerously purgative, but no information was found concerning the activity of the copey clusia against pain of a toothache or fracture.
Toxicity: The fruit is considered poisonous (Lewis 1977:34).

Cnidoscolus chayamansa McVaugh

Origin: New World
Common Names: tread-softly (Eng.); *chaya* (Sp.)
Uses: blood purifier; cholagogue
Constituents: The chemical composition of 100 g of fresh leaves is: moisture, 79 g; ash, 1.65 g; protein, 8.25 g; ether extract, 1.93 g; crude fiber, 1.94 g; total carbohydrates, 7.23 g; calcium, 421 mg; phosphorous, 63 mg; iron, 11.61 mg; carotene, 8.52 mg; thiamine, 0.23 mg; riboflavin, 0.35 g; niacin, 1.74 mg; and ascorbic acid, 274 mg (Morton 1981:430).
Activity: The tread-softly would not be effective as a "blood purifier" which referred to blood made impure by syphilis since no plant remedy is effective against that disease.

Cnidoscolus urens Anth.

Origin: New World
Common Names: drug tread-softly (Eng.); *tzitzicaztli* (Nah.)
Uses: diuretic; fatigue; gout; muscular cramps and pain; kidney stones

Coccoloba diversifolia Jacq.

Origin: New World
Common Names: pigeon plum (Eng.); *picuerero* (Sp.)
Uses: blood purifier

Cocos nucifera L.

Origin: Old World
Common Names: coconut (Eng.); *arbol de Nuez Indica* (Sp.); *coco* (Sp.)
Uses: antidote; diarrhea; dysentery; menstrual disorders; pain in the side; stomachic
Constituents: The fresh kernel, or meat, of the coconut contains 30 to 40% oil (Claus et. al. 1970:150). Coconut oil is the fixed oil obtained by expression or extraction from the seed kernels (Tyler et al. 1981:93). The oil consists of a mixture of glycerides, trimyristin (20%), trilaurin (50%), triolein, tristearin, tripalmitin, tripalmitic acid, and the glycerides of caprylic, capric, and caproic acids (Spoerke 1980:60; Stuart 1979:176). In the mixture of glycerides 80 to 85% of the acids are saturated (Tyler et al. 1981:93). The roots and husk fiber are rich in tannins (Morton 1981:53).
Activity: The water of the ripe nut irritates the bladder and urethra and is strongly diuretic. The water of the unripe nut is harmful only in excess, when it may induce diarrhea (Morton 1981:52–53). Since the roots of the coconut are astringent (Spoerke 1980:60), they could be useful in cases of poisoning, diarrhea, dysentery, pain in the side, and indigestion. Today the husk is also used to treat difficult menstruation (Rodríguez Rouanet 1971:252) and may be somewhat effective due to its astringent properties which cause contraction of tissues. The water of the ripe nut, a diuretic, would relieve water retention associated with the menstrual period.

Cosmos sulphureus Cav.

Origin: New World
Common Names: cambray (Eng.); *flor de muerto* (Sp.); *xochilpahtli* (Nah.)
Uses: colds; digestive disorders; flatulence; lack of appetite; pasmo; pectoral; tonic

Crataegus intricata J. Lange

Origin: New World
Common Names: thicket hawthorn (Eng.); *cañutillo* (Sp.); *espino real* (Sp.)
Uses: antidote; swollen eyelids
Activity: Perhaps the thicket hawthorn has sedative properties as does the related *Crataegus pubescens* Steud. If so, this would retard the progress of poison. No information was found concerning activity against swollen eyelids.

Crataegus pubescens Steud.

Origin: New World
Common Names: hawthorn (Eng.); *manzanilla* (Sp.); *texocotl* (Nah.)
Uses: coughs; diarrhea; fever; heart disorders; lung disorders; muscle cramps; tonic
Constituents: Hawthorn contains a number of saponins and glycosides. The flavonoid glycosides are thought to be the active constituents (Tyler et al. 1981:485). The plant also contains cratagolic acid, triterpene acids, purines, and anthocyanic-type pigments (glycosides) (Spoerke 1980:83). The fruit (haw) is rich in ascorbic acid, carotene, and pectin (Morton 1981:264).
Activity: Hawthorn acts on cardiac or circulatory problems by causing dilation of blood vessels, especially the coronary arteries, and by causing some reduction in blood pressure. It is used prophylactically in angina pectoris. Claims of cardiotonic activity are apparently false (Tyler et al. 1981:485).

It also produces a marked sedative effect which indicates action on the central nervous system (Tyler 1981:116). Due to its sedative properties, hawthorn would be of some use in alleviating muscle cramps, coughs, and lung problems. Because of the vitamin C content of the fruits, it may also be useful for colds (Latour 1977:27–28). Clinical reports have appeared claiming that flavonoids have a beneficial effect on common upper respiratory infections by virtue of their supposed capacity to increase capillary resistance. However, the data presented do not justify this indication for the use of bioflavonoids (Goodman and Gilman 1970:1670).

No pharmacologic information was found as to hawthorn's ability to decrease fever and diarrhea, but those problems often accompany colds and may have been alleviated as cold symptoms were reduced.

Toxicity: The action of hawthorn develops slowly, and its toxicity is low, becoming evident only in large doses (Tyler 1981:115–16).

Crescentia alata HBK.

Origin: New World

Common Names: crossleaf calabash tree (Eng.); *morro* (Sp.); *jícaro* (Sp.); *ayacahtecomatl* (Nah.)

Uses: bruises; coughs; fractures; headaches; influenza

Constituents: The pulp contains water, 11.702%; mineral salts, 1.213%; fatty oil, 8.000%; solid grease, 0.323%; acidic resin soluble in alcohol, 0.250%; acidic resin soluble in ether, 0.620%; glucose, 7.383%; tannic acid, 0.117%; pectic principles, 4.327%; dextrin, 0.823%; cellulose, woody, and unassayed principles, 65.233% (Martínez 1944:96–97).

Activity: Martínez reported that the pulp has been used as a pectoral so the plant may have some use in cases of influenza or coughing (1944:97). Due to the presence of tannin, the crossleaf calabash tree is astringent and antiseptic and would be useful for headaches and for fractures and bruises that involved abraded tissues.

Cymbopetalum penduliflorum Baill.

Origin: New World

Common Names: Mexican earflower (Eng.); *orejuela* (Sp.); *teonacaztli* (or *hueynacaztli*) (Nah.)

Uses: diarrhea; lack of appetite

Cyperus articulatus L.

Origin: New and Old Worlds

Common Names: jointed flatsedge (Eng.); *cañutillo* (Sp.); *apoyomahtli* (Nah.)

Uses: mange; sores; stomachache

Constituents: The jointed flatsedge contains furanoquinones and sesquiterpinols (Alejandro Domínguez 1978:236).

Activity: The root is antiemetic and possesses aromatic properties, diffusing a feeling of warmth throughout the system. It acts as a sedative in dyspeptic disorders and is particularly useful in vomiting due to pregnancy (Wren 1973:7).

Derivatives of furan (a flammable liquid) possess antimicrobial activity (Goodman and Gilman 1970:1052) and would be useful in treating sores and mange.

Datura stramonium L.

Origin: New World

Common Names: jimson weed (Eng.); *vuélvete loco* (Sp.); *tlapatl* (Nah.); *toloatzin* (Nah.)

Uses: asthma; epilepsy; malaria; rheumatism; swelling; trembling; tumors

Constituents: All parts of jimson weed contain the alkaloids hyoscyamine and scopolamine (hyoscine). The roots also possess cuscohygrine and 3,6-ditiglylteloidine (alkaloids) (Morton 1981:794). The plant also contains atropine (another alkaloid) (Stuart 1979:182). The total alkaloid content is approximately 0.25 to 0.7% (Spoerke 1980:101). The seeds contain about 0.2% of mydriatic alkaloids and about 15 to 30% of fixed oil. The roots contain a higher proportion of alkamines than the aerial portions (Trease and Evans 1983:551).

Activity: Jimson weed is a dangerous plant. It contains several very powerful hypnotic and hallucinogenic alkaloids, any of which in even quite modest doses can be fatal. The quantity of alkaloids depends on the particular species, season, and plant so it is difficult to know in advance how large a dose is being taken (Moerman 1982:105, 108).

The dried plant and seeds were formerly officially drugs in the U.S. and were used as anodynes and antispasmodics. The leaves have been widely used in cigarettes to relieve asthma (Morton 1981:794). The active alkaloids are volatile and pass with the smoke into the lungs. They then exert their effect by relaxing the smooth muscle of the lungs, which is constricted during an asthmatic attack (Weiner 1980:113). Atropine paralyzes the vagus nerve ending in the pulmonary branch, thus reducing bronchospasms (Spoerke 1980:101).

Jimson weed is also a narcotic and has been applied externally to reduce local pain (Stuart 1979:182). Due to its narcotic and anodyne properties, jimson weed would alleviate rheumatism, epilepsy, swellings, trembling, and perhaps chills and shaking associated with malaria. It may also have reduced the pain and swelling of skin tumors.

Toxicity: All parts of the plant contain the toxic agent, but the highest concentration is in the seeds. Ingestion of the plant can be fatal (Spoerke 1980:101). The chief toxic symptoms of smoking or ingesting large amounts of jimson weed are those of atropine poisoning: dilated pupils, impaired vision, dry skin and absence of secretions, extreme thirst, hallucinations, high temperature, skin rash, convulsions, and ultimately, loss of consciousness.

In small doses, atropine and the other anticholinergic alkaloids inhibit saliva production, sweating, and bronchial secretions, dilate the bronchi, and abolish vagal action. By smoking jimson weed, perhaps some symptomatic relief is obtained for asthma, but there is danger of toxic side effects (Lewis 1977:296–97).

The harmful properties of the plant were recognized in colonial times, and Fuentes y Guzmán said that it was seldom used (1969:1:246). According to the *Relacion Geográfica Atitlán,* upon drinking a tea made of jimson weed leaves or eating the seeds, Indians went crazy, lost their memory, or even died (1964:104). Hernández said that when jimson weed (tlapatl) was taken in abundance, it brought about insanity (1959:3:67). In the *Florentine Codex* it was said:

> He who eats it will no longer desire food until he shall die. And if he eats it moderately, he will forever be disturbed, maddened; he will always be possessed, no longer tranquil (Sahagún 1962:11:129).

Such behavior was caused by the plant's toxic effects on the central nervous system.

Dictamnus albus L.

Origin: Old World
Common Names: gasplant dittany (Eng.); *dictamo real* (Sp.); *fresnillo* (Sp.)
Uses: passions of the heart

Dieffenbachia seguine Schott

Origin: New World
Common Names: dumbcane (Eng.); mother-in-law plant (Eng.); *hierba de sapo* (Sp.)
Uses: bites; rheumatism
Constituents: The plant contains calcium oxalate and the proteolytic enzyme, dumbain (Claus et. al. 1970:458).
Activity: Ingestion of the leaves of dumbcane results in severe corrosive burns of the oral cavity, esophagus, and stomach (Tyler et al. 1981:453). The sap causes severe dermatitis and paralyzes the tongue. If swallowed, the sap causes temporary sterility in men (Morton 1981:58–59). Its paralyzing properties may help alleviate pain when used externally on rheumatism or bites.
Toxicity: A report of severe poisoning that resulted merely from the biting of *Dieffenbachia* included these manifestations: severe corrosive burns of the mouth, oropharynx, esophagus, and stomach (Goodman and Gilman 1970:828). The toxic effects have long been attributed to calcium oxalate crystals. More careful investigations suggest that calcium oxalate is probably not the major reason for the toxicity and points to a "proteinaceous" agent. Subsequent investigations have implicated the calcium oxalate crystals (perhaps merely as piercing agents), the proteolytic enzyme dumbcane, a cyanogenic glycoside, and the alkaloids asparagine and protoanemonin, the latter causing swelling of the pharynx and larynx (Arditti and Rodríguez 1982:296–97).

Disciphania calocarpa Standl.

Origin: New World
Common Names: *bejuco chirriarte* (Sp.)
Uses: blood purifier; kidney disorders

Dorstenia contrajerva L.

Origin: New World
Common Names: contrayerva torus herb (Eng.); *contrahierba* (Sp.); *tozpahtli* (Nah.)
Uses: antidote; colds; diarrhea; dysentery; stomach disorders; tonic
Activity: Contrayerva is a stimulant and a sudorific tonic (Vogel 1973:410). Contrahierba in Spanish means counter poison or antidote (Wren 1973:94). It was used as an antidote in Guatemala during the colonial period (*RGA* 1964:104; *RGZ* 1955:77). Its stimulant and diaphoretic activity would have aided in sweating out venom. These properties may also account for the plant's use as a tonic. No information was found which specifically describes the activity of the contrayerva torus herb for the other uses mentioned.

Epiphyllum strictum Brit. & Rose

Origin: New World
Common Names: epiphyllum (Eng.)
Uses: fractures

Eryngium campestre L.

Origin: Old World
Common Names: snakeroot eryngo (Eng.); *lechuguilla* (Sp.)
Uses: hemorrhoids
Constituents: The root contains saponins (Schauenberg and Paris 1977:201).
Activity: The root is the part of the plant ordinarily used. It has been mainly used to combat uterine irritation, bladder diseases, and painful urination (Lewis 1977:315; Wren 1973:115). Cortisone

is a derivative of the steroidal saponins (Claus et. al. 1970:109), and it has anti-inflammatory properties (Gilman et al. 1980:1479). This may be the basis of its use for hemorrhoids.

Eryngium carlinae Delar.

Origin: New World
Common Names: eryngo (Eng.); *escorcionera* (Sp.); *ocopiaztli* (Nah.)
Uses: diarrhea; emmenagogue; erysipelas; medicinal; menstrual disorders; pain; urinary disorders

Erythrina berteroana Urb.

Origin: New World
Common Names: type of coralbean tree (Eng.); *pito* (Sp.); *tz'ite* (Q.)
Uses: hemostatic
Constituents: The seeds contain the alkaloids erysodine, erysopine, erysothiopine, erysothiovine, erysovine, α- and β-erythroidine, and hypaphorine. The wood contains α- and β-erythroidine.
Activity: *Erythrina* species possess alkaloids that have curarelike action (Lewis 1977:43). The plant has narcotic properties which may also cause diminished blood flow (Morton 1981:316).
Toxicity: Death may result from ingesting the bark or seeds of any *Erythrina* species (Lewis 1977:43).

Erythrina corallodendron L.

Origin: New World
Common Names: coralbean tree (Eng.); *pito* (Sp.); *tz'ite* (Q.)
Uses: emmenagogue; fractures
Activity: The coralbean tree is an effective sedative. It may or may not be an emmenagogue but would be useful for menstrual pain. Its pain relieving abilities may account for the use of the coralbean tree to wrap up fractures.

Erythrina folkersii Krakoff & Moldenke

Origin: New World
Common Names: coralbean tree (Eng.); *pito* (Sp.); *tzompamitl* (Nah.); *tz'ite* (Q.)
Uses: asthma
Constituents: The seeds contain the alkaloids erysopine, erysovine, and hypaphorine.
Activity: Eating the cooked flowers causes drowsiness which makes the plant effective for asthma and hysteria.
Toxicity: The seeds are sometimes used for poisoning noxious animals (Morton 1981:318).

Eucalyptus globulus Labill.

Origin: Old World
Common Names: (Tasmanian blue gum) eucalyptus (Eng.); *eucalipto* (Sp.)
Uses: colds; fever; headaches; hemostatic; influenza
Constituents: The leaves contain tannin, a bitter, a flavonoid pigment, eucalyptine, a balsamic essential oil containing mainly cineole or eucalyptol (a syrupy liquid having a camphorlike odor), and a bitter resin (Schauenberg and Paris 1977:290). The leaf oil contains 70 to 80% eucalyptol. Other constituents include terpineol (a terpenoid alcohol), sesquiterpene alcohols, aliphatic aldehydes, isoamyl alcohol, ethanol, and terpenes.
Activity: The leaf oil is a mild local irritant and antiseptic (Morton 1981:623). Terpineol has disinfectant properties, and cineole has antimicrobial activity (Reynolds and Prasad 1982:673; 684). Eucalyptus contains tannin which protects abraded tissue (Goodman and Gilman 1970:992) and may therefore help stop bleeding. As eucalyptus is also an astringent, it would tend to close blood vessels and aid in alleviating a headache.

The vapor of eucalyptus is also inhaled to relieve coughs, colds, sore throat, chronic bronchitis, asthma, and tuberculosis (Stuart 1979:187; Weiner 1980:83; Wren 1973:116). Eucalyptus arrests excessive secretion by the bronchi (Schauenberg and Paris 1977:290). Bathing in water containing eucalyptus would also soothe a person who had influenza or fever due to the plant's cooling properties. The leaves and oil may be used internally or externally for fevers. Eucalyptus was sometimes used as a substitute for quinine in treating malaria and intermittent fevers (Weiner 1980:83).

Toxicity: Large doses of eucalyptus are toxic, leading to delirium, convulsions, and death (Stuart 1979:187).

Eupatorium ligustrinum Lag.

Origin: New World
Common Names: Mexican eupatorium (Eng.)
Uses: intestinal and stomach inflammation; liver disorders

Euphorbia hirta L.

Origin: New and Old Worlds
Common Names: asthma weed (Eng.); *golondrina* (Sp.)
Uses: asthma; diarrhea; skin parasites
Constituents: The plant contains leucocyanidol, quercitol (an alcohol), camphol (an alcohol), quercitrin (a glycoside), and a quercitol derivative containing rhamnose (a sugar) and a chlorophenolic acid. The triterpenoids and steroids taraxerol, taraxerone, α- and β-amyrin, capesterol, stigasterol, and sitosterol have been found in the latex of the plant (Morton 1981:425–26).

Activity: Asthma weed is an irritant and contains carcinogenic compounds (Lewis 1977:37). The latex resin, or sap, is highly irritating and often produces blistering from contact and emesis and purgation from ingestion. These effects are attributed to an acrid principle believed to be present in the sap (Tyler et al. 1981:454). In experimental animals, the plant produced bronchial dilation but depressed respiration and heart action (Morton 1981:426). The plant is antiamoebic, expectorant, and antiasthmatic. It is effective in treating bronchitic asthma and laryngeal spasm because it causes relaxation of the bronchi by central depressant action. The sap is applied externally for warts (Stuart 1979:189).

Asthma weed would seem to be a more effective purge than

antidiarrhetic due to its irritant properties. In this case, Cosminsky, who said that it was used for diarrhea, may have been referring to another plant called golondrina (1972:369), but asthma weed does contain tannin which acts to alleviate diarrhea. Perhaps the effect obtained depends upon the part of the plant used and the dosage administered.

Toxicity: The sap contains toxic principles which cause severe poisoning if ingested in quantity. The toxic principles are the complex esters related to diterpene phoabol (Lewis 1977:37).

Euphorbia lancifolia Schlect.

Origin: New World
Common Names: spurge (Eng.); *sapillo* (Sp.); *ixbut* (Maya)
Uses: galactagogue
Activity: In Yucatán, according to the *Ritual of the Bacabs,* ancient physicians believed in curing like with like: a vine that looked like a serpent was used to cure snake bite; a yellow fruit was given as medicine to cure jaundice; red plants or fruits were prescribed for patients who vomited blood or suffered from dysentery (Roys 1965). The fact that this type of spurge exudes sticky, milky sap from the broken stems and leaves may have led to its use to increase milk flow in nursing mothers (Rosengarten 1982:96). It is not clear if the Maya practice of treating like with like was an aboriginal custom, or if it originated from the European doctrine of signatures (see Vogel 1973:33).

The plant decoction is given to new mothers as a galactagogue. It is reputed to cause the flow of milk to resume and to induce flow even in women who are not mothers. In 1949, a study by a noted Guatemalan botanist and chemist reported that of 86 postpartum women tested, 54 showed an abundant increase in the production of milk after taking the plant. Another study made between 1949 and 1951 was not as conclusive and found that the lactogenic properties of the plant have been considerably exaggerated. However, the first study referred mainly to use during the first days after delivery when lactation starts. The second was carried out from 2 to 14 months after childbirth (Rosengarten 1982:98–103). The effect has been confirmed by other physicians in Guatemala and El Salvador who have administered the fluid extract of the plant in doses of 8 g to wet nurses (Morton 1981:443). In 1950, a Mexican doctor also found in experiments that intraveneous injections of the plant caused a fall of blood pressure and a marked slowing of the heart in lactating women (Rosengarten 1982:110).

Toxicity: Spurge has a reputation as being fatally toxic to grazing horses and cattle. Although it is often assumed this toxicity is due to the ingestion of seeds and herbage, it is probably attributable to the quantity consumed. The plant is undoubtedly toxic, like other species of *Euphorbia* (Morton 1981:442–43).

Ficus glabrata HBK.

Origin: New World
Common Names: deer fig (Eng.); *higuera india* (Sp.); *amatl* (Nah.)
Uses: scalp ringworm; toothache
Constituents: The latex contains ficin, a proteolytic enzyme (Morton 1981:150).

Activity: Ficin has tissue-dissolving properties and can irritate the skin and eyes. Living worms such as roundworms and whipworms are dissolved by ficin, and it has been used therapeutically as an ascaricide and in trichuriasis. Its value as a toothache remedy may be due to the fact that it is a protein digestant (Claus et al. 1970:352). Perhaps it was used to loosen a painful tooth for removal.

In the last thirty years or so the latex has become a standard treatment for worms in Central American hospitals. In Guatemala, it is collected and prepared for export and therapeutic use by a branch of a German pharmaceutical company.

Toxicity: The use of ficin in crude form is dangerous. Experimental administration of 10 to 15% solutions have been fatal to rats, guinea pigs, and cats within twenty-four hours (Morton 1981:150).

Foeniculum vulgare Mill.

Origin: Old World
Common Names: fennel (Eng.); *hinojo* (Sp.)
Uses: birth aid; cathartic (after birth); eye pain; galactagogue

Constituents: Fennel contains 2 to 6.5% volatile oil and 12% fixed oil (Spoerke 1980:70). The volatile oil of the seeds contains d-pinene (a terpene hydrocarbon), camphene (a terpene), d-α-phellandrene, dipentene, 50 to 60% anethole (a phenolic ether), fenchone (an oily terpeonod ketone), methyl chavicol (a liquid ether), aldehydes, and anisic acid (Morton 1981:648).

Activity: The dried, ripe fruits of fennel are used. Since they are rather small, they are often referred to as seeds. Fennel is a stomachic and carminative, and its desirable properties are attributed primarily to the volatile oil. Producing the same actions as the fruits, the oil has been shown to relieve spasms of the smooth muscles of experimental animals. This may partially explain fennel's effectiveness as a carminative (Tyler 1981:95). This use was not mentioned, however, in any of the Guatemalan sources.

Fennel is also aromatic, a weak diuretic, and a mild stimulant (Stuart 1979:191). It is also an expectorant and a galactagogue (Schauenberg and Paris 1977:234). As fennel is effective against spasms and is a weak diuretic, it would be useful during the birth process. During the colonial period, a decoction of fennel was used as an eyewash (Fuentes y Guzmán 1969:1:244), and it is good for inflamed eyelids (Thomson 1978:124).

Toxicity: Fennel fruit and oil may be safely taken in the very small amounts required to flavor food, beverages, etc. Fennel fruit, in quantities normally used for medicinal teas, is relatively innocuous, except for producing an occasional allergic response. Fennel oil, however, in quantities as small as 1 to 5 ml, has caused skin irritations, vomiting, seizures, and respiratory problems such as pulmonary edema (Tyler 1981:95). Very large doses disturb the nervous system (Stuart 1979:191).

Fumaria parviflora Lam.

Origin: Old World

Common Names: fumitory (Eng.); *fumaria* (Sp.)

Uses: bitter tonic; medicinal

Constituents: The leaves contain chlorophyll, vegetable albumin, bitter extract mixed with nitrogeneous material, bland resin, gum, lime and potassium salts, fumarin, an alkaloid, and fumaric acid (Martínez 1944:134).

Activity: Its use as a bitter tonic stems from its bitter principle.

Gaultheria odorata Willd.

Origin: New World

Common Names: wintergreen (Eng.); *flor de cumbre* (Sp.)

Uses: rheumatism

Constituents: The main ingredient of gaultheria or wintergreen oil is methyl salicylate, a colorless, yellow or red liquid that has the characteristic odor and taste of wintergreen (Tyler et al. 1981:142).

Activity: Other related species have been used for rheumatism. For example, *Gaultheria acuminata* Schlect. & Cham. has analgesic, antirheumatic, and antiseptic properties (Martínez 1944:45), and *Gaultheria odorata* Willd. probably has those properties as well.

Toxicity: Large doses of wintergreen oil have produced toxic symptoms. Ingestion of 10 ml by children has caused death. Symptoms of poisoning include nausea, vomiting, pulmonary edema, and convulsions (Tyler et al. 1981:142).

Genipa americana L.

Origin: New World

Common Names: marmalade box genipa (Eng.); *irayol de montaña* (Sp.); *xahualli* (Nah.)

Uses: eye disorders

Constituents: The pulp of the plant is high in iron and riboflavin and contains phenol. It has a high level of tannin, especially in the bark.

Activity: The pulp shows some antibiotic activity, probably due to the phenol (Morton 1981:863–64). Phenol is bacteriostatic, bactericidal, and fungicidal. When applied locally, it exerts an anesthetic action. It is also very irritating to exposed tissue and may cause necrosis. When taken orally, it causes extensive corrosion of the mucous membranes, severe pain, and vomiting. Brief stimulation occurs, and perhaps this was the basis for using the plant as a tonic in some areas although no information was found to indicate the plant was used that way in Guatemala (Gilman et al. 1980:967). The unripe rind is astringent. The marmalade box genipa is effective for some eye disorders due to its antibiotic, anesthetic, and antiseptic properties (Morton 1981:863–64).

Gliricida sepium Steud.

Origin: New World
Common Names: sweet-pea tree (Eng.); *madre de cacao* (Sp.); *cuauhyaoxochitl* (Nah.); *k'ante* (Q.)
Uses: fever; skin disorders
Constituents: The heartwood of the sweet-pea tree contains isoflavenes, butin 2 (a flavanone), a phenolic isoflavan, and isoflavone (gliricidin 6a), a dihydroflavonol (sepinol 7a), and a rare β-hydroxy-dihydrochalcone (gliricidol 9a).
Activity: In one pharmacologic assay, the bark has shown antiatherogenic activity. The leaf decoction is an expectorant. No information was found regarding the plant's activity against fevers or skin disorders.
Toxicity: The roots, seeds, and leaves are toxic to the mouse but not to the rat. The leaves are toxic to horses (Morton 1981:319–20).

Gnaphalium attenuatum DC.

Origin: New World
Common Names: cudweed (Eng.); *hierba del pastor* (Sp.); *sanaltodo* (Sp.); *viravira* (Sp.)
Uses: colds; diarrhea; healing agent; hemostatic; pasmo; skin disorders

Gouania lupuloides Urb.

Origin: New World
Common Names: chaw-stick (Eng.); *jaboncillo* (Sp.)
Uses: throat disorders
Constituents: The chaw-stick contains saponin (Morton 1981:499).

Guaiacum sanctum L.

Origin: New World
Common Names: guaiacum (Eng.); holywood lignumvitae (Eng.); *guayacán* (Sp.); *matlacuahuitl* (Nah.)
Uses: syphilis; urinary disorders

Guaiacum was the "miracle drug" of the Renaissance, the sure-cure which swept through Europe in the wake of syphilis. The Fuggers, an Augsburg trading concern, cornered the world market on guaiacum. They waged an intensive campaign on behalf of the cure, and even founded a model hospital in Augsburg to administer their product (Bettmann 1962:99). Spaniards began using it around 1508, and it was used in Italy and the rest of Europe by 1517 (Guerra 1966b:38).

Constituents: Guaiacum contains 18 to 25% resin, of which 70% is guaiaconic acid. It is 10% guaiaretic acid and 15% vanillin (Spoerke 1980:82). The bark and wood contain saponin. The resin contains guaiaretic acid and other phenolic compounds of the lignan group (Morton 1981:367).

Activity: The resin of guaiacum has a local irritant effect on the gastrointestinal tract and causes nausea (Spoerke 1980:82). The resin also has mild laxative and diuretic actions which probably accounts for the plant's use in urinary disorders (Reynolds and Prasad 1982:315). None of the plant remedies, including guaiacum, were effective against syphilis.

Toxicity: The resin in the wood and fruit is poisonous if eaten in quantity (Lewis 1977:46).

Hapophyton cinereum A.D.C.

Origin: New World
Common Names: *hierba mata cucaracha* (Sp.)
Uses: insect repellent

Heliotropium angiospermum Murr.

Origin: New World
Common Names: white clary (Eng.); *flor de alacrán* (Sp.)
Uses: gum infections

Toxicity: In Barbados, children have been fatally poisoned by overdoses of the plant decoction (Morton 1981:720–21).

Hordeum vulgare L.

Origin: Old World
Common Names: barley (Eng.); *cebada* (Sp.)
Uses: fever; measles; smallpox
Constituents: Barley is composed of proteins, fat, vitamins B and E, and mucilage (Stuart 1979:202). It also contains 60 to 68% starch, 8 to 17% pentosans (polysaccharides), 7 to 14% nitrogeneous substances, 4 to 5% cellulose, 1.5 to 2.5% sucrose, 4% lignin (a by-product of the pulp industry), some pectin, sugar, ash, and malt. Barley contains hordein, a protein related to gliadin, and the alkaloid hordenine (Spoerke 1980:29).
Activity: Barley is a nutritive and demulcent. Barley water is a soothing preparation for inflammations of the gastrointestinal system. Cooked barley is a useful poultice for sores and this probably accounts for its use in measles and smallpox. Hordenine is useful in bronchitis (Stuart 1979:202) and also stimulates peripheral circulation by causing constriction of the vessels. Barley may have been given to those with colds or bronchitis who also had fever.
Toxicity: Hordenine is slightly toxic but has a wide range of therapeutic properties (Schauenberg and Paris 1977:271).

Hura crepitans L.

Origin: New World
Common Names: sandbox tree (Eng.); *habilla* (Sp.); *cuauhtlalatzin* (Nah.)
Uses: cathartic
Constituents: The seeds contain the protein hurin or crepitin.
Activity: The sap is highly irritating to the skin and eyes. The seeds contain a purgative oil and hurin, which has been found to be a potent lymphatic mitogen.
Toxicity: The sap has been used as a fish poison and an ingredient in arrow poison. Ingestion of the raw seeds may cause violent vom-

iting and diarrhea (Morton 1981:446–47). The toxic principle is the irritant and carcinogenic diterpene huratoxin (Lewis 1977:38).

Hura polyandra Baill.

Origin: New World
Common Names: hura (Eng.); *habilla* (Sp.)
Uses: antidote
Activity: The powdered seeds are sometimes used as a purgative in Guatemala (Morton 1981:447), but no information was found as to whether hura is an effective antidote.
Toxicity: The seeds are used in Mexico to poison coyotes (Lewis 1977:38).

Hymenaea courbaril L.

Origin: New World
Common Names: West Indian locust (Eng.); *guapinol* (Sp.); *cuauhpinolli* (Nah.)
Uses: liver disorders; vermicide
Constituents: The bark and leaves contain tannin. The main constituent in the trunk resin is the deterpene Labd-13-en-8-ol-15-acid. The main sesquiterpene hydrocarbons of the leaf pocket resins are carophyllene and α- and β-selinene (Morton 1981:322).

Hyperbaena guatemalensis Standl.

Origin: New World
Common Names: *granadilla* (Sp.)
Uses: fever; pneumonia

Indigofera suffruticosa Mill.

Origin: New World
Common Names: anil indigo (Eng.); *añil* (Sp.); *xoicpoxihuitl* (Nah.)
Uses: bacteria; bladder inflammation; hosa; kidney infection; measles

Constituents: Anil indigo is composed of ammonia, green material, white indigo, extract, gum, red resin, blue indigo, carbonate of lime, iron peroxide, albumin, and silica.

Activity: In experiments performed by the Instituto Médico Nacional de Mexico, the only well determined physiological effect of the plant was purgative. In biologic assays, the wood has shown androgenic and some antibiotic activity. Therefore, it may be effective against kidney infection, bladder inflammation, and other conditions caused by bacteria. The stems showed central nervous system depression. They also showed hypotensive, antiatherogenic, and antiandrogenic activity. Mexican physicians have declared that the dried, powdered plant is antispasmodic and an effective treatment for epilepsy (Martínez 1944:38–40; Morton 1981:323–24). It is not clear what the illness called hosa was, but if it was a form of paralysis (see page 112), anil indigo was probably not effective. It is probably not effective against measles.

Toxicity: The crushed plant has been used as a fish poison, and the roots are insecticidal (Morton 1981:324).

Ipomoea batatas Lam.

Origin: New World
Common Names: sweet potato (Eng.); *camohtli* (Nah.)
Uses: galactagogue

Ipomoea purga Hayne

Origin: New World
Common Names: jalap (Eng.; Sp.); *matlalitztic* (Nah.)
Uses: cathartic; rheumatism

Constituents: Jalap yields not less than 9% resins (Tyler et al. 1981:148). The root contains 8 to 12% of the glycosidal resin called both jalapine or convolvuline. A volatile oil, starch, gum, and a sugar are also found in the herb (Spoerke 1980:97). The resin from the root contains a number of glycosides, β-methyl esculetin, and palmitic and stearic acids (Tyler et al. 1981:148). From jalapine, a new β-D-quinovoside has been obtained (Morton 1981:701).

Activity: The Spanish learned of the uses of jalap from Mexican Indians and introduced it into Europe around 1565 (Vogel 1973:411). Jalap is a drastic purgative (Tyler et al. 1981:148) which acts on the small intestine but is very irritating and should no longer be used as a cathartic (Goodman and Gilman 1970:1029). It produces profuse, watery diarrhea (Spoerke 1980:97). No information was found regarding its activity against rheumatism.

Jatropha curcas L.

Origin: New World

Common Names: Barbados nut (Eng.); *piñon* (Sp.); *tempachtli* (Nah.)

Uses: cathartic; fractures; galactagogue; gout; leprosy; loose teeth; measles; medicinal; toothache

Constituents: The leaves and twigs of the Barbados nut contain α-amyrin (a triterpene), a mixture of β-sitosterol, stigmasterol, campesterol, 7-keto-β-sitosterol, stigmast-5-ene-3β, 7α-diol and stigmast-5-ene-3β, and 7β-diol. The seeds contain about 40% oil and the protein curcin, a tannin. The bark contains a steroidal sapogenin.

Activity: The seed oil is drastically purgative. The leaves and twigs have shown activity against P-388 lymphocytic leukemia (Morton 1981:448–49; Trease and Evans 1983:332). The oil may be of some use for fractures, gout, and toothache due to the tannin content of the seeds and counter-irritant properties of the sap. It may have helped to heal gums, thereby strengthening teeth.

The Barbados nut was probably used to alleviate the rash and sores associated with measles and leprosy but would not be effective against those diseases. The galactagogue property of the plant is probably due to the steroidal sapogenin contained in the bark.

Toxicity: Curcin is a toxic protein, and the seeds have shown strong cocarcinogenic activity. Raw seeds cause violent vomiting and diarrhea. Roasted seeds may produce sores in the mouth. The sap is irritating to the skin and is toxic when ingested (Morton 1981:448).

Jatropha podagrica Hook.

Origin: New World
Common Names: tartago nettlespurge (Eng.); *ruibarbo de Guatemala* (Sp.)
Uses: cholagogue

Juglans pyriformis Liebm.

Origin: New World
Common Names: walnut (Eng.); *nogal* (Sp.)
Uses: blood purifier; skin disorders; tonic

Lantana camara L.

Origin: New World
Common Names: yellow sage (Eng.); *cinco negritos* (Sp.); *corronchocho* (Sp.)
Uses: cathartic; eczema; rheumatism
Constituents: Yellow sage contains the triterpene lantadene A, which is broken down in the liver. The essential oil of the plant and flowers contains α-phellandrene, dipentene, α-terpeneol, geraniol, linalool (an alcohol), cineole, eugenol (a phenol), citral (a liquid aldehyde), furfural, and phellandrone. The plant also contains the triterpenes α-amyrin, β-sitosterol, lantadene B, and an acidic triterpenoid substance. Terpene acids occurring in the leaves include lantanolic acid, lantic acid, 3-ketoursolic acid, and lantanilic acid (Morton 1981:739–40).
Activity: Cineole has antimicrobial properties (Reynolds and Prasad 1982:673) and may account for the use of yellow sage in cases of eczema. Eugenol has been used in dentistry for disinfecting root canals, as a local anodyne for relief of hypersensitive dentine, pain and irritation (Osol and Pratt 1973:517). This may be why the plant is used for rheumatism.
Toxicity: Lantadene A, the toxic principle, produces phyloerythrin (a rose-red pigment), which goes into the bloodstream causing photosensitization and later jaundice, kidney congestion, and death. Yellow sage is highly toxic to grazing animals. Green berries in

quantity have poisoned children in Florida, one fatally. Effects include vomiting, diarrhea, lethargy, cyanosis, labored respiration, dilated pupils, ataxia, and coma (Morton 1981:739–40). If enough berries are eaten, constipation would be relieved, but this would be a dangerous remedy.

Leonurus sibericus L.

Origin: Old World
Common Names: Siberian motherwort (Eng.)
Uses: blood purifier
Constituents: The entire plant contains leonurine. Leonurinine is reported in the seeds. The leaves possess Alkaloid A and another unnamed alkaloid (Morton 1981:766).

Liquidambar styraciflua L.

Origin: New World
Common Names: American storax (Eng.); American sweet gum (Eng.); *liquidámbar* (Sp.); *ocotzocuahuitl* (Nah.)
Uses: diarrhea; dysentery; emmenagogue; menstrual pain; uterus infections; wounds
Constituents: The balsam is liquid at first but hardens when exposed to the air. It contains 20 to 30% water, 30 to 50% alcoholic resin (storesin), 5 to 15% free cinnamic acid, 5 to 10% styracin (cinnamyl cinnamate), about 10% phenylpropyl cinnamate and small quantities of ethyl and benzyl cinnamate, and styrene (a hydrocarbon). It also contains an aromatic liquid which has been called styrocamphene, and traces of vanillin. The leaves are rich in tannin (Morton 1977:129–30), and probably the bark as well.
Activity: The balsam is of great value as an external application in skin disorders, and is also a well-known stimulating expectorant (Harris 1972:175). American storax is effective for diarrhea, dysentery, menstrual pain, and wounds due to the tannin content. It is a good healing agent due to its antiseptic and astringent qualities and to the soothing properties inherent in balsam. This probably accounts for its use in treating uterus infections. Its stimulating qualities would cause it to be effective as an emmenagogue.

Collection: Storax is a balsam obtained from the trunk of the tree. Most is produced in Central America where large forests of it are found. The balsam exudes excrescences on the outside of the bark. These pockets are tapped with gutters, and the balsam is led into containers (Tyler et al. 1981:159).

Lycopodium dichotomun Jacq.

Origin: Old World

Common Names: club moss (Eng.); *cabello de sacerdote* (Sp.); *tzonpilihuizpahtli* (Nah.)

Uses: dropsy; epilepsy; evacuate all of the humors; heart disorders; joint pain; syphilis

Constituents: The plant contains three toxic alkaloids: lycopodine, clavatine, and clavotoxine. The spores are non-toxic and contain sporonine, a sugar, and an oil which is 50% of their content.

Activity: The spores can be used for healing wounds and for disease of the urinary system (Schauenberg and Paris 1977:44). This may be why it was used for dropsy and to evacuate the humors. The plant is not useful for syphilis but was probably applied to sores resulting from that disease and may have helped to heal them. No information was found as to whether club moss is effective against epilepsy, heart disorders, or joint pain.

Manilkara zapota Van Royen

Origin: New World

Common Names: *chicozapote* (Sp.); *sapodilla* (Sp.); *chichiltzapotl* (Nah.)

Uses: anemia

Constituents: The bark is said to contain the alkaloid sapotine. Methyl salicylate, HCN (hydrocyanic acid), and benzaldehyde (a colorless liquid aldehyde) have been reported in the leaves.

Activity: Abdominal pain and vomiting may result if more than six seeds are consumed. Due to its astringent qualities, the plant may be somewhat useful in treating anemia.

Toxicity: The seeds possess sufficient HCN to be toxic in quantity (Morton 1981:659–60).

Marrubium vulgare L.

Origin: Old World
Common Names: white horehound (Eng.); *marrubio* (Sp.)
Uses: coughs; emmenagogue
Constituents: White horehound contains tannins, volatile oil which contains marrubiol, mucilage, resin, sterols, marrubiin, and vitamin C (Stuart 1979:219). A volatile oil fraction and marrubiin, a hydroxyditerpenoid lactone bitter principle, give the distinctive taste to horehound preparations (Tyler et al. 1981:487). Marrubiin is now known to be an artifact which does not pre-exist in the plant but is formed from the closely related premarrubiin during the isolation procedure (Tyler 1981:122).
Activity: White horehound is useful in many respiratory disorders, but specifically in bronchitis and coughs. Premarrubiin stimulates secretions of the bronchial mucosa which accounts for the expectorant quality of white horehound. In fact, according to Varro Tyler, its use in extracts for coughs and colds appears to be the only use that can be presently justified (1981:122–23). White horehound has a high concentration of mucilage which would be expected to ease irritation accompanying sore throat (Weiner 1980:107).

It promotes bile flow, stimulates the appetite, and is considered beneficial in disorders of the gall bladder and stomach. It has a weak sedative action and causes purgation in large doses (Stuart 1979:219). It is also said to be a carminative (Spoerke 1980:89). Perhaps these characteristics explain horehound's use as an emmenagogue.

Marrubic acid has been shown to stimulate the flow of bile in rats. This might account for the cathartic properties observed with large doses, but it is difficult to evaluate since the marrubic acid content of the plant is not yet known (Tyler 1981:122–23).

Mesechites trifida Muell. Arg.

Origin: New World
Common Names: *rehilete de flores rojas* (Sp.)
Uses: bites and stings

Montanoa tomentosa Cerv.

Origin: New World
Common Names: *cihuapahtli* (Nah.)
Uses: birth aid; emmenagogue; headaches; malaria; pain in the side; reduce phlegm and coldness in the stomach; skin disorders; syphilis; tumors; women's disorders
Constituents: Cihuapahtli contains kauradienoic acid, monoginoic acid, zoapatlin, and monginol. Tomentosine is contained in the leaves and flowers, and montanol and zoapatanol in the leaves. Betain (an ammonium salt) of glicine (an amino acid) is in the root.
Activity: The kauradienoic acid in the leaves has uteroconstricting activity and is capable of inducing abortion if administered orally. Montanol and zoapatanol lack action on the uterus although they manifest ill-defined biodynamic properties on other tissues (Lozoya and Lozoya 1982:218). Cihuapahtli is capable of aiding birth in appropriate dosages. It is not clear if the plant has any other activity.
Toxicity: Cihuapahtli is dangerous when it is not administered in the proper dosage and at the right moment. Serious occurrences of intense and frequent pains without birth, fatigue, thirst, labored breathing, and in some cases, death have resulted (Martínez 1944:333).

Mucuna argyrophylla L.

Origin: New World
Common Names: cowitch (Eng.); *habillas de Tampico* (Sp.); *ojo de venado* (Sp.)
Uses: goiter; hemostatic

Murraya paniculata Jack

Origin: Old World
Common Names: Chinabox jasmine orange (Eng.); *boj de China* (Sp.); *limoncillo* (Sp.)
Uses: colic and stomach pain; syphilis
Constituents: The bark, leaves, and seeds possess unnamed alkaloids. The leaves contain the flavonoid pigment exoticin and a coumarin, 7-methoxy-8-(3-butenyl-3-methyl-2-oxo) coumarin. The ripe fruits

yield coumurrayin (5,7-dimethoxy-8-(3,3-dimethylallyl) coumarin).

Activity: The Chinabox jasmine orange has been confirmed as useful in treating toothache by Colombian and Panamanian physicians. Chewing the shoots numbs the tongue (Morton 1981:377). If the plant has analgesic properties, then it may also be effective for colic and stomach pain. It is not effective against syphilis but may have been used for pain of syphilitic sores.

Musa sapientum L.

Origin: Old World

Common Names: banana (Eng.); *platano de Guinea* (Sp.); *cuauhxilotl* (Nah.); *sak'ul* (Q.)

Uses: cataracts; dysentery; inflamed or injured gums

Constituents: The plant and unripe fruit are high in tannin. The ripe fruit and peel contain serotonin (a crystalline phenolic amine), levarterenol, and dopamine (a monoamine).

Activity: The plant and unripe fruit have antibiotic activity (Morton 1981:101) and would help inflamed or injured gums. Due to the high tannin content, the banana would be useful for dysentery. No information was found concerning its activity against cataracts.

Myroxylon balsamum Harms.

Origin: New World

Common Names: tolu balsam (Eng.); *balsamo de tolu* (Sp.); *huitziloxitl* (Nah.)

Uses: skin parasites

Constituents: Tolu balsam contains about 80% resin derived from resin alcohols combined with cinnamic and benzoic acids. The drug is rich in free aromatic acids and contains about 12 to 15% free cinnamic and about 8% free benzoic acid. Other constituents are esters such as benzyl benzoate, benzyl cinnamate, and vanillin (an aldehyde). Recent investigations have shown the presence of additional esters as well as styrene (a hydrocarbon), eugenol, ferulic acid, 1,2-diphenylethane, mono- and sesquiterpene hydrocarbons, and alcohols. The balsam also contains numerous triterpenoids.

The plant contains from 35 to 50% total balsamic acids calculated on the dry alcohol-soluble matter (Trease and Evans 1983:325).

Activity: Tolu balsam is mainly used as a flavoring for expectorants in syrup form (Hatcher and Batton 1944:55). It has antiseptic (Harris 1972:182) and soothing properties and may have some usefulness against skin parasites, but Mellen, who mentioned this use (1974:133), may have meant Myroxylon *balsamum* var. *pereirae* Harms.

Collection: Tolu is a balsam obtained by incision from the trunk of the tree of *Myroxylon balsamum* Harms. It is collected by making V-shaped incisions in the bark. The secretion flows into a gourd placed in the angle of the V. Each tree secretes enough to fill many such gourds (Trease and Evans 1983:325).

Myroxylon balsamum var. *pereirae* Harms.

Origin: New World

Common Names: Peru balsam (Eng.); *balsamo de Peru* (Sp.); *huitziloxitl* (Nah.)

Uses: bronchitis; colds; respiratory problems; wounds

Constituents: Peru balsam contains the volatile oil cinnamein (about 60%) which consists mainly of benzyl cinnamate and a lesser amount of benzyl benzoate. It also contains resin esters (30 to 38%) which are composed mostly of peruresinotannol cinnamate and benzoate (the salt or ester of benzoic acid), vanillin, free cinnamic acid, peruviol, and other substances in small amounts (Tyler et al. 1981:160). The seed balsam contains 0.39% coumarin and 0.40% tannin (Morton 1981:335).

Activity: Peru balsam is applied as an ointment, or undiluted, as a stimulant to wounds and ulcers to promote healing and the process of scarring. It is used as a parasiticide in skin diseases, such as scabies (Hatcher and Batton 1944:55). It also has antiseptic properties with the action being due primarily to the high content of benzoic acid and related substances (Weiner 1980:42).

It is a rubefacient and is used for its astringent properties in various hemorrhoid preparations (Tyler et al. 1981:160). Guatemalans still apply the trunk balsam to itching skin as it irritates and sensitizes it. This activity can cause dermatitis (Morton 1977:167).

The essential oil is stimulating and expectorant and is useful in cases of chronic mucous, catarrh, diarrhea, dysentery, asthma, and chronic bronchitis (Weiner 1980:42–43; Wren 1973:235).

Collection: Peru balsam comes from Mexico and Guatemala, but in colonial times it was shipped from Peruvian ports which accounts for the name (Guerra 1966b:38). Montero de Miranda said that there were some balsam trees in Verapaz but not many, and the Indians did not know how to collect the resin (1954:345).

The balsam is a pathologic product and is formed by injury to the trees. The tree is beaten on four sides and then scorched to cause the bark to separate from the trunk. Four intermediate strips of bark are left uninjured to prevent killing the tree. Within a week, the bark drops from the trunk and the balsam begins to exude freely from the exposed wood. The areas are wrapped with rags which are subsequently removed as they become saturated with balsam. The rags are boiled and, as the water cools, the balsam settles out, is recovered, and strained (Tyler et al. 1981:160).

Nicotiana spp.

Origin: New World

Common Names: rustica: wild tobacco (Eng.); *picyietl* (Nah.); *sic'* (Q.); *tabacum:* Mexican tobacco (Eng.); *cuauhyetl* (Nah.)

Uses: asthma; bites; cathartic; chills; colds; fatigue; flatulence; fractures; fright; headaches; hunger; indigestion; medicinal; pain; respiratory disorders; rheumatism; snake in abdomen; swellings; thirst; toothache; wounds

Constituents: Tobacco contains various alkaloids, mainly the highly toxic nicotine and anabasine, and the less toxic nornicotine (Morton 1981:796). The leaves contain a series of secondary alkaloids related to nicotine (nicoteine, nicotelline, nicotimine, nicotoine, nornicotine, nicotyrine, anabasine, anatalbine, and others). Also present are betaine, asparagine, tannins, resins, and enzymes (Schauenberg and Paris 1977:46). Tobacco leaves contain 0.6 to 9% nicotine and an aromatic principle known as tobacco camphor. The roots of *N. tabacum* contain the pyridine alkaloids anabasine and anatabine (Lewis 1977:392).

Activity: Nicotine is primarily responsible for tobacco's physiological action (Emboden 1979:35). Tobacco is a narcotic, sedative, diaphoretic, and emetic (Vogel 1973:384).

Nicotine can increase heart rate by excitation of sympathetic cardiac ganglia or paralysis of parasympathetic cardiac ganglia, and it can slow heart rate by paralysis of sympathetic or stimulation of parasympathetic cardiac ganglia. Nicotine tends to produce a discharge of epinephrine from the adrenal medulla, and this hormone accelerates cardiac rate and raises blood pressure. The major action of nicotine consists initially in transient stimulation of all autonomic ganglia.

Nicotine stimulates a number of sensory receptors. It also markedly stimulates the central nervous system and would alleviate fatigue. Stimulation of the central nervous system is, however, followed by depression. This may be why tobacco was used to treat the snake in abdomen illness, which was probably some form of hysteria. Nicotine also excites respiration and has an antidiuretic action. It causes vasoconstriction as well (Goodman and Gilman 1970:588–89).

Europeans believed that tobacco cured the Indians of many illnesses. They used it against syphilis as an analgesic which took "the afflicted out of their minds so they did not feel pain" (Bettmann 1962:129). Tobacco was used on poisonous bites in Guatemala. It caused sweating and vasoconstriction and would have impeded the progression of poison and swelling. Nicotine is also a contact insecticide (Lewis 1977:366).

Tobacco can alleviate pain due to its analgesic properties. This would account for its use for fractures, swellings, toothache, headaches, wounds, and other pain. By stimulating the central nervous system, it could counteract chills. It acts on the appetite and alleviates hunger and indigestion (and perhaps flatulence). Nicotine, when inhaled, inhibits hunger contractions of the stomach and slightly increases blood sugar levels. These actions, along with the deadening of sense buds, probably account for a decrease in hunger after smoking (Lewis 1977:392). Its narcotic and sedative properties allow it to alleviate asthma, rheumatism, respiratory problems, and perhaps thirst.

Toxicity: Nicotine can cause vomiting, diarrhea, slow pulse, collapse, and respiratory failure. Death from eating the leaves as boiled greens is known (1977:54–55). Appropriate doses produce tremors in humans and animals. With larger doses the tremors are followed by convulsions (Goodman and Gilman 1970:588). It is one of the most toxic of all drugs. Use of tobacco infusions against intestinal parasites has caused death (1970:590).

Tobacco is poisonous to grazing animals. The leaves and their products have caused fatal poisoning, whether applied internally or externally, as nicotine is absorbed through the skin. The dried leaves are carcinogenic (Morton 1981:796–97).

Nopalea cochenillifera Salm-Dyck

Origin: New World
Common Names: cochineal cactus (Eng.); *nopal* (Sp.); *tuna* (Sp.); *nochtli* (Nah.); *nopalli* (Nah.)
Uses: colds; coughs

Ocimum basilicum L.

Origin: Old World
Common Names: sweet basil (Eng.); *albahaca* (Sp.)
Uses: hijillo; vermicide
Constituents: The plant varies in chemistry with the variety and location. The seed mucilage contains the sugars *D*-glucose, *D*-galactose, *D*-mannose, *L*-arabinose, *D*-xylose, and *D*-rhamnose as well as *D*-galacturonic acid and *D*-mannuronic acid (Morton 1981:773–74). The essential oil mainly consists of estragol and also contains eugenol, lineol, and linalool. It sometimes contains thymol, tannins, basil, and camphor.
Activity: Basil is antispasmodic, a galactagogue, a stomachic, carminative, and a mild sedative. It may be used in simple gastrointestinal complaints, particularly for stomach cramps and vomiting (Stuart 1979:229). It has been taken as a vermifuge in Guatemala (Morton 1981:773), but this would not be effective. Hijillo is a native-defined illness having several symptoms (see pp. 34–35), and perhaps some of them may be alleviated by using basil.

Ophioglossum vulgatum L.

Origin: New World
Common Names: adder's tongue fern (Eng.); *lengua de serpeinte* (Sp.)
Uses: expectorant

Oxalis corniculata L.

Origin: Old World
Common Names: creeping oxalis (Eng.); sorrel (Eng.); *corazón acedo* (Sp.); *cuauhtla xoxocoyolin* (Nah.); *lotz* (Q.)
Uses: burns; cataracts; colds; dry mouth; eye disorders and injuries; inflamed or injured gums; throat inflammation and sores
Constituents: The plant contains oxalic acid.
Toxicity: Creeping oxalis has been linked to fatalities in sheep and rabbits in Africa (Morton 1981:361). In dilute solution oxalic acid is toxic, and strong solutions are corrosive. In acute poisoning from ingestion there is local irritation and corrosion of the mouth, esophagus, and stomach, with pain and vomiting, followed shortly by muscular tremors, convulsions, and collapse. Death may occur within a few minutes (Reynolds and Prasad 1982:787). Many of the uses of the plant are associated with problems involving inflammation, sores, and burns. Perhaps this was another example of using like to treat like. As the creeping oxalis caused burning, it may have been used to treat such complaints.

Pachira aquatica Aubl.

Origin: New World
Common Names: Guiana chestnut pachira (Eng.); *zapotón* (Sp.); *palo gordo* (Sp.)
Uses: liver disorders
Constituents: The seeds contain 58% white, inodorous fat. The bark yields 2.7% tannin and yellow dye which are used to tint sails, fishing nets, and lines.
Activity: In pharmacologic assay, the bark has shown some antibiotic activity so the plant may be useful for some liver disorders (Morton 1981:545).

Paullinia fuscescens HBK.

Origin: New World
Common Names: rusty paullinia (Eng.); *bejuquillo* (Sp.); *chilmecatl* (Nah.)
Uses: skin disorders

Persea americana Mill.

Origin: New World
Common Names: avocado (Eng.); *ahuacaxihuitl* (Nah.); *ōj* (Q.)
Uses: bites; bruises; diarrhea; fractures; pasmo; rashes; sores
Constituents: The leaves of the avocado contain methyl-chavicol and d-α-pinene and produce hydrocyanic acid. The ripe fruit and its peel contain large amounts of chlorophyll (Morton 1981:236–37). The pulp and seeds are rich in oleic, linoleic, palmitic, stearic, linolenic, capric, and miristic acids. The oil of the seed contains abundant tocopherol (a phenolic compound). Esculin (a crystalline glucoside) is also present and a group of saturated aliphatic hydrocarbons, alcohols, terpenes, and sterols.

The following amino acids are in the pulp: aspartic and glutamic acid, accompanied by leucin, valine, and lecine. Gamma aminobuturic acid is in the fruit. Proto-cyanidine, carnitine, and a high content of carotenoids are very abundant in the seeds (Lozoya and Lozoya 1982:25–26).

Activity: The husk of the fruit and the seeds have shown some antibiotic activity (Lozoya and Lozoya 1982:18). This would make it useful for treating sores, rashes, bites, bruises, and fractures. There have been reports of the seeds alleviating neuralgia and rheumatism which, if true, would indicate analgesic properties (Martínez 1944:26–27). The husk of the fruit is good for diarrhea (Lozoya and Lozoya 1982:17) and is well known in Mexico for its antihelmintic properties (Martínez 1944:27), but this activity has not been experimentally verified (Lozoya and Lozoya 1982:18). It is difficult to say whether the avocado would help alleviate any symptoms of the native-defined illness pasmo.

Toxicity: The unripe fruit is poisonous. The ground-up seed is mixed with cheese to poison rats and mice. The leaves have caused poisoning in cattle in California (Morton 1981:236).

Perymenium grande Greenman

Origin: New World
Common Names: *tatascamite* (Sp.)
Uses: eye disorders

Petiveria alliacea L.

Origin: New World
Common Names: garlic guineahen weed (Eng.); *apacín* (Sp.); kispar (Q.)
Uses: antispasmodic; diarrhea; emmenagogue; liver disorders; menstrual pain; throat disorders; vermicide
Constituents: The plant contains the triterpenes isoarborinol, isoarborinol acetate, and isoarborinal cinnamate.
Activity: The weed gives a garlic flavor to the milk and meat of cows that graze on it and causes abortion in cattle (Morton 1981:198). Therefore, it may be of some value as an emmenagogue in humans. A Mexican physician reported that it was useful as an antispasmodic and as a diaphoretic (Martínez 1944:439). This probably explains its use for menstrual pain. No information was found regarding the plant's activity for the other uses mentioned.

Phlebodium aureum John Smith

Origin: New World
Common Names: garden polypody (Eng.); *calaguala* (Sp.)
Uses: diuretic; emmenagogue; expectorant; fever; hemostatic; liver disorders
Constituents: The rhizome contains ecdysterone and two ecdysones, one of which has been named polypodoaurein (Morton 1981:12).

Picramnia antidesma Sw.

Origin: New World
Common Names: bitterwood (Eng.); Jamaica bitterbush (Eng.); *chilillo* (Sp.)
Uses: erysipelas

Constituents: The plant contains moisture, ash, volatile oil, the alkaloid picramnia, soluble and insoluble resins (in alcohol), wax, tannin, organic acids, coloring material, traces of glucoside, and extractive materials.

Activity: Claims have been made for the plant's effectiveness for chronic eczema and tumors (Martínez 1944:64). It may have been of some help in erysipelas.

Pimenta dioica Merr.

Origin: New World

Common Names: allspice pimenta (Eng.); *pimenta gorda* (Sp.)

Uses: rheumatism

Constituents: Allspice pimenta contains volatile oil comprised mainly of eugenol, cineole, phellandrene, and caryophyllene (a liquid sesquiterpene).

Activity: The plant is a carminative and an aromatic stimulant. The powdered berries are of benefit in flatulence and dyspepsia. They may be incorporated in stimulant lotions and plasters (Stuart 1979:239) which may be useful in cases of rheumatism. Cineole is a counter-irritant and has antimicrobial properties (Reynolds and Prasad 1982:673).

Pinus montezumae Lam.

Origin: New World

Common Names: montezuma pine (Eng.); *piño* (Sp.); *ocotl* (Nah.); *chaj* (Q.)

Uses: cold illnesses; coughs; evil eye; expectorant; fractures; medicinal; muscle cramps; stomach disorders

Constituents: Turpentine (an oleoresin) contains 64% α-pinene and 33% β-pinene. Pine oil contains 65% α-terpineol, 10% methyl chavicol and related phenol ethers, 9% borneol, 8% fenchol, and 4% menthols.

Activity: Turpentine has counter-irritant properties. It would be effective when rubbed on muscle cramps; possibly including a cramping somach. Pine oil is a disinfectant and a deodorant (Tyler et al. 1981:114–15). Pine tar, a product obtained by the destructive distillation of the pine wood, is a local irritant and an antibacterial agent and would be useful for fractures. It also possesses expectorant properties and would help colds and coughs (1981:132–33). Some of the symptoms associated with evil eye may be alleviated by the Montezuma pine.

Collection: Turpentine is secreted in ducts located directly beneath the cambium in the sapwood. During springtime, bark is chipped from the tree and following removal of a rounded chip, a spray of 50% solution of sulfuric acid is applied to the freshly cut surface. As the turpentine flows, it is guided by metal gutters into containers attached directly to the tree trunk (Tyler et al. 1981:154).

Piper aduncum L.

Origin: New World
Common Names: pepper (Eng.); *cordoncillo* (Sp.); *achiotlin* (Nah.)
Uses: stomach disorders

Piper auritum HBK.

Origin: New World
Common Names: pepper (Eng.); *cordoncillo* (Sp.)
Uses: rheumatism
Constituents: The plant contains 80.40 g water, 2.48 g ash, 4.25 g protein, 1.82 g fat (ether extract), 2.80 g fiber, 8.25 g total carbohydrate, 317 mg calcium, 49 mg phosphorous, 4.80 mg iron, 5.95 mg carotene, 0.12 mg thiamine, 0.28 mg riboflavin, 1.97 mg niacin, 49 mg ascorbic acid, per 100 g. It yields 0.47% to 0.58% yellow essential oil which contains safrole (an ether). The aporphone-type alkaloids cepharadione A and B are present in small amounts (Morton 1981:125–26).
Activity: As with most peppers, this plant probably has counter-irritant properties which would make it useful for rheumatism.

Piscidia piscipula Sarg.

Origin: New World
Common Names: Jamaica fishfuddle tree (Eng.); *barbasco* (Sp.)
Uses: toothache

Constituents: All parts of the plant, but especially the root bark, contain ichthynone, piscidin (an anodyne), or piscidic acid, and rotenone (a crystalline compound).

Activity: The dried bark, particularly of the root, is pungent. Pharmaceutical preparations from this tree have been used successfully against neuralgia, whooping cough, insomnia, hysteria, chronic bronchitis, and chronic alcoholism. They have proven useful in relieving headache and abdominal pain during pregnancy and menstruation, and also the pain associated with bone fractures and surgical operations. Preparations from all parts of the plant have been found to be potent uterine depressants. The active properties seem to be related to those of opium or *Cannabis sativa* L., but the latter is more powerful (Morton 1981:340–41). Since it has analgesic properties, the plant is effective for toothache.

Toxicity: Ichthynone, piscidin, and rotenone are the toxic principles. The leaves, bark, and wood of this plant have all been much used as a fish poison. Extracts are toxic to various insects. The fruits have been used in compounding arrow poisons (1981:340–41).

Pluchea odorata Cass.

Origin: New World

Common Names: fleabane (Eng.); wild tobacco (Eng.); *salvia* (Sp.)

Uses: paralysis

Plumeria rubra var. *acutifolia* Poir.

Origin: New World

Common Names: Mexican frangipani (Eng.); *flor de mayo* (Sp.); *cacaloxochitl* (Nah.)

Uses: cathartic; headache; pain in side; sore chest

Constituents: The bark of plumeria contains 0.96% of the glycoside plumierid, whereas the wood, leaves and roots contain only 0.20 to 0.52%. None is in the latex.

Activity: The latex causes dermatitis in sensitive individuals. The plant is a mucilaginous sedative and a sudorific. A weak flower infusion has been taken as a pectoral in chest complaints and as an especial remedy for hoarseness (Morton 1981:677–78). Mexican frangipani would be useful for pain in the side, due to its sedative properties. Fuentes y Guzmán said that the leaves were put on the temples to alleviate a headache (1972:2:114), but it is doubtful if this would have any effect. No pharmacologic information was found respecting the plant's purgative properties, but the latex may cause diarrhea due to its irritant qualities.

Toxicity: Plumerid is slightly toxic (Morton 1981:677).

Polygala floribunda Benth.

Origin: New World
Common Names: milkwort (Eng.); polygala (Eng.)
Uses: strengthen teeth
Constituents: Polygala species contain saponins and methly salicylate.
Activity: The saponins have anti-inflammatory properties. Methyl salicylate is readily absorbed through the skin (Lewis 1977:225) and is used as an anodyne in lumbago, sciatica, and rheumatic conditions (Reynolds and Prasad 1982:264). The plant may tighten, or strengthen, the teeth by healing gum infections.

Pouteria viridis Pitt.

Origin: New World
Common Names: green sapota (Eng.); *injerto verde* (Sp.)
Uses: destroy phlegm and bad humors; vermicide

Proboscidea triloba Schlect. & Cham.

Origin: New World
Common Names: martynia (Eng.); *flor de aromo* (Sp.)
Uses: throat disorders

Prunus capuli Cav.

Origin: New World
Common Names: black cherry (Eng.); *cerezo* (Sp.); *capolcuahuitl* (Nah.)

Uses: diarrhea; fever

Constituents: The leaves contain amygdalin (a cyanogenic glycoside), essential oil, fat acidic resin, tannin, glucose, a brown pigment, and mineral salts. The bark contains tannin, gallic acid, starch, fat, salts of calcium, potassium, and iron. The leaves, bark, and seeds release hydrocyanic acid when they come in contact with water.

Activity: In pharmacologic assay, the leaves have shown central nervous system depression, antiatherogenic, and anti-inflammatory activity (Morton 1981:265). It is effective against diarrhea (Martínez 1944:61) due to the tannin content. It is also effective against fever resulting from an inflammation due to its anti-inflammatory properties.

Toxicity: The fresh leaves taken in decoction can be toxic. Vertigo, respiratory and cardiac disorders, and even death can result because of the toxic action of the hydrocyanic acid. Cyanogenic glucosides characterize the genus *Prunus*. When collected and dried, the leaves lose toxicity by gradually losing amygdalin. The seeds retain their cyanogenic components for a long time (Lozoya and Lozoya 1982:80, 92). A dose of only two drops of the bark's essential oil produced the death of a cat in less than five minutes (Martínez 1944:60).

Psidium guajava L.

Origin: New World

Common Names: guava (Eng.); *guayaba* (Sp.); *xoxocotl* (Nah.)

Uses: cramps; diarrhea; hepatitis; indigestion

Constituents: The flowers contain tannin, and the leaves contain 9 to 10%. The bark has 12 to 30% tannin, and the roots are also rich in it. The leaves contain β-sitosterol, maslinic acid, guaijavolic acid, and unidentified neutral products.

The essential oil of the leaves consists mainly of caryophylene (a liquid sesquiterpene), β-bisabolene (an oily sesquiterpene), aromadendrene (a sesquiterpenoid hydrocarbon), β-selinene, nerolidol (a liquid sesquiterpenoid alcohol), caryophyllene oxide, and sel-11-en-4α-ol. Triterpenoids in the leaves include oleanolic, ursolic, crategolic, and guaijavolic acids. The ripe fruit is high in ascorbic acid.

Activity: The leaves and flowers have shown antibiotic activity (Morton 1981:629–30). Guava is effective against diarrhea and accompanying cramps and indigestion due to the tannin content and is useful for hepatitis due to its antibiotic activity.

Rhus terebinthifolia Schlect. & Cham

Origin: New World
Common Names: terebinth sumac (Eng.); *sal de venado* (Sp.)
Uses: rheumatism

Ricinus communis L.

Origin: Old World
Common Names: castor plant (Eng.); *higuerillo* (Sp.)
Uses: bruises; cathartic; cold illnesses; colic; cramps; deafness; earache; fractures; headaches; indigestion; pain; pinched nerves; skin disorders; sores; tumors; vermicide
Constituents: The leaves of the castor plant are rich in potassium nitrate and, in smaller amounts, ricin (a toxalbumin). A polyacetylenic compound, trans-dehydromatricaric ester, has been isolated from extracts of the leaves of the plant. In the leaves, stem, and seed hydrocyanic acid is present. From root extracts a polyacetylenic derivative can be isolated (Scarpa and Guerci 1982:119–20). Castor seeds contain from 45 to 55% fixed oil, about 20% protein substances consisting of a globulin (a protein), albumin, nucleoalbumin, glycoprotein, and ricin, an alkaloid, ricinine, and several enzymes. Castor oil is the fixed oil obtained from the seed and is a mixture of triglycerides, about 75% of which is triricinolein. The remainder consists of diricinoleoglycerides with the third acyl group representing either oleic, linoleic, dihydroxystearic, or a saturated (palmitic or stearic) acid (Tyler et. al. 1981:88–89).
Activity: Castor oil is a stimulant cathartic (Tyler et al. 1981:88–89). The cathartic action of the oil is said to be due to free ricinoleic acid and its stereoisomer (Trease and Evans 1983:332). Its use is

not recommended during menstruation or pregnancy and is dangerous in cases of intestinal obstruction and appendicitis (Morton 1977:196).

Castor oil is used locally on the skin for its emollient properties and would be useful in treating bruises (Gilman et al. 1980:1008). It has been recommended for itch, ringworm, and cutaneous complaints (Wren 1973:70). Undecylenic acid, which is prepared from castor oil, is used in fungistatic preparations (Trease and Evans 1983:332). The seed contains vitamin E and nicotinic acid which, due to its irritant action, could act as a hemostatic and cicatrizing agent, especially for burns, wounds, and sores (Scarpa and Guerci 1982:129). The seed oil mixed with turpentine has been used in Guatemala to expel tapeworm (Morton 1981:464). The plant was probably not effective for deafness.

Ricin inhibits tumor formation in rats. It most probably provides a barrier, though weak, with an immunological action that seems to be effective against tumors. The extract of the leaves is active against some microbes, such as *Mycobacterium tuberculosis*. Local application of the leaves causes hyperthermia (and would therefore relieve pain). This probably explains the use of the plant for headache, earache, fractures, colic, cramps, indigestion, and pinched nerves. It has anti-inflammatory action which may be due to the toxic action of ricin which causes vasodilation followed by an increase of platelets.

The vitamins and enzymes present in large quantities in the seeds and ricin, which causes production of antibodies endowed with a specific immunological action, could account for the use of the plant in infectious diseases (Scarpa and Guerci 1982:121, 125–26, 129). Fuentes y Guzmán said the castor plant was good for illnesses coming from cold causes, and perhaps some of these, like colds or influenza, could have been alleviated by using this plant (1972:3:35).

Toxicity: The entire plant is poisonous, but most of the toxic protein ricin is concentrated in the seeds and is a potent allergen. There have been many cases of poisoning in humans and animals (Morton 1981:464–65). If chewed, nausea, muscle spasms, purgation, convulsions, and death may result. Kidney dysfunction is common. Usually two to four seeds are poisonous to humans; eight are fatal (Lewis 1977:39). When the oil is expressed from the seeds, the poisonous ingredients are left behind in the cake (Wren

1973:70). The pulp of the seeds also contains allergens which in sensitive persons can promote strong allergic reactions such as conjunctivitis, dermatitis, eczema, and bronchial asthma (Scarpa and Guerci 1982:121).

Rosmarinus officinalis L.

Origin: Old World

Common Names: rosemary (Eng.); *romero* (Sp.)

Uses: diarrhea; influenza; stomachache

Constituents: Rosemary contains essential oil (to 2%) which contains 2 to 5% esters (mainly bornyl acetate) and 10 to 20% free alcohols (mainly borneol and linalool), organic acids, choline, saponosides, heterosides, and tannins (Stuart 1979:254). The leaves contain a number of flavonoid pigments.

Activity: Whatever physiological activity the plant possesses is attributed to the volatile oil. It has antibacterial properties, and one of the flavonoid pigments contained in the leaves, diosmin, is reported to decrease capillary permeability and fragility (Tyler 1981:188). Rosemary oil is a flavor and is used in perfumes. It possesses carminative properties and would help in cases of diarrhea accompanied by gas (Claus et al. 1970:198). It is antispasmodic, stimulates the flow of bile, and would help a stomachache (Schauenberg and Paris 1977:252–53; Stuart 1979:254). The leaves would also make a soothing bath for those suffering from influenza. Rosemary has insecticidal activity, and the plant decoction is astringent (Morton 1981:779–80).

Toxicity: Although consumption of the leaf rarely causes death, extremely large doses are toxic and can induce abortions or convulsions (Stuart 1979:254). Large doses of the oil produce irritation of the stomach, intestines, and kidneys (Tyler 1981:189).

Rourea glabra HBK.

Origin: New World

Common Names: rourea (Eng.); *canjura* (Sp.)

Uses: skin disorders

Toxicity: The fruit and seeds are poisonous (Lewis 1977:41).

Ruellia geminflora HBK.

Origin: New World
Common Names: ruellia (Eng.); *maravillita* (Sp.)
Uses: bruises; cathartic; fright; intestinal inflammation; liver disorders; pneumonia; tumors

Ruta graveolens L.

Origin: Old World
Common Names: rue (Eng.); *ruda* (Sp.)
Uses: abortifacient; emmenagogue; epilepsy; evil eye; fright; heart disorders; hemostatic; pain; pinta
Constituents: Rue contains volatile oil (to 0.6%), containing various ketones, but mainly methylnonylketone (to 90%), also limonene, cineole, methyl acetate, resin, tannins, the rhamno-glucoside, rutin, coumarin, fixed oil, bergapten (a crystalline lactose), xanthotoxin, alkaloids, ascorbic acid, furocoumarins, and several other active substances (Stuart 1979:257). The leaves contain volatile oil and tannins (Spoerke 1980:151).
Activity: A number of animal experiments have shown that various types of rue extracts will cause abortion, and this is probably due to a direct stimulant effect on the uterine muscles. The agent responsible for this effect is the furoquinoline alkaloid skimmianine (Weiner 1980:166). Rue is also an emmenagogue (Morton 1981:378).

Rue exerts a vasoconstrictor effect on the capillaries (Claus et al. 1970:121). Rutin has been called vitamin P (along with hesperidin) and is a permeability factor. It has been used in the treatment of conditions characterized by capillary bleeding and increased capillary fragility. However, evidence for the therapeutic efficacy of rutin and related compounds is not conclusive, and products containing them are no longer marketed for medicinal purposes in the U.S. (Tyler et al. 1981:73). Therefore, rue may not be an effective hemostatic.

Rue increases blood flow to the gastrointestinal system, aids in colic, and acts as a stomachic. It may alleviate some of the symptoms associated with evil eye and fright. It is of value in certain autonomic nervous system disorders, and traditionally has been used for epilepsy (Stuart 1979:257). No information was found concerning rue's effectiveness on heart disorders, pain, or pinta.

Toxicity: A number of cases of human poisoning have been reported when extracts were used to induce menses and/or abortion. To cause this effect large doses must be taken. Evidently, in large doses, some clinical constituent other than skimmianine has a predominant toxic effect (Weiner 1980:166).

The furocoumarins, such as bergapten and xanthoxanthin, confer a significant toxicity, especially on fresh rue, causing it to blister the skin following contact and exposure to sunlight (Tyler 1981:192). Besides inducing various types of skin rashes, rue produces kidney irritation and degeneration of the liver (Spoerke 1980:152). There is appreciable doubt about the utility and safety of rue, especially in the fresh state (Tyler 1981:193).

Salix chilensis Mol.

Origin: New World

Common Names: Humboldt's willow (Eng.); *sauce* (Sp.); *huexotl* (Nah.); *tz'oloj che* (Q.)

Uses: fever; liver disorders; malaria; rheumatism

Constituents: The bark yields the glucoside salicin (Morton 1981:132).

Activity: Today salicin is used as an antirheumatic drug. Salicin is readily hydrolyzed to saligenin (salicyl alcohol), which has some use in medicine as an analgesic. Salicylic acid is a disinfectant and is antipyretic (Lewis 1977:151). It is also antiseptic and a stimulant (Hatcher and Batton 1944:204). It is a mild irritant and application of salicylic acid preparations on the skin may cause dermatitis. It has bacteriostatic and fungicidal actions. No information was found concerning the plant's activity for liver disorders.

Toxicity: Symptoms of acute systematic salicylate poisoning have been reported after the application of salicylic acid ointments and solutions to large areas of the body (Reynolds and Prasad 1982:277).

Salmea scandens DC.

Origin: New World

Common Names: *barbasco* (Sp.); *verbesina* (Sp.)

Uses: rheumatism; stomach inflammation
Activity: Chewing the root numbs the tongue and lips (Morton 1981:963) so the plant may have some effect on rheumatism and the pain of stomach inflammation.

Salvia hispanica L.

Origin: New World
Common Names: Mexican chía (Eng.); *chía* (Sp.); *chían* (Sp.); *chiyantli* (Nah.); *aq'* (Q.)
Uses: medicinal; stimulant
Activity: Sage has carminative properties (Reynolds and Prasad 1982:683). This may account for its use as a medicinal. It may also have stimulant activity.

Salvia involucrata Cav.

Origin: New World
Common Names: roseleaf sage (Eng.); *salvia* (Sp.)
Uses: throat disorders
Activity: No specific information was found on the activity of this type of sage, but the related red sage is an effective antiseptic gargle (Stuart 1979:258). Perhaps this plant is also effective for throat disorders.

Sambucus mexicana Presl. ex A.DC.

Origin: New World
Common Names: Mexican elder (Eng.); *sáuco* (Sp.); *xometl* (Nah.)
Uses: cathartic; coughs; diarrhea; dropsy; emetic; medicinal
Constituents: The fruits are rich in tannin. The leaves, flowers, roots, and uncooked fruits are said to contain a cyanogenetic glucoside (Morton 1981:880) called sambunigrin. The bark and leaves of elder contain a cathartic resin called sambucine. The cyanogenic glucoside yields about 0.16% hydrocyanic acid from the fresh

leaves. The berries contain viburnic acid, a volatile oil, potash, lime, tyrosin (an amino acid), and coloring matter used as a dye.

The flowers contain approximately 0.23% volatile oil, and a glycoside called rutin. Mexican elder also contains a soft resin, albumin, wax, and tannic acid.

Activity: The bark, berries, and leaves have some laxative properties. The volatile oils may have some diuretic and diaphoretic properties. This may account for the plant's use in cases of dropsy. The inner bark is a strong cathartic and emetic (Spoerke 1980:68–69). Mexican elder probably aggravates diarrhea in some instances due to its cathartic properties, but it also contains tannin so the effect produced may depend on the dosage and part used. Since the related *Sambucus nigra* L. is used for colds and nasal catarrh (Stuart 1979:259), it is possible that Mexican elder has those capabilities as well and may alleviate coughs.

Sechium edule Sw.

Origin: New World
Common Names: vegetable pear (Eng.); *chayohtli* (Nah.)
Uses: fractures; wounds
Constituents: The new shoots are a moderately good source of iron, carotene, thiamine, riboflavin, and niacin.
Activity: Peeling the raw fruits may cause skin inflammation and numbness in the hands and arms if many are peeled (Morton 1981:894–95). Perhaps the inflammatory or numbing properties of the plant contain an effective constituent active against pain. This probably accounts for the plant's use for fractures and wounds.

Sedum dendroideum Moc. & Sessé ex DC.

Origin: New World
Common Names: stonecrop (Eng.); *siempreviva* (Sp.); *tetzmitl* (Nah.); *pashl'q* (Q.)
Uses: burning mouth; diarrhea; fractures; hemorrhoids
Constituents: The plant contains pyridine and piperdine.
Activity: The juice is astringent and is used to harden the gums, shrink hemorrhoids, relieve chilblains, and halt dysentery and nosebleed.

It is also put into the eyes to alleviate irritation (Morton 1981:261). It seems to have some pain-killing properties which may explain its use for burning mouth and fractures.

Selaginella lepidophylla Spring

Origin: New World
Common Names: resurrection selaginella (Eng.); *doradilla* (Sp.)
Uses: antispasmodic; diarrhea; diuretic; emmenagogue; kidney disorders; medicinal
Constituents: The resurrection selaginella contains chlorophyll, glucose, gum, pigment, albumin, carbonic acid, silicic acid, sulphuric acid, hydrochloric acid, phosphoric acid, potassium, sodium, calcium, magnesium, and iron (Morton 1981:6).

Senecio vulgaris DC.

Origin: Old World
Common Names: common groundsel (Eng.); *lechuguilla* (Sp.); *nanahuapahtli* (Nah.)
Uses: syphilis
Constituents: The common groundsel contains pyrrolizidine alkaloids, including senecionine, mucilage, tannins, resin, various mineral salts, and unknown substances.
Activity: The common groundsel is a vulnerary and a hemostatic but is rarely used today, except externally as a wash for cuts (Stuart 1979:263). It is not effective against syphilis but may have helped alleviate syphilitic sores.
Toxicity: The herb appears to have low therapeutic value and has produced toxic necrosis of the liver (Spoerke 1980:108–109). Senecionine is poisonous, irritates the liver, and causes lesions and cirrhosis (Schauenberg and Paris 1977:52).

Simaba cedron Planch.

Origin: New World
Common Names: cedron simaba (Eng.); *cedron* (Sp.)
Uses: bites and stings; colds; stomach disorders; tonic

Constituents: The fruits, leaves, and bark contain the glucoside cedrine (simarubine).

Activity: In large doses the seeds causes intestinal pain and drastic purgation (Morton 1981:390–91). This may account for the plant's use in stomach disorders. No pharmacologic information was found on its effectiveness for stings but in Guatemala the seed powder is taken to combat bites of all poisonous animals (1981:390). No information was found as to whether the cedron simaba has value as a tonic or alleviates colds.

Siparuna nicaraguensis Hemsl.

Origin: New World
Common Names: *hormiguillo* (Sp.)
Uses: colds; headaches; influenza; wounds

Smilax aristolochiaefolia Mill.

Origin: New World
Common Names: greenbrier (Eng.); Mexican sarsaparilla (Eng.); *zarzaparrilla* (Sp.); *mecapahtli* (Nah.)
Uses: hepatitis

Constituents: Greenbrier contains a mixture of saponins derived mainly from sarsapogenin and smilagenin (steroidal aglycones) (Tyler 1981:199). It also contains other phytosterols, resin, volatile oil, starch, and calcium oxalate (Claus et al. 1970:111).

Activity: Greenbrier is currently recognized as having potential value only as a flavoring agent and as a source of sarsapogenin and smilagenin (Tyler et al. 1981:495). The saponins, however, do have a strong diuretic action as well as some diaphoretic, expectorant, and laxative properties (Tyler 1981: 199). While its mode of action is obscure, it may stimulate absorption of other drugs (Trease and Evans 1983:485). None of these properties would make the plant effective against hepatitis.

Collection: There are several types of greenbrier or sarsaparilla. Sarsaparilla, the more general name for *Smilax* spp., is obtained from the roots of several woody climbing plants native to Central and South America. In Verapaz, sarsaparilla was exploited for profit. Montero de Miranda said that the hills there were full of it

(1954:354). Vázquez de Espinosa said, however, that the best sarsaparilla came from Honduras (1968:244). By 1574, sarsaparilla was being processed in five towns in Verapaz, as well as in the surrounding mountains. Although merchants in Seville questioned its value, sarsaparilla was much esteemed in Central America (Sherman 1979:255). It was imported into Europe steadily from 1568 (Guerra 1966b:38).

Smilax cordifolia Humb. & Bonpl.

Origin: New World
Common Names: greenbrier (Eng.); sarsaparilla (Eng.); *cozolmecatl* (Nah.)
Uses: emmenagogue; sterility
Constituents: Chlorine, phosphates, carbonates, sulphates, salts of potassium, salts of sodium, magnesium, calcium, iron oxide, and silica were found in the ashes. Several methods of analysis revealed such constituents as gallic acid, resin, tannin, malic acid, saponin, mucilage, glucose, calcium oxalate, and an alkaloid with saponin being the principal active constituent (Martínez 1944:73–74).
Activity: Since the related *Smilax ornata* Hook. is a diuretic (Stuart 1979:265), *Smilax cordifolia* Humb. & Bonpl. may also aid in menstruation by helping to eliminate water and by its hemolytic action. A Mexican physician also noted the diuretic effect of this plant (Martínez 1944:74). No information was found concerning its activity against sterility.

Smilax officinalis L.

Origin: New World
Common Names: greenbrier (Eng.); sarsaparilla (Eng.); *zarzaparrilla* (Sp.); *cuauhmecatl* (Nah.)
Uses: syphilis

Smilax spinosa Mill.

Origin: New World
Common Names: greenbrier (Eng.); sarsaparilla (Eng.); *zarzaparrilla* (Sp.)
Uses: blood purifier; hepatitis; malaria

Solanum mammosum L.

Origin: New World
Common Names: nipplefruit (Eng.); *chichitia* (Nah.)
Uses: clean kidneys; elephantiasis; hepatitis; kidney disorders; scrofula; skin eruptions
Constituents: The fruit contains the alkaloids solanidine and solasodine and the glycoalkaloids solasonine, solamargine, and β-solamargine (Morton 1981:806–807).

Solanum nigrum L.

Origin: Old World
Common Names: black nightshade (Eng.); *hierba mora* (Sp.); *tonchichi* (Nah.); *imut* (Q.)
Uses: blood purifier; erysipelas; evil eye; fever
Constituents: The black nightshade contains steroidal glycoalkaloids such as solanine, demissine, and others in the green shoots, leaves, and fruits (Tyler et al. 1981:457).
Activity: Solanine is used as a stimulant for the central nervous system (Vogel 1973:342). The intact glycoalkaloid is irritant, and the steroid alkamine is responsible for the major nervous symptoms (Lewis 1977:55). The black nightshade is a diaphoretic, which may explain its use for fevers. The leaves have been used on skin problems since the time of Dioscorides (Weiner 1980:140–41), and this probably accounts for its use for erysipelas. It is possible that some of the symptoms associated with evil eye are alleviated by the black nightshade. The black nightshade is not effective as a blood purifier.
Toxicity: Solanine, demissine, and other steroidal glycoalkaloids contained in the plant are toxic (Tyler et al. 1981:457). Effects of irritation include nausea, vomiting, abdominal pain, constipation or diarrhea. Nervous effects are apathy, drowsiness, salivation, weakness or paralysis, circulatory and respiratory depression, unconsciousness, and death. The most poisonous part of the plant is the unripe fruit, but stems, leaves, and roots are also dangerous (Lewis 1977:55).

Spigelia humboldtiana Schlect. & Cham.

Origin: New World
Common Names: spigelia (Eng.); *lombricera* (Sp.)
Uses: vermicide
Activity: No pharmacologic information concerning the action of this type of spigelia was found, but the related *Spigelia marilandica* L. was an effective anthelmintic when accompanied by a purgative (Stuart 1979:266).
Toxicity: High doses may prove fatal (Morton 1981:666).

Spondias mombin L.

Origin: New World
Common Names: yellow mombin (Eng.); *jocote amarillo* (Sp.); *macaxocotl* (Nah.)
Uses: anemia
Constituents: The bark contains tannin, and the leaves evidently also do because the leaf decoction is astringent (Morton 1981:476). No information was found regarding the plant's value in alleviating anemia.

Spondias purpurea L.

Origin: New World
Common Names: purple mombin (Eng.); *jocote de corona* (Sp.); *atoyaxocotl* (Nah.); *k'inom* (Q.)
Uses: anemia; diuretic
Constituents: The purple mombin contains a great deal of tannin. The leaves and bark are very astringent (Morton 1981:478). No information was found as to the plant's value in treating anemia.

Sweetia panamensis Benth.

Origin: New World
Common Names: billywebb sweetia (Eng.); *chichipahtli* (Nah.)
Uses: cathartic; malaria; syphilis; tight chest
Constituents: The bark contains the alkaloid sweetinine.

Activity: In pharmacologic assays, the bark has shown antiatherogenic activity and central nervous system depression. This may explain its use for a tight chest. It was included in the *National Formulary,* Fifth Edition, as a bitter and alterative, under the name *cascara amarga,* in 1926 (Morton 1981:349–50). It was probably used for malaria and fever due to its bitter principles. No information was found concerning the plant's cathartic activity, and it is not effective against syphilis.

Tagetes erecta L.

Origin: New World

Common Names: Aztec marigold (Eng.); *flor de muerto* (Sp.); *cempohualxochitl* (Nah.)

Uses: abdominal disorders; chills; cold illnesses; diuretic; dropsy; emmenagogue; fever; hemorrhoids; pinched nerves; tight chest; wounds

Constituents: The flowers are rich in xanthophyll esters. Both the petals and the root contain α-terthienyl (Morton 1981:969). The Aztec marigold also contains essential oil, resin, and tannin (Martínez 1944:69).

Activity: The constituent α-terthienyl has nematocidal properties (Morton 1981:969). In the *Farmacopea Mexicana* it was stated that it was an emmenagogue and antihelmintic (Martínez 1944:69). It is also antispasmodic and would alleviate chills, cold illnesses, a tight chest, and pinched nerves. The plant's alleged ability to remedy abdominal problems may have been due to the tannin if a person had diarrhea or to its antihelmintic properties if worms were present. Due to the tannin content, the Aztec marigold would also have been helpful for wounds and hemorrhoids. No information was found on the plant's ability to aid dropsy sufferers or to allay fever. Nothing was found regarding any diuretic activity.

Tagetes lucida Cav.

Origin: New World

Common Names: sweet marigold (Eng.); *pericon* (Sp.); *hierba de San Juan* (Sp.); *yaoxochitl* (Nah.); *iya'* (Q.)

Uses: diarrhea; diuretic; inflammation; indigestion; neuralgia; stomachache

Constituents: The plant contains three acidic resins, gallic acid, tannin, glucose, dextrin, pectin, gum, and mineral salts. The seed contains an unnamed alkaloid.

Activity: In one pharmacologic assay, the leaves and stems showed central nervous system depression and some hypotensive activity (Morton 1981:971). Although the sweet marigold has been reported to be a narcotic, chemical analyses are incomplete. However, reports are too numerous in favor of the plant as a Huichol narcotic to deny the worth of continuing chemical and ethnobotanical inquiry (Emboden 1979:99). The sweet marigold's narcotic properties would work to relieve neuralgia and pain associated with inflammation. At the Instituto Médico Nacional in Mexico, trials gave no positive results in treating malaria or diarrhea (Martínez 1944:214). However, it does contain pectin which is used effectively for the latter problem (Reynolds and Prasad 1982:958). Morton confirmed that the decoction is commonly used to relieve indigestion, upset stomach, and nausea (1981:971). The pectin and tannin would be effective for these problems. No information was found on the diuretic activity of the sweet marigold.

Talauma Mexicana Don.

Origin: New World

Common Names: Mexican talauma (Eng.); *anonilla* (Sp.); *yollohxochitl* (Nah.)

Uses: fever; heart disorders

Constituents: The seeds contain 56% fatty material, resins, essential oil, colored material, talaumine, a resinous glucoside, salts of potassium and soda, oxalic and malic acids, and iron (Martínez 1944:322).

Activity: In pharmacologic assays, the leaves have hypotensive, antiatherogenic, and central nervous system depressant activity (Morton 1981:220). Extracts of the leaves and flowers administered to animals produced intravenously vasoconstriction, arterial hypertension, and increased the force of contraction and muscle tone of the heart (Lozoya and Lozoya 1982:122). According to the *Farmacopea Mexicana,* the bark was used for fevers (Martínez 1944:323), but it is not known if the plant is effective or not.

Tamarindus indica L.

Origin: Old World
Common Names: tamarind (Eng.); *tamarindo* (Sp.); *cuauhmochitl* (Nah.)
Uses: cathartic; erysipelas; measles; hot illnesses
Constituents: The ripe pulp contains up to 10.86% or as much as 15.23% of tartaric acid. It also contains acetic, citric, malic, and succinic acids, sugars, and pectin. The seed coat is high in tannin.
Activity: The main use of the pulp is as a laxative, and the tartaric acid may be responsible for the purgative effect (Morton 1981:350). When in the intestinal tract, the sugars in the fruit are not absorbed to a very high degree. Because of this, they cause the intestines to expand, which results in a nonirritant type of bowel movement. The pulp also has refrigerant effects (Weiner 1980:189) which may account for its use in measles, erysipelas, and hot illnesses.

Thalictrum hernandezii Tauch.

Origin: New World
Common Names: meadowrue (Eng.); *cozticpahtli* (or *poztecpahtli*) (Nah.)
Uses: dislocations; fractures
Constituents: The dried root contains water 26.938%, ash 5.660%, resin 4.290%, glucose 16.936%, alkaloid 3.264%, coloring material 5.176%, extractive materials 13.940%, and vegetable fiber 23.796%. The ash contains potassium, soda, lime, magnesium, iron, carbonic, sulphuric, and phosphoric acid (Martínez 1944:88).

Theobroma cacao L.

Origin: New World
Common Names: cocoa (Eng.); *cacao* (Sp.); *cacahuatl* (Nah.); *kako* (Q.)
Uses: burning mouth and other parts; cathartic; fatigue; fever; galactagogue; heat of the liver and lungs; lack of appetite; digestive disorders; toothache
Constituents: The seeds of the plant contain 45 to 50% fatty oil. Their essential oil contains about 50% linalool and aliphatic acids and

various esters. The leaves, roots, and seeds contain the alkaloids caffeine and theobromine (Morton 1981:556–57). The seeds also contain about 15% starch and 15% proteins. Caffeine is present from 0.07 to 0.36% and theobromine 1 to 4% (Tyler et al. 1981:96). A relatively recent high-performance liquid chromatographic study revealed the presence of four biogenic amines, one of which was 2-phenylethyl-amine (Stone 1984:72). Cacao also has a high tannin content (Goodman and Gilman 1970:368).

The fat of the seed is called cocoa butter and consists of the glycerides of stearic, palmitic, arachidic, oleic, and other acids. These acids are combined with glycerol partly as triglycerides and partly as mixed glycerides (Trease and Evans 1983:335).

Activity: Cacao products are used chiefly as beverages and flavoring agents (Vogel 1973:409). Theobromine is a diuretic and smooth muscle relaxant but has little stimulant action on the central nervous system (Tyler et al. 1981:261). In large doses, theobromine causes nausea and anorexia (Reynolds and Prasad 1982:348). Any medicinal actions of the seed products are due to their theobromine and caffeine content, which act as a mild stimulant and diuretic (Stuart 1979:271). Cacao may, therefore, stimulate the appetite and relieve fatigue. Caffeine produces many undesirable side effects such as: nervousness, insomnia, rapid and irregular heartbeats, elevated blood sugar and cholesterol levels, excess stomach acid, and heartburn, especially if taken in large amounts (Tyler 1981:57–58).

The 2-phenylethyl-amine present in cacao is a source of energy and also influences the nervous system. If taken in large quantities, it can have numerous side effects. It is known to be a stimulant not unlike amphetamine in action, and it has also been reported to cause hallucinations (Stone 1984:72).

Cacao may help to relieve burning mouth, heat of the liver and lungs, toothache, and chills associated with fever because of its nervine, emollient, and muscle relaxant properties. It may also be used in treating the pain of acute biliary colic. Although cacao was considered healthful in colonial times and to be good for the stomach, it can irritate the stomach as already mentioned.

Cocoa butter is an emollient and nutritive and is much used in suppositories and ointments (Stuart 1974:271). Cacao butter is a mild cathartic and due to its emollient properties protects the gastrointestinal tract (Goodman and Gilman 1970:988). No information was found regarding cacao's activity in stimulating milk flow.

Toxicity: Cacao fruit waste products may cause theobromine poisoning with death resulting from sudden heart failure (Lewis 1977:36). Theobromine is toxic to horses in doses exceeding 5 g per day (Morton 1981:557).

Thevetia peruviana Schum

Origin: New World
Common Names: yellow oleander (Eng.); *chilindron* (Sp.); *yoyotli* (Nah.)
Uses: antidote; paralysis; toothache
Constituents: The latex and seeds contain thevetin and several other glycosides (Morton 1981:683) such as cerebrin and neriifolin (Lewis 1977:52).

In colonial Guatemala yellow oleander was a commonly used antidote (Ximénez 1967:253). This may have been due to the doctrine of signatures which led to the using of a poisonous plant like yellow oleander to combat poison. The root decoction has also been taken as an antidote for snakebite in Venezuela (Morton 1981:684). However, it may also have been due to the fact that yellow oleander does have analgesic properties (Martínez 1944:75) and would soothe the pain of bites. It is also effective for toothache. No information regarding its activity against paralysis was found.

Toxicity: Thevetin is highly toxic (Morton 1981:683). Along with cerebrin and neriifolin it produces symptoms similar to those of fatal digitalis poisoning. All parts of the plant are dangerous (Lewis 1977:52). Ingestion of even one seed of yellow oleander causes burning and dryness in the mouth and throat, dilated pupils, vomiting, purging, headache, cardiac depression, and sometimes death (Morton 1981:683).

Tibouchina longifolia Baill.

Origin: New World
Common Names: glorybush (Eng.); *nitro dulce* (Sp.)
Uses: eye disorders

Tillandsia usneoides L.

Origin: New World
Common Names: treebeard tillandsia (Eng.); *musgo blanco* (Sp.); *cuauhpachtli* (Nah.); *ek* (Q.)
Uses: hemorrhoids
Activity: The *Farmacopea Mexicana* said that the treebeard tillandsia has astringent properties (Martínez 1944:439). It would therefore reduce hemmorrhoidal swelling.

Tithonia diversifolia Gray

Origin: New World
Common Names: Mexican sunflower (Eng.); *mirasol* (Sp.)
Uses: eczema; malaria; sores

Trichilia havanensis Jacq.

Origin: New World
Common Names: bitterwood (Eng.); *lagarto* (Sp.); *limoncillo* (Sp.); *xopilcuahuitl* (Nah.)
Uses: malaria; rheumatism
Activity: The seeds are purgative and emetic. It may have been used for malaria due to its bitter properties. No information was found concerning bitterwood's activity against rheumatism.
Toxicity: The sap of the tree is violently poisonous (Morton 1981:407).

Tridax procumbens L.

Origin: New World
Common Names: tridax (Eng.); *hierba del toro* (Sp.)

Uses: cholagogue; emmenagogue; inflammation; insecticide; vermicide

Constituents: The leaves and seeds contain an unnamed alkaloid (Morton 1981:974).

Vanilla planifolia Andr.

Origin: New World

Common Names: vanilla (Eng.); *vainilla* (Sp.); *cuauhmecaexotl* (Nah.); *tlilxochitl* (Nah.)

Uses: cathartic; flatulence; stimulant; tonic

Constituents: The cured pods contain aromatic principles and vanillin, glucovanillin, vanillic acid, anisic acid, and aldehyde (Morton 1981:115). Vanillin is the aldehydic aglycone developed during the curing of vanilla beans and is its chief component.

Vanilla, or vanilla bean, is the cured, full-grown, unripe fruit of the plant. Green vanilla contains two glycosides, glucovanillin (avenein), and glucovanillic alcohol. Vanilla also contains about 10% sugar, 10% fixed oil, and calcium oxalate (Tyler et al. 1981:74–75).

During curing the glycosides in green vanilla are acted upon by an oxidizing and hydrolyzing enzyme which occurs in all parts of the plant. Glucovanillic alcohol yields glucose and vanillic alcohol. The latter is converted into vanillic aldehyde (vanillin). Glucovanillin yields glucose and vanillin.

Activity: Vanilla was discovered in Mexico by the Spaniards where it was used for flavoring the cacao beverage (Tyler et al. 1981:74). It is an aromatic carminative (Stuart 1979:278). Vanilla calms digestive organs and the stomach and has diuretic properties which probably accounts for its use as a tonic. It stimulates the brain and has direct action on the motor nerves and spinal column (Harris 1972:186). No information was found concerning any cathartic activity.

Veratrum sabadilla Retz.

Origin: New World

Common Names: false hellebore (Eng.); *cebadilla* (Sp.); *cuimichpahtli* (Nah.)

Uses: elephantiasis; head lice; loose teeth; skin disorders; sores; toothache; vermicide; wounds

Activity: The veratrum alkaloids possess hypotensive action through reflex inhibition of pressure receptors in the heart and carotid sinus. They also have emetic action and may cause nausea in hypotensive dosage (Sim 1965:155).

Since the related green hellebore (*Veratrum viride* Ait.) was once used to get rid of head lice, it is possible that false hellebore has that effect as well. Green hellebore has antiparasitic properties (Stuart 1979:278). False hellebore may also be antiparasitic, and that would explain its use for elephantiasis, skin disorders, wounds, and sores. False hellebore has analgesic properties (Reynolds and Prasad 1982:1769) so it would be useful in alleviating a toothache and pain of wounds and sores. No information was found regarding the plant's value as a vermicide.

Toxicity: All veratrum preparations have a narrow therapeutic margin, and it is difficult to obtain a significant reduction in blood pressure without side effects. Nausea and vomiting are the most common side effects. Other complications are muscle cramps, salivation, sweating, gastric distress, hiccough, blurred vision, and mental confusion (Goodman and Gilman 1970:735).

Veratrine, a mixture of alkaloids, would not be used internally. It was formerly applied externally for its analgesic properties and as a parasiticide, especially for head lice. However, there is a danger of systemic poisoning from absorption even when veratrine is used externally. It is an intense local irritant and has powerful direct stimulating action on all muscle tissues (Reynolds and Prasad 1982:1769).

Verbena litoralis HBK.

Origin: New World

Common Names: vervain (Eng.); *verbena fina* (Sp.); *tzopelicxihuitl* (Nah.); *chachalbe* (Q.)

Uses: colds; diarrhea; malaria; smallpox; stomachache

Activity: In Chile, the leaves are used as poultices and the leaf juice, mixed with lard, is applied in hospitals on decomposing wounds with great success (Morton 1981:755). This may be why vervain was used for smallpox. No information was found concerning its activity against colds, diarrhea, malaria, or stomachache.

Vernonia deppeana Less.

Origin: New World
Common Names: ironweed (Eng.)
Uses: antispasmodic; gastric disorders; hemorrhoids; hemostatic; inflammation; tonic

Verticillaria acuminata Ruiz et Pavon

Origin: Old World
Common Names: *arbol de María* (Sp.); palo de aceite (Sp.)
Uses: tumors; wounds

Vitis tiliifolia Humb. & Bonpl.

Origin: New World
Common Names: wild grape (Eng.); *bejucode agua* (Sp.); *uva* (Sp.)
Uses: eye disorders
Constituents: The plant contains oxycinamic acids, flavonoids, polyphenols, and cyanogenic glucosides.
Activity: The wild grape is a diuretic (Alejando Domínguez 1978:235) and an astringent (Morton 1981:507). It would be effective for some eye disorders due to its astringency.

Waltheria americana L.

Origin: New World
Common Names: Florida waltheria (Eng.); *escobillo blanco* (Sp.)
Uses: eye inflammation; rheumatism; toothache

Yucca elephantipes Reg.

Origin: New World
Common Names: bulbstem yucca (Eng.); *iczotl* (Nah.); *cuauhcamohtli* (Nah.)
Uses: coughs; diuretic; influenza; scars
Constituents: *Yucca* species, together with other agaves, are known to contain large quantities of saponins, which are steroid derivatives (Tyler 1981:235). The flowers contain as much as 560 mg ascorbic

acid per 100 g and moderate amounts of niacin and thiamine. The hearts are very high in calcium. The young leaves yield up to 2,150 mg per 100 g of ascorbic acid. The mature leaves yield up to 3,220 mg.

Activity: The specific identity and amounts of the numerous saponins in bulbstem yucca have been found to vary markedly depending on the part of the plant tested and the season in which it was collected (Tyler 1981:235). It is therefore difficult to determine the effectiveness of the plant for the uses given above.

Zea mays L.

Origin: New World

Common Names: corn (Eng.); maize (Eng.); *trigo indio* (Sp.); *tlaolli* (Nah.); *ixīm* (Q.)

Uses: asthma; cathartic; colds; decongestant; diarrhea; diuretic; dysentery; emmenagogue; expel and destroy the pituitary humor; fever; flatulence; galactagogue; measles; menstrual disorders; ringworm

Constituents: Corn silk contains saponin, salts of potassium, tannin, sterols, allontoin (a crystalline oxidation product of uric acid), L-arabinose, arabinose, and galactose (sugars), maizenic acid, phlobaphene, betaine (an ammonium salt), galactose, maizenic acid, phlobaphene and in some types, an alkaloid. The leaves contain the alkaloid hordenine and an unnamed alkaloid is in the seeds. The husks, silk, and other parts of highly pigmented strains are high in tannin and other phenols (Morton 1981:43). The styles of the female flowers contain saponins, a fatty oil, and potassium salts. The stigmas contain tannin, steroids, and allantoine (Schauenberg and Paris 1977:213). Corn oil consists largely of triglicerides of the unsaturated oleic and linolic acids with smaller proportions of palmitic and stearic acids (Trease and Evans 1983:329).

Activity: Corn products have been accepted as drugs. Corn smut (*Ustilago zeae*), a fungus, was used to hasten childbirth by increasing the severity of labor. It was also given to stop hemorrhage after childbirth and for abdominal lochial discharge (Vogel 1973:294). This probably accounts for corn's use as an emmenagogue and for menstrual problems. Corn silk was also used as a diuretic. It was formerly a remedy in the United States for cystitis and urethritis (Morton 1981:43).

Corn starch is a nutrient, demulcent, protective, and absorbent. It was used to allay itching and as a dusting powder (Vogel 1973:294). This ability to alleviate itching may explain the plant's use for measles. It has been recommended in many urinary and bladder problems (Wren 1973:97).

Corn oil is a mild cathartic and acts as a protective for the gastrointestinal tract in cases of corrosive poisoning. When applied externally, it is an emollient to the skin and mucous membranes (Gilman et al. 1980:952). Corn has been used in many illnesses in highland Guatemala which probably stems from the fact that it is a staple food with nutritive qualities. No specific information was found regarding corn's activity against the other uses mentioned.

Toxicity: The young seedlings and the wilted plants, under certain conditions, contain a sufficient cyanogenic glycoside level to cause fatalities in grazing animals. Corn may also accumulate toxic levels of nitrate (Morton 1981:43).

Zebrina pendula Schnizl.

Origin: New World

Common Names: wandering Jew (Eng.); *cañutillo* (Sp.); *hierba de pollo* (Sp.); *acaxaxan* (Nah.)

Uses: cathartic; dysentery; mange; sores

Activity: In Florida, the watery sap is a frequent cause of skin inflammation, rash, small blisters, and itching (Morton 1981:73). These irritant qualities may account for the plant's use as an enema for constipation. Since the irritant qualities would appear to aggravate dysentery, perhaps another part of the plant was used to combat dysentery. Wandering Jew causes sores, and according to the doctrine of signatures, it would have been used to heal mange and sores, probably with negative results.

Zingiber officinale Rosc.

Origin: Old World
Common Names: ginger (Eng.); *jengibre* (Sp.)
Uses: colds; throat disorders; tonic
Constituents: Ginger is the dried rhizome of the plant (Tyler et al. 1981:156). It contains about 1 to 2% volatile oil and from 5 to 8% resinous matter, starch, and mucilage (Trease and Evans 1983:458). The rhizome contains the ketone zingerone and gingerol. The sesquiterpenes, farnesine, methyl-heptenone, cineole, borneol, geraniol, and linalool are found in the essential oil (Morton 1981:106). It also contains bisabolene, zingiberene, and zingiberol (sesquiterpenes). The characteristic pungency is attributed to ginger oleoresin from which the aromatic ketones zingerone and shogaol have been isolated. Ginger also contains more than 50% starch.
Activity: Ginger is a flavor and is used as a condiment, an aromatic stimulant, and a carminative (Tyler et al. 1981:156–57). It is very valuable in flatulent colic, dyspepsia, and atonic dyspepsia. It is often used as an adjunct to other remedies for general tonic or stimulant purposes, or in purgatives to prevent griping. It is a rubefacient when applied externally in the fresh state. Large doses should be avoided by patients suffering from any skin complaint (Stuart 1979:283). No information was found regarding ginger's activity against throat disorders or colds.
Collection: Ginger was introduced into Jamaica and other West Indian Islands by the Spaniards (Trease and Evans 1983:457). It became an important export product and by 1547, four million pounds of it arrived in Seville (Guerra 1966b:38).

The plant is sterile and is grown by vegetative means. Pieces of rhizome each bearing a bud are planted in holes or trenches during March or April. When the stems wither, in about December or January, the rhizomes are ready for collection.

CHAPTER EIGHT

Conclusion

There is no native work which describes aboriginal or colonial Indian medicine in the Guatemala highlands. However, it has been possible to reconstruct some of the past practices and knowledge by referring to the ethnohistoric, ethnographic, and botanical sources written primarily by non-Indians.

In pre-Columbian times illness was attributed to a variety of supernatural and natural causes. Religion, medicine, and morality were closely interwoven. Diagnosis often involved discovering which supernatural entity or sorcerer was responsible for the illness, and treatment involved restoring the sick individual's balance with the gods or spirits which had been offended or counteracting the sorcery. Many of the beliefs regarding illness present in ancient Mexico seem to have existed in the Guatemala highlands as well. The soul, or teyolía, associated with the heart, could be harmed by immoral sexual conduct, illnesses that covered the heart with phlegm, and by sorcery.

The life force of an individual, the tonalli, which was associated with the head, could also cause illness. This mainly occurred when the tonalli left the body. If it was not restored, the individual died. A primary cause of the tonalli leaving the body was fright, and this is still seen as a common cause of illness in the Guatemala highlands today. The contemporary illness fallen fontanel is also related to ancient beliefs concerning the tonalli as are beliefs in the tona, or companion animal, and the nagual who can cause illness due to supernatural power.

A luminous gas, called the ihíyotl, was associated with the liver and was believed to emanate from persons, animals, or objects. Some of these, such as immoral persons and corpses, gave off harmful emanations that could cause illness. Today hijillo is a native-defined illness that is probably derived from ancient beliefs associated with the ihíyotl.

Ancient Mexican concepts of equilibrium and disequilibrium have also formed an important part of illness etiology in highland Guatemala. Many factors could produce disequilibrium and cause a person to become ill, such as sex, age, overworking, becoming overtired, and committing a sin. Today this concept particularly survives in the strength-weakness principle where a weak body, due to weak blood, is deemed to be particularly susceptible to illness. The contemporary illness called evil eye is related to the strength-weakness principle and is believed to be caused in weak individuals by hot-blooded persons. In ancient times it was also thought that cold and heat had to be in equilibrium for health. This is probably the basis for the belief that evil or bad wind or air could cause illness as too much heat or cold is believed to enter the body from exposure to such air.

Various gods were also believed to send illnesses. The *Popol Vuh* contains several references to gods whose function it was to cause illness. Other gods, such as Grandfather and Grandmother, seem to have had curing roles. Ix Chel, the moon goddess, was prominent in ancient Maya medicine. Lineage gods, such as those of Chiya', also seem to have figured significantly in predicting epidemics although they do not seem to have brought them. Certain other supernatural beings, or sprites, are also believed able to send illness among contemporary Indians.

Evil sorcerers were feared for their ability to cause illnesses. Witchcraft existed in ancient as well as modern times. If witchcraft were suspected as a cause of illness, a person would go to a good sorcerer to counteract the evil magic believed to be making him sick.

Treatment for illness involved individual and community rituals, going to a medical practitioner, and using herbal medicines. Many individual and community rituals were aimed at preserving or restoring health. Divination, usually by lots, was carried out by important priests if the health of the community was at stake, or by a curer for an individual patient. Bathing in the sweatbath and using medicinal waters were common practices both for regular personal hygiene and treatment of illness.

There were many types of medical practitioners in ancient times, and some of these, such as the physician of noble birth, did not survive long after the Conquest. Various types of ancient specialists died out while others combined, merging their roles. Today bite specialists, bonesetters, herbalists, midwives, and surgeons remain, but much of the specialized knowledge of the elite physicians was lost in early colonial times due to the decline of the nobility and the system of offices. The native medicine observed in colonial times probably represented that employed by commoners since time immemorial.

The native medical system emphasized herbology. Due to the shortage of trained European physicians and to the Spanish interest in herbal medicine, that portion of native medicine survived. Some European plant remedies were also assimilated into Indian medicine. What was found to be useful and/or compatible with Indian beliefs and practices was adopted. It is clear from the analysis of many of the plant remedies that they do contain active constituents which often aided in curing or alleviating illnesses in accordance with native practice. Unfortunately, it was sometimes not possible to get information regarding the active principles of some of the plants used by Guatemalan Indians, but in the future some of these may also prove to be medically useful. Some of the plants were incorrectly used according to modern scientific medical practice, but it is clear that much of the herbal treatments employed in the Guatemala highlands in colonial and contemporary times were useful.

The aboriginal medical system must have been developed by trial and error over a long period of time. It is not known whether the pre-Columbian Indian physicians conducted the same type of experimental research with plants that their counterparts in Mexico did. It is possible that Guatemalan physicians shared in such medical knowledge due to the gradual spread of ideas from Mexico. The congruence of some plant remedies found in the Guatemalan and Mexican sources suggests that, in some instances, this may have been the case.

The most important immediate effect of the Conquest as far as native health was concerned was the introduction of several Old World epidemic diseases. While Europeans also contracted New World diseases as well, the toll was far less severe than that suffered by the Indians. Smallpox, plague, typhus, and measles were important early epidemics. Many Indians died and neither native nor Spanish medicine had any effect on the mortality. Epidemics continued to occur with regularity during the entire sixteenth to eighteenth centuries. Mumps, fevers, and pneumonia were mentioned in the seventeenth century sources in addition to those which began earlier and continued to ravage the Indians.

While epidemics occurred from time to time and were the most serious threat to native health, other introduced diseases, which became endemic to certain areas, also affected the population. Erysipelas, leprosy, malaria, and onchocerciasis became health problems in Guatemala after the Conquest.

The Spaniards, primarily churchmen, attempted to deal with the catastrophic Indian mortality as best they could. Hospitals were built in the capital of Santiago for both Indians and Spaniards. Trained

European physicians resided only in the capital and treated mainly Europeans. It is clear from the information contained in the sources that Indians had to rely primarily on their own curers or their priests for medical treatment. The cofradías were important in assisting local priests in caring for the sick and in providing sacraments for the dying. At some point in time, probably the mid-seventeenth century when few priests lived in remote Indian areas, native treatment specialists probably began to exercise their curing functions through the cofradías as they do today in many Indian towns.

After the Conquest, native beliefs began to merge with those of the Spaniards. Many pre-Columbian ideas concerning medicine and illness causation were compatible with Catholicism and European medical theory. Saints were substituted for ancient gods as patrons of various illnesses, and some pilgrimage centers, such as Esquipulas, assumed Catholic characteristics and continued to have curing functions. European humoral theory also proved to be compatible with aboriginal beliefs concerning illness, especially those relating to equilibrium and disequilibrium.

Although European ideas were blended with Indian beliefs, native illness etiology remained primarily intact. In fact, in many of the conservative, remote Indian areas Spanish influence was not strong enough to cause significant change. The indigenous population continued to view illness as resulting from sorcery, sin, and violation of the moral order. The Spaniards were unsuccessful in their attempts to stamp out such practices as nagualism, divination, sorcery, and bathing. They did, however, make a successful assault on native gods, and this resulted in the substitution of Catholic religious figures for aboriginal ones in causation of illness. Many rituals and incantations must also have disappeared. Medical rituals, as opposed to herbal remedies, were rarely described by the colonial chroniclers, but this may have been due to the fact that Indians soon learned to keep such behavior secret. Medical rituals are carried out in the highlands today but may differ significantly from those of earlier times.

The story of Indian medicine in highland Guatemla is a fascinating one, and it is to be lamented that there are no lengthy Indian-written documents dating from the early post-Conquest period dealing with the subject. It is difficult to know how much medical knowledge has been lost forever, and it can only be hoped that someday documents will be brought to light that will reveal more about the system of healing used by ancient highland Guatemalan physicians in pre-Columbian and early colonial times.

Appendix

Names of Medicinal Herbs in Cakchiquel, Spanish, and Latin*

Cakchiquel	*Spanish*	*Latin*
nap:Yuk ruvach	el arbol de coyol	*Acrocomia vinifera* Oerstd.
kux:chichip	el culantrillo	*Adiantum capillus-veneris* L.
met (from Nah.)	el maguey	*Agave americana* L.
pak	el arbol de anona	*Annona reticulata* L.
sakiqix	el carro santo; o chicalote	*Argemone mexicana* L.
sakixak	los ajenjos	*Artemisia absinthium* L.
rucheel quxu	el arbol del achiote	*Bixa orellana* L.
ruqum maria	la leche de maría	*Calophyllum brasiliense* var. *rekoi* Standl.
cañavixte	el arbol de cañafistula	*Cassia fistula* L.
quiq; lazquiq	el arbol de hule	*Castilla elastica* Sessé
chulbalam	una yerba que cura el mal de orina	
xan:ruvach	el arbol de cocos	*Cocos nucifera* L.
muc	el arbol de orejuela	*Cymbopetalum penduliflorum* Baill.
amisakul chamahij	la contrayerba	*Dorstenia contrajerva* L.
paharqix	escorcionera	*Eryngium carlinae* Delar.
rakanxmukur	la yerba de la golondrina	*Euphorbia hirta* L.
kux	el arbol de amate	*Ficus glabrata* HBK.
quylaj akorn	el ynojo	*Foeniculum vulgare* Mill.
koxte	el arbol madre de cacao	*Gliricida sepium* Steud.
sakmacar	la birabira	*Gnaphalium attenuatum* DC.
vaylajche	el arbol de guayacán	*Guaiacum sanctum* L.
kopinol	el arbol de cuapinol	*Hymenaea courbaril* L.
chichuy runak	el piñon	*Jatropha curcas* L.
okob	el arbol de liquidámbar	*Liquidambar styraciflua* L.
moysaput	el arbol de chicosapote	*Manilkara zapota* Van Royen

*This list of names in Cakchiquel and Spanish is taken from Pantaleón de Guzmán (1704). Latin binomials of the plants he listed are taken from Chapter 7. Because Pantaleón de Guzmán's work is not widely available, his list of medicinal plants is included separately in this appendix. His spellings are given for Spanish names and sometimes differ from modern terminology.

Cakchiquel	*Spanish*	*Latin*
saqul	el platanal: o platano	*Musa sapientum* L.
vchmalanche	el arbol de balsamo	*Myroxylon balsamum* spp.
may	el tabaco de narices: o polbos tabaco bobo: el medicinal	*Nicotiana* spp.
sik	el tabaco de humar	
nimakmay	el tabaco bobo grande	
lotzijmay	el tabaco bobo pequeño	
noxtiy	la penca o la tuna	*Nopalea cochenillifera* Salm-Dyck
lotz	la yerba acedera (corazón acedo)	*Oxalis* spp.
cupumchuche	arbol:o palo gordo	*Pachira aquatica* Aubl.
oj	el arbol aguacates	*Persea americana* Mill.
chaj	el arbol de piño de ocote	*Pinus montezumae* Lam.
kankaj	el arbol de cacaloxuchit	*Plumeria rubra* var. *acutifolia* Poir
chimayatulul	el arbol de sapote injerto	*Pouteria viridis* Pitt.
capilin	el arbol de capulines	*Prunus capuli* Cav.
qiak	el arbol guayabas	*Psidium guajava* L.
ruxak àxeite	la higuerilla	*Ricinus communis* L.
rora	ruda	*Ruta graveolens* L.
sikab	el arbol de sauce	*Salix* spp.
tzolij	la salbia	*Salvia* spp.
tunayche	el arbol de sáuco	*Sambucus mexicana* Presl. ex A.DC.
paxlak	siempreviba	*Sedum dendroideum* Moc. & Sessé ex DC.
rukuxil ruvachabaj	la doradilla	*Selaginella lepidophylla* Spring
ruxequl	la sarsaparilla o palo de la vida	*Smilax* spp.
mahcujychaj	la yerbamora (hierba mora)	*Solanum nigrum* L.
kenum	el arbol de xocotes	*Spondias purpurea* L.
qaylajche	el arbol de chichicpacti	*Sweetia panamensis* Benth.
kana cotzij eyan	el pericón	*Tagetes lucida* Cav.
tamarimbo	el arbol de tamarindos	*Tamarindus indica* L.
cacouj	el arbol de cacao	*Theobroma cacao* L.
taxuchit cotzij	el arbol de baynillas	*Vanilla planifolia* Andr.
cuchcuy	la cebadilla	*Veratrum sabadilla* Retz.
recha qahol chicop	la berbena	*Verbena litoralis* HBK.
rucheel maria	el arbol de maría	*Verticilaria acuminata* Ruiz et Pavon
chachalbey	la escobilla	*Waltheria americana* L.

Glossary

abortifacient	An agent that induces abortion
acids	Compounds often found in plant tissues (especially in fruit tissues) which have astringency as a common property.
aglycone	The nonsugar component of the glycosides.
aguardiente	(Spanish) Strong rum made from brown cane sugar.
aldehydes	A class of very reactive organic compounds typified by acetaldehyde and characterized by the group CHO.
aliphatic	Of, relating to, or derived from fat.
alkaloids	Organic nitrogeneous compounds. They affect the nervous sytem and blood vessels. Alkaloids are toxic and potentially fatal if the dose is excessive.
alkamine	An alcohol which contains an amine group.
alterative	An agent presumed to correct a disordered bodily function.
amine	A compound derived from ammonia
analgesic	A substance that relieves pain (See anodyne).
androgenic	Pertaining to the male sex hormone testosterone which is responsible for masculine characteristics.
anodyne	Analgesic.
anorexia	Lack of appetite.
anthelmintic	An agent destructive to worms.
anthraquinones	Glycosides with aglycones related to anthracene and employed as cathartics.

Glossary

aperitive	A substance that stimulates the appetite.
aromatic	A substance with a spicy fragrance and stimulant qualities.
asthma	A respiratory disorder characterized by severe paroxysms of difficult breathing usually followed by a period of complete relief. Attacks recur at more or less frequent intervals.
astringent	A substance that causes contraction and constriction of a tissue. It also causes a thin layer of coagulation to form on wounds and mucus. It is effective when used as a compress, or for bathing inflammations and swellings.
ataxia	The inability to coordinate voluntary muscular movements that is symptomatic of any of several disorders of the nervous system.
atherosclerosis	Hardening of the inner lining of the arteries.
atolli	(Nahua) A thick beverage made with corn meal soaked in water. It is then strained and boiled until it reaches the consistency of porridge.
atonic dyspepsia	Caused by lack of bodily tone or muscle tone.
audencia	(Spanish) 1. Court or governing body of a region, or the area of the court's jurisdiction. 2. In colonial times, an advisory and judicial body that ruled on behalf of the crown. It was composed of judges (*oidores*) and was subordinate judicially to the Council of the Indies in Spain.
balsam	An aromatic resinous substance containing benzoic or cinnamic acid in addition to resin and usually essential oil.
bechic	A substance that soothes a cough.
bioflavonoids	A group of compounds which contribute to the maintenance of normal blood vessel conditions by decreasing capillary permeability and fragility.
bitter	A medicinal agent that has a bitter taste. Its action is usually local and is exerted on the gastrointestinal tract. Other bitters have a diuretic action or stimulate the liver by activating the secretion and flow of bile. At one time, bitters were extensively used in liquid medicaments to stimulate the appetite.

cambrium — A formative layer one cell thick occurring between the xylem and phloem of most vascular plants.

capillaries — Very small blood vessels from which nourishment is fed directly to the tissues.

carcinogen — Any substance which stimulates the formation of cancer.

carminative — An agent that aids in expelling gas from the gastrointestinal tract so as to relieve colic or griping.

carotenoids — Any of several highly unsaturated pigments, most of which are yellow, orange, or red.

cataract — Opacity of the lens of the eye.

catarrh — Inflammation associated with free discharge of mucous membranes especially those of the upper respiratory tract.

cathartic — A strong laxative.

cholagogue — A substance which stimulates the release of bile from the gall bladder.

choleretic — A substance that stimulates the production of bile.

circumcision — Removal of the foreskin of the penis or excision of a circular piece of the prepuce.

cirrhosis — An inflammatory disease of the liver involving replacement of liver cells by fibrous tissue.

cofrade — (Spanish) Member of a religious brotherhood of laymen, called cofradía in Spanish, which is dedicated to the care of a patron saint.

colic — Acute abdominal pain.

copal — (Spanish from the Nahua word *copalli.*) The common name given to a variety of resins used as incense.

corregidor — (Spanish) The official in charge of an administrative-judicial unit or district called a corregimiento in Spanish.

counterirritant — An agent applied to the skin to produce an irritation, in order to counteract a deep inflammation.

curare — (Spanish) A poison which paralyzes nerves and muscles.

Cyanogenic glycoside	A glycoside which yields hydrocyanic acid as one of the products of hydrolysis.
decoction	Plant parts are immersed in cold water and placed in a covered vessel. The mixture is then cooked for 5 to 30 minutes. The vessel is removed from the heat and left to sit for a few minutes before being strained. This method is good for making teas from husks, roots, or stems.
depolymerization	To decompose by various means into relatively simple compounds.
dermatitis	Skin irritation or inflammation.
diaphoretic	A substance that promotes perspiration.
disinfectant	A strong, toxic preparation or procedure that destroys microorganisms.
dissepiment	A separating membrane or partition, as that between adjacent carpels of a compound ovary.
diuretic	A substance that increases the amount of urine produced.
divination	The practice aimed at obtaining factual knowledge about the future by various ways which have no empirical connection to the information being sought.
dysentery	A term given to a number of disorders marked by inflammation of the intestines, especially of the colon, and accompanied by abdominal pain and frequent stools containing blood and/or mucus.
dyspepsia	An impairment in the powers or function of digestion.
eczema	An inflammatory disease of the skin.
edema	Excessive accumulation of fluid in the tissues, which causes swelling.
emetic	A substance that causes vomiting.
emic	The inside or native view of a culture.
emmenagogue	A substance that facilitates and regularizes menstrual flow.
emollient	Any agent that softens or soothes. It reduces inflammations and irritations, e.g., fats and oils which are used for their local action on the skin and, occasionally, the mucous membranes.

endemic — A disease, usually contagious, which occurs in one locality.

enzyme — A substance manufactured by living tissue which stimulates specific chemical changes.

epidemic — A disease which affects large numbers of people.

epizöötic — Epidemic among animals.

erythema — A patch of redness of the skin.

erythrocyte — A red blood cell.

essential oils — Aromatic, volatile compounds obtained by distillation; they may possess antiseptic properties.

ester — 1. Compound that on hydrolysis yields an organic or inorganic acid and an alcohol or phenol. 2. Any compound formed from an alcohol and an acid.

ethnography — A description of a culture.

etic — The outsider's view of a culture.

etiology — Determinant or cause of a disease.

exanthematic — An eruptive disease or its symptomatic eruption, used especially of eruptions accompanied by fever.

expectorant — An agent that tends to decrease viscosity and promote discharge of mucus from the respiratory tract.

febrifuge — A substance that counteracts fever.

fibrillation — An irregular heart action due to abnormal spread of impulses from one portion of the heart to another; it usually indicates a failing heart.

fistula — An abnormal canal which often occurs in or around the anus.

flatulence — A distention of the stomach or intestines by air or other gases.

flavonoids — A group of aromatic oxygen compounds. Anthocyanins are one subgroup and account for the majority of yellow, red, and blue pigmentation. Flavonoids are grouped in order of increasing oxidation state: catechins; leucoanthocyanidins and flavanones, flavanols, flavones, and anthocyanidins; and flavonols. See bioflavonoids.

fontanel — (or fontanelle) The soft space in between the bones of newborn and infant skulls.

fulminating — A severe and rapidly progressing illness which reaches its full severity within a few hours or days.

furocoumarins — A group of antifungal dyestuffs which on contact with the skin cause photosensitization.

galactagogue — A substance that increases milk production.

gastroenteritis — Inflammation of the stomach and intestines which is characterized by pain, nausea, and diarrhea.

glaucoma — An eye disease associated with increased pressure within the eyeball.

glucoside — See glycoside.

glycoside — A compound yielding one or more sugars among the products of hydrolysis. When the sugar formed is glucose, the substance may be called a glucoside. Nonsugars are called aglycones.

gout — Painful disease involving joint inflammation and chalky deposits—the result of a purine metabolic disturbance (high blood levels of uric acid).

gums — Translucent, amorphous substances which are frequently produced in higher plants as a protective after injury. They are soluble or swell up in water.

gynecology — Branch of medicine which deals with diseases of the female reproductive organs.

hallucinogen — Substance which produces changes in perception, thought, and mood in nontoxic doses.

hechícero — (Spanish) Witch, wizard, sorcerer.

hematoma — Hemorrhage under the skin which forms a blood clot.

hemolysis — The breaking down or destruction of red blood cells.

hemorrhoid — Dilation of veins around the anus.

hemostatic — Any substance that prevents bleeding or promotes clotting of blood.

hepatitis — Inflammation of the liver.

herpes — Acute inflammation of the skin, caused by a virus, characterized by the formation of small pustular areas.

hydrocarbons	A large class of organic compounds containing only carbon and hydrogen.
hypertensive	A substance that causes an increase in blood pressure.
hyperthermia	Producing a high fever by artificial means.
hypocalcemia	A condition caused by too little calcium in the blood.
hypotensive	A substance that reduces blood pressure.
influenza	An acute infectious disease which usually occurs in epidemics and pandemics. It is characterized by sudden onset, fever, and generalized aches and pains.
infusion	Teas are usually made by infusion. The dried plant is placed in a cup, boiling water is added, the mixture is covered and left to stand for 5 to 10 minutes before it is strained. This method is best for preparing leaves and flowers.
ketones	A class of organic compounds containing the carbonyl group C=O whose carbon atom is joined to two other carbon atoms; that is, with the carbonyl group occurring within the carbon chain.
k'ucumatz	(Quiché) Pneumonic plague.
lactone	An aromatic liquid, $C_{10}H_8O_4$, prepared by distillation from lactic acid.
lipids	Fixed oils, fats, and waxes. Esters of long-chain fatty acids and alcohols, or of closely related derivatives.
maceration	Plants with a high proportion of volatile oils are best prepared by maceration which involves steeping them in cold water. A teaspoon of dried plant material is put into a cupful of cold water and left to stand for 12 to 24 hours. It is then heated and strained.
manta	(Spanish) Blanket composed of strips of cotton cloth woven on a backstrap loom and sewn together along the edges.
marasmus	Progressive emaciation, especially in the young because of malnutrition and due chiefly to faulty assimilation and utilization of food.

melena	1. Black, tarry stools caused by the presence of altered blood, often occurring from bleeding from the stomach or small intestine. 2. Black vomit.
milpa	(Spanish from Nahua *milli*) 1. Corn field, often containing other interspersed crops. 2. In Guatemala, any cultivated land.
mitogen	Any substance which induces mitosis.
mucilage	A gelatinous substance that contains protein and polysaccharides and is obtained especially from the seed coats of various plants. It is similar to plant gums but swells in water without dissolving and forms a slimy mass. It forms a protective and soothing preparation.
nagual	(Spanish) Person with the magical powers needed to transform into animal forms.
narcotic	A drug that produces sleep or stupor and relieves pain.
necrosis	Death of tissue, usually in localized areas of individual cells or small cell groups.
neuralgia	Nerve pain.
ocote	(Spanish from Nahua *ocotl*) Pitchpine splints, used for torches and for starting fires.
osteitis	Inflammation of the bone.
oxytocic	An agent that hastens childbirth.
pathology	The study of diseases.
pectin	A purified carbohydrate product obtained from the dilute extract of the inner rind of citrus fruits.
pectoral	Drug used internally for problems of the chest and lungs.
peste	(Spanish) 1. Pneumonic plague. 2. Any epidemic.
pharmacology	The science dealing with the nature and action of drugs and medicines.
phenol	a soluble crystalline acidic compound that turns pinkish upon exposure to light and air and has a characteristic odor. It is a powerful caustic poison and is a useful disinfectant in dilute solution.
phlebotomy	bloodletting.

pleurisy — Inflammation of the lining of the chest cavity.

pneumonia — Lung inflammation associated with alveolar exudate or cavitation.

prosthesis — The artificial replacement for an amputated or missing part of the body.

proteolytic — Referring to the destruction of proteins.

pulque — (Spanish) A beverage obtained by fermenting the sap of the century plant.

purge — Cathartic.

regidor — (Spanish) Officer of the town council.

resins — Any of various solid or semisolid viscous, organic substances exuded from various plants and trees. They are usually clear or translucent, or yellowish or brownish.

rubefacient — An agent that reddens the skin by producing active or passive increases of blood to the skin.

sapogenin — An aglycone yielded by saponins upon hydrolysis, or in a few cases, found free in plants.

saponins — Agents which produce a lathering effect such as emulsions, and colloidal solutions capable of increasing the permeability of membranes. They can cause hemolysis by destroying the membranes of red blood cells and have a local irritant effect. Some are diuretic and others aid digestion.

sarampión — (Spanish) Measles.

scrofula — Tuberculosis of the lymphatic glands or of bones and joint surfaces which usually produces marked irregular superficial ulcers. It results from the infection of various organs with a bacillus *Mycobacterium tuberculosis.*

sedative — A drug given to calm the nerves.

shaman — Part time magico-religious specialist who practices divination and curing and derives his or her power from a supernatural source.

sialogogue — A medication which promotes saliva secretion.

spasmolytic — Any agent that decreases spasms.

steroid — A drug of hormone origin, especially from the pituitary and adrenal glands (also plant steroids).

sterol — A solid complex cyclic alcohol found in the lipid fractions of many tissues.

stimulant — A substance which temporarily stimulates nervous or muscular activity.

stomachic — An agent which stimulates the appetite and promotes digestion.

strabismus — Cross-eye, squint, and other muscle defects which result in lack of alignment of the eyes.

sudorific — A medication given to induce sweating.

suerte — (Spanish) Luck or destiny.

tabardete — (Spanish) Exanthematic typhus. Epidemic disease characterized by fever.

tabardillo — See tabardete.

tannins — A group of complex phenolic compounds which coagulate albuminous substances and lead to rapid clotting of blood. They are astringent, disinfectant and antiseptic. They neutralize many poisonous alkaloids and are found in bark, roots, stems, and leaves. Tannins rapidly become corrosive and care must be taken in applying them in cases of severe diarrhea or burns.

terpenes — A class of hydrocarbons found in many essential oils, especially from conifers, but also in resins and other vegetable aromatic products. Included are monoterpenes, sesquiterpenes, diterpenes, triterpenes and others.

terpenoids — Compounds characterized by a structure similar to that of the terpenes and often including these hydrocarbons as well as oxygenated derivatives.

terpineol — (or terpinol) Any of three fragrant unsaturated low-melting crystalline terpenoid alcohols or a viscous liquid commercial mixture.

therapy — Treatment.

tona — (Spanish, from Nahua *tonalli*) Companion animal which is thought to be born when a person is born and to share that person's fate.

tonic — Preparations believed to have the power of stimulating a person who feels below par. Today more is known, and it is often possible to treat the underlying cause so that tonics are seldom required.

trepanning — An operation in which a hole is bored in the skull.

triglycerides — Triesters of glycerol with one, two, or three different acids.

tzolkin — (Yucatec) The 260-day sacred calendar consisting of 13 months and 20 days.

uremia — A serious illness caused by the inability of the kidneys to eliminate metabolic wastes. Unless kidney function is restored, death from uremic poisoning occurs.

uterotropic — Having a special affinity for or exerting its principle influence upon the uterus.

vahos — (Spanish) Vapors, fumes, emanations, or odors.

vasoconstrictor — Any agent that constricts blood vessels.

vasodilator — Any agent that causes a widening of the lumen, or passageway, of the blood vessels.

vena cava — (Latin) Either of two large veins conveying blood to the right atrium of the heart.

ventosa — (Spanish) Cupping.

vermifuge — An agent which destroys or expels worms or intestinal animal parasites.

vessicant — An agent which causes blistering.

viruelas — (Spanish) Pimpled, pustuled appearance usually referred to as smallpox.

volatile oils — See essential oils.

vulnerary — An agent that promotes the healing of wounds.

xibalba — (Quiché) Maya underworld.

Abbreviations

AGC	Archivo General de Centroamérica
Annals	*Annals of the Cakchiquels*
LV	*Libro Viejo*
PV	*Popol Vuh*
RGA	*Relación Geográfica Atitlán*
RGAG	*Relación Geográfica Aguacatepec*
RGSA	*Relación Geográfica San Andrés*
RGSF	*Relación Geográfica San Francisco*
RGZ	*Relación Geográfica Zapotitlán y Suchitepéquez*

See *Bibliography for complete references.*

Bibliography

Ackerknecht, Erwin H.

1972 *History and Geography of the Most Important Diseases.* New York: Hafner Publishing Company, Inc.

Adams, Richard N.

1952 *Un análisis de las creencias y prácticas médicas en un pueblo indígena de Guatemala.* Instituto Nacional Indígena, Publicaciones Especiales, 17. Guatemala.

1957 *Cultural Surveys of Panama-Nicaragua-Guatemala-El Salvador-Honduras.* Washington, D.C.: Pan American Sanitary Bureau. Scientific Publication 33.

——— and Arthur J. Rubel

1967 Sickness and Social Relations. In *Social Anthropology,* edited by Manning Nash. Handbook of Middle American Indians vol. 6:333–56. Austin: University of Texas Press.

Adams, Ruth

1976 *The Complete Home Guide to All the Vitamins.* New York: Larchmont Books.

Aguilar, Girón, José Ignacio

1966 *Relación de unos aspectos de la flora útil de Guatemala.* 2d ed. Guatemala.

Aguirre, Gerardo G.

1972 *La cruz de Nimajuyú: Historia de la Parroquia de San Pedro la Laguna.* Guatemala.

Alejandro Domínguez, Dr. Xorge

1978 Conocimientos medicos de los mayas, aztecas, tarascos y la herbolaria medica mexicana. *Guatemala Indígena* vol. 13:no. 2, 220–38.

Alonso Pedraz, Martín

1958 *Enciclopedia del idioma: diccionario histórico y moderno de la lengua española (siglos XII al XX), etimológico, tecnológico, regional e hispanoamericano.* Madrid: Aguilar.

Bibliography

Alvarado, Pedro de

1954 *Relación hecha por Pedro de Alvarado a Hernando Cortés, en que se refieren las guerras y batallas para pacificar las provincias del antiguo reino de Goathemala (1524).* Mexico: José Porrua e Hijos.

Anderson, Arthur J. O. and Charles E. Dibble

1950–69 *See* Sahagún.

Andrews, J. Richard and Ross Hassig.

1984 *See* Ruíz de Alarcón.

Annals of the Cakchiquels (Annals)

1967 *The Annals of the Cakchiquels.* Translated from the Cakchiquel Maya by Adrián Recinos and Delia Goetz. *Title of the Lords of Totonicapán.* Translated from the Quiché text into Spanish by Dionisio José Chonay, English Version by Delia Goetz. Norman: University of Oklahoma Press.

Archivo General de Centroamérica (AGC)

In citations to works in this archive the letter A refers to colonial documents, *exp.* refers to *expediente* (proceedings), *leg.* to *legajo* (file), and *fol.* to *folio* (page).

Arditti, Joseph and Eloy Rodríguez

1982 Dieffenbachia: Uses, Abuses and Toxic Constituents. *Journal of Ethnopharmacology* vol. 5:293–302.

Arriola Jorge Luís

1973 *El libro de las geonimias de Guatemala.* Seminario de Integración Social Guatemalteca. Guatemala: Editorial José de Pineda Ibarra.

Ashburn, Percy M.

1947 *The Ranks of Death: A Medical History of the Conquest of America,* edited by Frank D. Ashburn. New York: Coward-McCann, Inc.

Asturias, Francisco

1958 *Historia de la medicina en Guatemala.* Guatemala: Editorial Universitaria.

Bailey, Liberty Hyde and Ethel Zoe Bailey

1976 *Hortus third: A Concise Dictionary of Plants Cultivated in the United States and Canada.* Revised and expanded by the staff of the Liberty Hyde Bailey Hortorium. New York: Macmillan.

Barefoot Doctor's Manual

1974 *A Barefoot Doctor's Manual.* Geographic Health Studies Program of the John E. Fogarty International Center for Advanced Study in the Health Sciences. Washington, D.C.: U.S. Department of Health, Education, and Welfare. Public Health Service. National Institute of Health.

Bettmann, Otto L.

1962 *A Pictorial History of Medicine.* Springfield, Ill.: Charles C. Thomas Publisher.

Bible.

1340 *Bible.* Manuscripts, Latin. O.T. *Psalms. Luttrell.* Additional MS 42130. London: The British Library.

Borhegyi, Stephan F. de
1959 Culto a la Imagen del Señor de Esquipulas en Centro America y Nuevo México. *Antropología y historia de Guatemala* vol. 11:no. 1, 44–49. Guatemala.

Bremme de Santos, Ida
1963 Aspectos hispánicos e indígenas de la cultura cakchiquel. *Anales de la Sociedad de Geografía e Historia de Guatemala* vol. 36:517–63. Guatemala.

Brintnall, Douglas E.
1979 *Revolt Against the Dead: The Modernization of a Maya Community in the Highlands of Guatemala.* New York: Gordon and Brach.

Broussard, Ray, trans.
1952 *Atitilán and Its Dependencies* (1585). Translated by Ray Broussard. Master's thesis, University of Texas.

Bruce-Chwatt, L. J.
1965 Paleogenesis and Paleo-Epidemiology of Primate Malaria. *Bulletin. World Health Organization* vol. 32:no. 3, 363–87.

Bunzel, Ruth
1967 *Chichicastenango: A Guatemalan Village.* Seattle: University of Washington Press.

Carmack, Robert M.
1973 *Quichean Civilization: The Ethnohistoric, Ethnographic, and Archaeological Sources.* Berkeley and Los Angeles: University of California Press.
1981 *The Quiché Mayas of Utatlán: The Evolution of a Highland Guatemala Kingdom.* Norman: University of Oklahoma Press.

——— and Dwight T. Wallace
1977 Ethnohistory of the Central Quiché: The Community of Utatlan. In *Archaeology and Ethnohistory of the Central Quiche,* edited by Dwight T. Wallace and Robert M. Carmack. Institute for Mesoamerican Studies, State University of New York, Publication no. 1, 1–19. Albany.

———, Juan Fox, and Rosalio Stewart
1975 *La formacion del reino quiché.* Instituto de Antropología e Historia. Ministerio de Educación Pública. Publicación Especial no. 7. Guatemala.

Chickering, Carol Rogers
1973 *Flowers of Guatemala.* Norman: University of Oklahoma Press.

Chinchilla Aguilar, Ernesto
1963 Las yerbas medicinales en el mundo indígena, descrito por Fuentes y Guzmán. In *La danza del sacrificio y otros estudios,* 39–64. Ministerio de Educación Pública. Guatemala: Central Editorial José de Pineda Ibarra.
1967 Forward to *Historia natural del reino de Guatemala,* by fray Francisco Ximénez, 5–9. Guatemala: Editorial José de Pineda Ibarra.

Cifuentes Aguirre, Oscar

1963 *Odontología y mutilaciones dentarias mayas.* Guatemala: Editorial Universitaria.

Claus, Edward P., Varro E. Tyler, and Lynn Brady

1970 *Pharmacognosy.* 6th ed. Philadelphia: Lea & Febiger.

Cline, Howard F.

1972 The Relaciones Geográficas of the Spanish Indies, 1577–1648. In *Guide to Ethnohistorical Sources,* edited by Howard F. Cline. Handbook of Middle American Indians 12:1, 183–242. Austin: University of Texas Press.

——— and Nicolau d'Olwer, Luís

1973 Sahagún and His Works. In *Guide to Ethnohistorical Sources,* edited by Howard F. Cline and John B. Glass. Handbook of Middle American Indians 13:2, 186–207. Austin: University of Texas Press.

Cochran, Doris M.

1943 *Poisonous Reptiles of the World: A Wartime Handbook.* Washington, D. C.: Smithsonian Institution. Wartime Background Studies, no. 10.

Codex Vaticanus B (Codex Vaticanus 3773)

1939 *Codice Vaticano B.* Ms. pictorico mexicano no. 3773 de la biblioteca Vaticana. Libreria Anticuaria. Mexico: A. M. Echaniz.

Coe, Michael C.

1975 *Classic Maya Pottery at Dumbarton Oaks.* Washington, D. C.: Dumbarton Oaks.

1982 *Old Gods and Young Heroes.* The Pearlman Collection of Maya Ceramics. Jerusalem: The Israel Museum.

Colby, Benjamin H. and Pierre L. van den Berghe

1969 *Ixil Country: A Plural Society in Highland Guatemala.* Berkeley and Los Angeles: University of California Press.

——— and Lore M. Colby

1981 *The Daykeeper: The Life and Discourse of an Ixil Diviner.* Cambridge, Mass.: Harvard University Press.

Comas, Juan

1954 Influencía indígena en la medicina Hipocrática en la Nueva España del siglo XVI. *América Indígena* vol. 14:no. 4, 327–61.

Cook, Sherburne F.

1946 The Incidence and Significance of Disease among the Aztecs and Related Tribes. *Hispanic American Historical Review* vol. 26:320–35.

Cortés y Larraz, Pedro

1958 *Descripción geográfico-moral de la diocesis de Goathemala (1768–1770).* 2 vols. Biblioteca Goathemala, vol. 20. Guatemala.

Cosminsky, Sheila

1972 *Decision Making and Medical Care in a Guatemalan Indian Community.* Ph.D diss., Brandeis University.

1975 Changing Food and Medical Beliefs and Practices in a Guatemalan Community. *Ecology of Food and Nutrition* vol. 4:183–91.

1976 The Evil Eye in a Quiche Community. In *The Evil Eye,* edited by Clarence Maloney, 163–74. New York: Columbia University Press.

1977a Alimento and Fresco: Nutritional Concepts and Their Implication for Health Care. *Human Organization* vol. 36: no. 2, 203–207.

1977b Childbirth and Midwifery on a Guatemala Finca. *Medical Anthropology* vol. 1:no. 3, 69–104.

1977c The Impact of Methods on the Analysis of Illness Concepts in a Guatemalan Community. *Social Science and Medicine* 11:5. 325–32.

1983 Medical Pluralism in Mesoamerica. In *Heritage of Conquest: Thirty Years Later,* edited by Carl Kendall, John Hawkins, and Laurel Bossen, 159–73. Austin: University of Texas Press.

——— and Mary Scrimshaw

1980 Medical Pluralism on a Guatemalan Plantation. *Social Science and Medicine* vol. 14B:no. 4, 267–78.

Crabtree, Don E.

1968 Mesoamerican Polyhedral Cores and Prismatic Blades. *American Antiquity* vol. 33:no. 4, 446–78.

Crosby, Alfred W., Jr.

1967 Conquistador y Pestilencia: The First New World Pandemic and the Fall of the Great Indian Empires. *Hispanic American Historical Review* vol. 47:no. 3, 321–37.

1972 *The Columbian Exchange: Biological and Cultural Consequences of 1492.* Westport, Conn.: Greenwood Publishing Company.

Cruz, Martín de la

1552 *Libellus de medicinalibus Indorum herbis.* Biblioteca Apostolica Vaticana, Rome. Codex Barberini Latin 241. Ex-Francisco Barberini and Diego de Cortavila collections. Colegio de Santa Cruz, Tlatelolco, D. F.

ca. 1700 *Libellus de medicinalibus Indorum herbis.* Copy in the Royal Library of Windsor Castle. *Ca.* late 16th or 17th century.

1939 *The De La Cruz-Badiano Aztec Herbal of 1552.* Translation and Commentary by William Gates. The Maya Society, Publication 23. Baltimore.

1940 *See* Emmart.

1952 *Libellus de medicinalibus Indorum herbis.* El manuscrito pictórico mexicano-latino de Martín de la Cruz y Juan Badiano de 1552. Mexico: Editorial Vargas Rea y El Diario Español.

1964 *Libellus de medicinalibus Indorum herbis,* manuscrito azteca de 1552. Según traducción latina de Juan Badiano, versión española con estudios y comentarios por diversos autores. Mexico: Instituto mexicano del Seguro Social.

Dieseldorff, Erwin P.
1940 Las plantas medicinales del departamento de Alta Verapaz. *Anales de la Sociedad de Geografía y Historia de Guatemala* vol. 16:192–206.

Douglas, William G.
1969 *Illness and Curing in Santiago Atitlán, A Tzutujil Maya Community in the Southwestern Highlands of Guatemala.* Ph.D diss., Stanford University.

Dunn, Frederick L.
1965 On the Antiquity of Malaria in the Western Hemisphere. *Human Biology* vol. 37:no. 4, 385–93.

Edmonson, Munro
1965 *Quiche-English Dictionary.* Middle American Research Institute, Tulane University, Publication no. 30. New Orleans.
1971 *The Book of Counsel: The Popol Vuh of the Quiche Maya of Guatemala (ca. 1554–1558).* Middle American Research Institute, Tulane University, Publication no. 35. New Orleans.

Emboden, William
1979 *Narcotic Plants.* New York: Macmillan.

Emmart, Emily Walcott, trans.
1940 *The Badianus Manuscript (Codex Barberini, Latin 241) Vatican Library: An Aztec Herbal of 1552.* Translated by Emily Walcott Emmart. Baltimore: The Johns Hopkins Press.

Estrada, Juan de
1955 Relación geográfica Zapotitlán y Suchitepéquez: Descripción de la provincia de Zapotitlán y Suchitepéquez (1579) por su alcalde mayor capitán Juan de Estrada y el escribano Fernando de Niebla. *Anales de la Sociedad de Geografía e Historia de Guatemala* vol. 28:68–83. Guatemala.

Farfán, Agustín
1579 *Tractado brebe de chirurgia y del conocimiento y cura de algunas enfermedades que en esta tierra mas comunmente suelen haber.* Mexico.
1592 *Tractado brebe de medicina, y de todas las enfermedades.* Mexico.
1944 *Tractado breve de medicina.* Obra impresa en Mexico por Pedro Ocharte en 1592, y ahora editada en facsimil. Madrid: Ediciones Cultura Hispanica.

Feldman, Lawrence H.
1971 *A Tumpline Economy: Production and Distribution Systems of Early Central-East Guatemala.* Ph.D. diss., Pennsylvania State University.

Figueroa Marroquín, Horacio
1957 *Enfermedades de los conquistadors.* San Salvador: Ministerio de Cultura. Departamento Editorial.

Florentine Codex
1950–69 *See* Sahagún.

Follett, P.H.F.
1932 War and Weapons of the Maya. *Middle American Research Institute,* Tulane University, Publication 4, 373–410. New Orleans.

Ford, Karen Cowan
1975 *Las yerbas de la gente: A study of Hispano-American medicinal plants.* Ann Arbor: University of Michigan, Anthropological Papers, no. 60.

Foster, George M.
1953 Relationships Between Spanish and Spanish-American Folk Medicine. *Journal of American Folklore* vol. 66:201–17.
1960 *Culture and Conquest: America's Spanish Heritage.* Chicago: Quadrangle Books.

Frampton, John
1925 *See* Monardes.

Frankenberg, Ronald
1980 Medical Anthropology and Development: A Theoretical Perspective. *Social Science and Medicine* vol. 14B:no. 4, 197–207.

Fuentes y Guzmán, Francisco Antonio de
1932–33 *Recordación Florida: Discurso historical y demostración natural, material, militar, y política del reyno de Guatemala (1690–1699).* Biblioteca Goathemala, vols. 6–8. Guatemala.
1969–72 *Obras históricas de don Francisco Antonio de Fuentes y Guzmán: Recordación Florida (1690–1699).* Edición y estudio preliminar de Carmelo Sáenz de Santa María. Biblioteca de Autores Españoles. Madrid: Ediciones Atlas.

Furst, Peter T.
1976 *Hallucinogens and Culture.* San Francisco: Chandler & Sharp Publishers, Inc.

Gage, Thomas
1648 *The English-American, his Travail by Sea and Land or, A new Survey of the West-India's.* London.
1958 *Thomas Gage's Travels in the New World.* Edited and with an introduction by J. Eric S. Thompson. Norman: University of Oklahoma Press.
1969 *Thomas Gage's Travels in the New World.* Edited by J. Eric S. Thompson. Norman: University of Oklahoma Press.

Garcés, Diego de
1973 Relación Garcés (1570–72). In *Quichean Civilization: The Ethnohistoric, Ethnographic, and Archaeological Sources,* edited by Robert M. Carmack, 379–85. Berkeley and Los Angeles: University of California Press.

García de Palacio, Diego
1860 *Carta dirigida al Rey de España por el Licenciado Dr. Don Diego García del Palacio, oidor de la Real Audencia de Guatemala, año 1576.* New York: E. G. Squier.

1866 Relación hecha por el Licenciado Palacio al Rey D. Felipe II, en la que describe la provincia de Guatemala, las costumbres de los indios y otras cosas notables (1574). Madrid: *Colección de Documentos Inéditos del Archivo de Indias,* vol. 6.

1927 Relación hecha por el Licenciado Palacio al Rey D. Felipe II, en la que describe la provincia de Guatemala, las costumbres de los indios y otras cosas notables (1574). *Anales de la Sociedad de Geografía e Historia de Guatemala* vol. 4:71–92.

Gates, William

1939 *See* Cruz.

Gersdorff, Hans von

1967 *Feldbuch der Wundarznei.* Wissenschaftliche Buchgesellschaft. Darmstadt.

Gillin, John

1951 *The Culture of Security in San Carlos: A Study of a Guatemalan Community of Indians and Ladinos.* Middle American Research Institute, Tulane University, Publication 16. New Orleans.

Gilman, Alfred Goodman, Louis Goodman, and Alfred Gilman, eds.

1980 *The Pharmacological Basis of Therapeutics.* New York: Macmillan Publishing Company.

Girón Mena, Dr. Manuel Antonio

1979 Itzamná y la medicina maya. *Guatemala Indígena* vol. 14:nos. 3–4, 1–81.

Glass, John B. and Donald Robertson

1975 A Census of Native Middle American Pictorial Manuscripts. *Guide to Ethnohistorical Sources,* edited by Howard F. Cline. Handbook of Middle American Indians, vol. 14:part 3, 81–252. Austin: University of Texas Press.

Goff, Charles Weer

1953 New Evidence of Pre-Columbian Bone Syphilis in Guatemala. In *The Ruins of Zaculeu,* edited by R. B. Woodbury and A. S. Trik, 312–19. Richmond, Virginia: The William Byrd Press.

1967 Syphilis. In *Diseases in Antiquity,* edited by Don Brothwell and A. T. Sandison, 279–94. Springfield, Ill.: Charles C. Thomas Publisher.

González Sol, Rafael

1939 Especímenes zoológicos utilizados por nuestros aborígines. *Anales de la sociedad de Geografía e Historia de Guatemala* vol. 16:68–73.

Goodman, Louis S. and Alfred Gilman, Eds.

1970 *The pharmacological basis of therapeutics: a textbook of pharmacology, toxicology, and therapeutics for physicians and medical students.* London: Macmillan.

Gordon, George B. and J. Alden Mason

1925–34 *Examples of Maya Pottery in the Museum and Other Collections.* Philadelphia: University Museum.

Guerra, Francisco
1961 *Nicolas Bautista Monardes: su vida y su obra, ca. 1493–1558.* Mexico: Compañia Fundidora de Fierro y Acero de Monterrey.
1964 Maya Medicine. *Medical History* vol. 8:no. 1, 31–43.
1966a Aztec Medicine. *Medical History* vol. 10:no. 4, 315–38.
1966b Drugs from the Indies and the Political Economy of the Sixteenth Century. *Analecta Medico-Historica* vol. 1:29–54.
1969 The Role of Religion in Spanish American Medicine. In *Medicine and Culture,* edited by F.N.L. Poynter, 179–88. London: Wellcome Institute of the History of Medicine.

Guzmán, Fray Pantaleón de
n.d. *Compendio de nombres en lengua cakchiquel y significado de verbos por imperativos y acusativos recíprocos (1704).* Photocopy from the Library of Congress.

Harris, Ben Charles
1972 *The Compleat Herbal.* Barre, Mass.: Barre Publishers.

Hatcher, Robert A. and Paul C. Batton
1944 *Useful Drugs: A Selected List of Essential Drugs.* Chicago: American Medical Association.

Hernández, Francisco
1635 De partibus septuaginta octo maximi templi Mexicani . . . In *Historia naturae maximae peregrinae,* by Juan Eusebio Nieremberg. Antwerp.
1651 *Rerum medicarum Novae Hispaniae thesaurus seu plantarum, animalium, mineralium mexicanorum historia . . . Regis collecta ac in ordinem digesta, a Ioanne Terrentio Lynceo . . . noti illustrata. Rome.*
1790 *Francisci Hernandi, medici atque historici Philippi II, Hisp. et Indiar . . . 3 vols. Madrid.*
1959–60 *Obras completas.* 3 vols. Mexico: Universidad Nacional de Mexico.

Hinshaw, Robert E.
1975 *Panajachel: A Guatemalan Town in Thirty-Year Perspective.* Pittsburg: University of Pittsburgh Press.

Jarcho, Saul
1957 Medicine in Sixteenth Century New Spain As Illustrated by the Writings of Bravo, Farfán, and Vargas Machuca. *Bulletin of the History of Medicine* vol. 31:425–41.

Jeanselme, Edouard
1931 *Histoire de la Syphilis.* Paris: Doin.

Joralemon, Donald
1982 New World Depopulation and the Case of Disease. *Journal of Anthropological Research* vol. 38:no. 1, 97–127.

Juarros, Domingos
1937 *Compendio de la historia de la ciudad de Guatemala.* Guatemala: Tipografía Nacional.

Kelsey, Harlan P. and William A. Dayton

1942 *Standardized Plant Names.* 2d ed., Harrisburg, Pa.: J. Horace McFarland Company.

La Farge, Oliver

1947 *Santa Eulalia: the religion of a Cuchumatan Indian town.* Chicago: University of Chicago Press.

Landa, Bishop Diego de

1966 *Landa's relación de las cosas de Yucatán (ca. 1566),* edited by Alfred M. Tozzer. Papers of the Peabody Museum of American Archaeology and Ethnology, Harvard University, vol. 18. Reprint. New York: Kraus Reprint Corp.

Landy, David

1978 Role Adaptation: traditional curers under the impact of Western medicine. In *Health and the Human Condition: Perspectives on Medical Anthropology,* edited by Michael H. Logan and Edward E. Hunt, Jr., 217–41. North Scituate, Mass.: Duxbury Press.

Las Casas, Bartolomé de

1909 Apologética historia de las Indias (*ca.* 1550). In *Historiadores de Indias* by Manuel Serrano y Sanz. 2 vols. Madrid.

1967 *Apologética historia sumaria,* edición preparada por Edmundo O'Gorman. 2 vols. Mexico: Instituto de Investigaciones Históricas, Universidad Nacional Autónoma de México.

Latour, John Paul

1977 *The ABC's of Vitamins, Minerals, and Natural Foods.* New York: Arco Publishing Company, Inc.

Lewis, Walter H.

1977 *Medical Botany.* New York: John Wiley & Sons.

Libro Viejo (LV)

1934 *Libro viejo de la fundación de Guatemala, y papeles relativos a don Pedro de Alvarado (1524).* Biblioteca Goathemala, vol. 12. Guatemala.

Logan, Michael H.

1973a Digestive Disorders and Plant Medicinals in Highland Guatemala. *Anthropos* vol. 68:nos. 3–4, 537–47.

1973b Humoral Medicine in Guatemala and Peasant Acceptance of Modern Medicine. *Human Organization* vol. 32:no. 4, 385–95.

1977 Anthropological Research on the Hot-Cold Theory of Disease: Some Methodological Suggestions. *Medical Anthropology* vol. 1:no. 4, 87–112.

1978 Digestive Disorders and Plant Medicinals in Highland Guatemala. In *Health and the Human Condition: Perspectives on Medical Anthropology,* edited by Michael Logan and Edward E. Hunt, Jr., 180–88, North Scituate, Mass.: Duxbury Press.

López Austin, Alfredo

1971 De las plantas medicinales y de otras cosas medicinales. *Estudios de Cultura Nahuatl* vol. 9:125–230. Mexico.

1972 Textos acerca de las partes del cuerpo humano y de las enfermedades y medicinas en los *Primeros Memoriales* de Sahagún. *Estudio de Cultura Nahuatl* vol. 10:129–53. Mexico.

1974a Descripción de medicinas en textos dispersos del Libro XI en los códices Matritense y Florentino. *Estudios de Cultura Nahuatl* vol. 11:45–135. Mexico.

1974b Sahagún's Work and the Medicine of the Ancient Nahuas: Possibilities for Study. In *Sixteenth Century Mexico: The Work of Sahagún,* edited by Munro S. Edmonson, 205–24. Albuquerque: University of New Mexico Press.

1980 *Cuerpo humano e ideologia: las concepciones de los antiguos Nahuas.* 2 vols. Mexico: Universidad Nacional Autónoma de Mexico.

Los Angeles Times

1983 Hot Peppers and Substance P. *Home Magazine* (October), p. 29.

Lothrop, Samuel K.

1928 Santiago Atitlán, Guatemala. *Indian Notes.* vol. 5:no. 4, 370–95. New York: Museum of the American Indian, Heye Foundation.

Lozoya, Xavier and Mariana Lozoya

1982 *Flora medicinal de Mexico. Primera parte: Plantas Indígenas.* Mexico: Instituto mexicano del Seguro Social.

Luttrell, Psalter See Bible.

Lutz, Christopher H.

1976 *Santiago de Guatemala, 1541–1773: The Socio-Demographic History of a Spanish-American Colonial City.* Ph.D. diss., University of Wisconsin.

Lyons, Albert S. and R. Joseph Petrucelli, II

1978 *Medicine: An Illustrated History.* New York: Harry N. Abrams, Publishers.

MacLeod, Murdo J.

1973 *Spanish Central America: A Socioeconomic History, 1520–1720.* Berkeley and Los Angeles: University of Wisconsin.

McElroy, Ann and Patricia K. Townsend

1979 *Medical Anthropology in Ecological Perspective.* North Scituate, Mass.: Duxbury Press.

McNeill, William H.

1977 *Plagues and Peoples.* Garden City, New York: Anchor Press/Doubleday.

Madsen, William

1955 Hot and Cold in the Universe of San Francisco Tecospa, Valley of Mexico. *Journal of American Folklore* vol. 68:123–39.

Martínez, Maximino

1939 *Las plantas medicinales de México.* 2d. ed. Mexico: Ediciones Botas.

1944 *Las plantas medicinales de México.* 3rd ed. Mexico: Ediciones Botas.

Martínez Durán, Carlos

1964 *Las ciencias médicas en Guatemala. Origin y evolución.* 3rd ed. Guatemala: Editorial Universitaria.

Mellen, George-Ann
1974 El uso de las plantas medicinales en Guatemala. *Guatemala Indígena* vol. 9:no. 12, 99–179.

Méndez Domínguez, Alfredo
1983 Illness and Medical Theory among Guatemalan Indians. In *Heritage of Conquest: Thirty Years Later,* edited by Carl Kendall, John Hawkins, and Laurel Bossen, 267–98. Albuquerque: University of New Mexico Press.

Miles, S. W.
1957 The Sixteenth-Century Pokom-Maya: A Documentary Analysis of Structure and Archaeological Setting. *Transactions of the American Philosophical Society* 47:731–81. Philadelphia.

Moerman, Daniel E.
1982 *Geraniums for the Iroquois.* Algonne, Mich.: Reference Publications.

Monardes, Nicolas
1565 *Historia medicinal de todas las cosas que se traen de nuestras Indias Occidentales, que sirven al uso de las medicina.* Seville.
1925 *Joyfull Newes Out of the Newe Founde Worlde* (1577). Translated by John Frampton. 2 vols. London: Constable and Company Ltd.

Mondloch, James L.
1978 *Basic Quiche Grammar.* Institute for Mesoamerican Studies, State University of New York, Publication no. 2. Albany.

Montero de Miranda, Fray Francisco
1954 Descripción de la provincia de la Verapaz (*ca.* 1574). *Anales de la Sociedad de Geografía e Historia de Guatemala* vol. 27:342–58. Guatemala.

Morton, Julia F.
1977 *Major Medicinal Plants: Botany, Culture and Uses.* Springfield, Ill.: Charles C. Thomas, Publisher.
1981 *Atlas of Medicinal Plants of Middle America: Bahamas to Yucatán.* Springfield, Ill.: Charles C. Thomas, Publisher.

Nash, Manning
1969 Guatemalan Highlands. In *Ethnology,* edited by Evon Z. Vogt. Handbook of Middle American Indians vol. 7:1, 30–45. Austin: The University of Texas Press.

Neuenswander, Helen L. and Shirley D. Souder
1980 El síndrome caliente-frío humedo-seco entre los quichés de Joyabaj: Dos modelos cognitivos. *Guatemala Indígena* vol. 15:nos. 1–2, 137–69.

Nicholson, H. B.
1973 Sahagún's Primeros Memoriales, Tepepolco. In *Guide to Ethnohistorical Sources,* edited by Howard F. Cline and John B. Glass. Handbook of Middle American Indians vol. 13:no. 2, 207–18. Austin: University of Texas Press.

Nicolau d'Olwer, Luís *See* Cline.

Nieremberg, Juan Eusebio
1635 *See* Hernández.

Oakes, Maud
1969 *The Two Crosses of Todos Santos: Survivals of Mayan Religious Ritual.* Bollinger series 27. Princeton, New Jersey: Princeton University Press.

Orellana, Sandra L.
1984 *The Tzutujil Maya: Continuity and Change, 1250–1630.* Norman: University of Oklahoma Press.

Ortíz de Montellano, Bernard
1975 Empirical Aztec Medicine. *Science* vol. 188:no. 4185, 215–20.
1980 Las hierbas de Tlaloc. *Estudios de Cultura Nahuatl* vol. 14:287–314. Mexico.

Osol, Arthur and Robertson Pratt
1973 *The U.S. Dispensatory.* Philadelphia: J. B. Lippincott Company.

Ossado Ricardo (el Judío)
1944 Descripción de los hombres y virtudes de los yerbas indígenas de Yucatán y las enfermedades a que se aplican (1834). In *Las plantas medicinales de Mexico* by Maximino Martínez, 527–78. Mexico: Ediciones Botas.

Paul, Lois
1974 The Mastery of Work and the Mystery of Sex in a Guatemalan Village. In *Women, Culture, and Society,* edited by Michelle Z. Rosallo and Louise Lamphere, 281–339. Stanford: Stanford University Press.
1975 Recruitment to a Ritual role: The Midwife in a Maya Community. *Ethos* vol. 3:no. 3, 449–67.

Paul, Benjamin D.
1976 The Maya Bonesetter as Sacred Specialist. *Ethnology* vol. 15:no. 1, 77–81.

Paul, Lois and Benjamin D. Paul
1975 The Maya Midwife as Sacred Specialist: A Guatemalan Case. *American Ethnologist* vol. 2:no. 4, 707–26.

Ponce, Fray Alonso
1873 *Relación breve y verdadera de algunas cosas de las muchas que sucedieron al padre fray Alonso Ponce en las provincias de la Nueva España* (1584). Madrid.

Popol Vuh (PV)
1929 *See* Ximénez
1971 *The Book of Counsel: The Popol Vuh of the Quiche Maya of Guatemala* (*ca.* 1554–1558). Translated by Munro S. Edmonson. Middle American Research Institute, Tulane University, Publication no. 35. New Orleans.

Recchi, Dr. Nardo Antonio
1651 *See* Hernández

Reina Ruben E.

1966 *The Law of the Saints: A Pokomam Pueblo and Its Community Culture.* Indianapolis and New York: The Bobbs-Merrill Company, Inc.

Relación geográfica Aguacatepec (RGAG)

1965 Descripción de San Bartolomé del Partido de Atitlán (1585), por Alonso Páez Betancor and fray Pedro de Arboleda. *Anales de la Sociedad de Geografía e Historia de Guatemala* vol. 38:262–76. Guatemala.

Relación geográfica Atitlán (RGA)

1964 Relación de Santiago Atitlán (1585), por Alonso Páez Betancor y fray Pedro de Arboleda. *Anales de la Sociedad de Geografía e Historia de Guatemala* vol. 37:87–106. Guatemala.

Relación geográfica San Andrés (RGSA)

1952 Ranch of San Andrés, Dependency of Atitlán, by Alonso Páez Betancor and fray Pedro de Arboleda. In *Description of Atitlán and Its Dependencies* (1585), translated by Ray Broussard, 101–21. Master's thesis, University of Texas.

Relación geográfica San Francisco (RGSF)

1952 San Francisco, Dependency of Atitlán, by Alonso Páez Betancor and fray Pedro de Arboleda. In *Atitlán and Its Dependencies (1585),* translated by Ray Broussard, 122–45. Master's thesis, University of Texas.

Relación geográfica Zapotitlán y Suchitepéquez (RGZ)

1955 Descripción de la Provincia de Zapotitlán y Suchitepéquez (1579), por su alcalde mayor capitán Juan de Estrada y el escribano Fernando de Niebla. *Anales de la Sociedad de Geografía e Historia de Guatemala* vol. 28:68–83. Guatemala.

Remesal, Antonio de

1932 *Historia general de las indias occidentales, y particular de gobernación de Chiapa y Guatemala* (*ca.* 1620). Biblioteca Goathemala, vols. 4–5. Guatemala.

1964 *Historia general de las indias occidentales y particular de la gobernación de Chiapa y Guatemala* (*ca.* 1620). Biblioteca de Autores Españoles, vol. 175. Madrid.

Reynolds, James E. F. and Anne B. Prasad, eds.

1982 *Martindale. The Extra Pharmacopoeia.* London: The Pharmaceutical Press.

Ritual of the Bacabs

1965 *See* Roys.

Robertson, Donald

1959 *Mexican Manuscript Painting of the Early Colonial Period: The Metropolitan Schools.* New Haven: Yale University Press.

Rodríguez Rouanet, Francisco

1969 Practicas medicas tradicionales de los indígenas de Guatemala. *Guatemala Indígena* vol. 4:no. 2, 51–86.

1971 Aspectos de las medicina popular en el area rural de Guatemala. *Guatemala Indígena* vol. 6:no. 1, 1–330. Guatemala.

Rosengarten, Frederic, Jr.

1982 A Neglected Mayan Galactagogue—Ixbut (*Euphorbia lancifolia*). *Journal of Ethnopharmacology* vol. 5:91–112.

Rothenberg, Robert E.

1968 *The New American Medical Dictionary and Health Manual.* Revised edition. New York: The New American Library.

Roys, Ralph L.

1931 *The Ethno-botany of the Maya.* Middle American Research Institute, Tulane University, Publication no. 2. New Orleans.

1965 *Ritual of the Bacabs.* Translated and edited by Ralph L. Roys.

1967 *The Book of Chilam Balam of Chumayel.* Norman: University of Oklahoma Press.

Rubel, Arthur J.

1964 The Epidemiology of a Folk Illness: Susto in Hispanic America. *Ethnology* vol. 3:no. 3, 268–83.

Ruíz de Alarcón, Hernando

1984 *Treatise on the Heathen Superstitions that Today Live among the Indians Native to this New Spain, 1629.* Translated and edited by J. Richard Andrews and Ross Hassig. Norman: University of Oklahoma Press.

Sáenz de Santa María, Carmelo

1940 *Diccionario Cakchiquel-Español.* Guatemala: Tipografía Nacional.

Sahagún, fray Bernardino de

ca. 1578–79 *Florentine Codex.* Códice Florentino. Historia general de las cosas de Nueva España. Biblioteca Medicea-Laurenziana, Florence, Italy. Palantine collection, Mss. 218–20.

1950–69 *Florentine Codex. General history of the Things of New Spain* (*ca.* 1578–79). Translated from the Aztec into English, with notes and illustrations, by Arthur J. O. Anderson and Charles E. Dibble. Santa Fe, New Mexico: School of American Research, Monograph 14.

Salazar, Ramón A.

1951 *Historia del desenvolvimiento intelectual de Guatemala (epoca colonial).* Tomo 1. Biblioteca de Cultura Popular. Guatemala: Ministerio de Educación Pública.

Saler, Benson

1964 Nagual, Witch, and Sorcerer in a Quiché Village. *Ethnology* vol. 3:no. 3, 305–28.

Scarpa, Antonio and Antonio Guerci

1982 Various Uses of the Castor Oil Plant (*Ricinus communis* L.). *Journal of Ethnopharmacology* vol. 5:117–37.

Schauenberg, Paul and Ferdinand Paris

1977 *Guide to Medicinal Plants.* Translated by Maurice Pugh Jones. Guildford & London: Lutterworth Press.

Schendel, Gordon

1968 *Medicine in Mexico.* Austin: University of Texas Press.

Schultze Jena, Leonhard

1933 Leben, Glaube und Sprache der Quiché von Guatemala. In *Indiana,* vol. 1. Jena: Verlag von Gustav Fischer.

Scultetus, Johannis

1693 *Armamentarium Chirurgicum.* London: Batav.

Shattuck, George Cheever

1938 *A Medical Survey of the Republic of Guatemala.* Washington, D.C.: Carnegie Institution. Publication no. 499.

Sherman, William L.

1979 *Forced Native Labor in Sixteenth-Century America.* Lincoln: University of Nebraska Press.

Shimkin, Demitri B.

1973 Models for the Downfall: Some Ecological and Culture-Historical Considerations. In the *Classic Maya Collapse,* edited by T. P. Culbert, 269–99. Albuquerque: University of New Mexico Press. School of American Research Advanced Seminar Series.

Sim, Stephen K.

1965 *Medicinal Plant Alkaloids.* Toronto: University of Toronto Press.

Simeon, George

1973 The Evil Eye in a Guatemalan Village. *Ethnomedizin* vol. 2:314, 437–41.

1977 *Illness and Curing in a Guatemalan Village: A Study in Ethnomedicine.* School of Public Health: University of Hawaii.

Solano Pérez-Lila, Francisco de P.

1963 Los mayas del siglo XVII. *Antropología e Historia de Guatemala* vol. 15:no. 2, 3–34. Guatemala.

Soustelle, Jacques

1974 *Daily Life of the Aztecs on the Eve of the Spanish Conquest.* Stanford, California: Stanford University Press.

Spoerke, David G., Jr.

1980 *Herbal Medications.* Santa Barbara: Woodbridge Press Publishing Company.

Standley, Paul C. and Julian A. Steyermark

1946–77 *Flora of Guatemala.* Fieldiana: Botany. Chicago: Field Museum of Natural History.

Stone, Doris

1984 Pre-Columbian migration of *Theobroma cacao* and *Manihot esculenta* Crantz from Northern South America into Mesoamerica: A Partially Hypothetical View. Pre-Columbian Plant Migration, edited by Doris Stone. *Papers of the Peabody Museum of Archaeology and Ethnology* 76:67–83.

Stuart, Malcolm, ed.

1979 *The Encyclopedia of Herbs and Herbalism.* New York: Grossett & Dunlap.

Tax, Sol and Robert Hinshaw
1969 The Maya of the Midwestern Highlands. In *Ethnology,* edited by Evon Z. Vogt, Handbook of Middle American Indians vol. 7:no. 1, 69–100. Austin: University of Texas Press.

Tedlock, Barbara
1982 *Time and the Highland Maya.* Albuquerque: University of New Mexico Press.

Tenzel, James H.
1970 Shamanism and Disease in a Mayan Indian Community. *Psychiatry* vol. 33:372–80.

Thompson, Sir J. Eric S.
1972a *A Commentary on the Dresden Codex: A Maya Hieroglyphic Book.* Philadelphia: American Philosophical Society.
1972b *Maya History and Religion.* Norman: University of Oklahoma Press.

Thomson, William A. R.
1976 *Black's Medical Dictionary,* edited by William A. R. Thomson. 31st ed. London: Adam & Charles Black.
1978 *Healing Plants: A Modern Herbal.* New York: McGraw Hill Book Company.

Title of the Lords of Totonicapán
1967 *See Annals of the Cakchiquels.*

Trease, George Edward and William Charles Evans
1983 *Pharmacognosy.* 11th ed. London: Baillière Tindall.

Tyler, Varro E.
1981 *The Honest Herbal: A Sensible Guide to the Use of Herbs and Related Remedies.* Philadelphia: George F. Stickley Company.

———, Lynn R. Brady, and James E. Robbers
1981 *Pharmacognosy.* 8th ed. Philadelphia: Lea & Febiger.

Valladares, Leon A.
1957 *El hombre y el maíz: Etnografía y etnopsicología de Colotenango.* Guatemala: Universidad de San Carlos.

Varela, Francisco
ca. 1600 *Calepino en lengua Cakchiquel* (*ca.* 1600). Guatemala.

Vázquez de Herrera, Francisco
1714–16 *Crónica de la provincia del Santíssimo Nombre de Jesús de Guatemala de el Orden de N. Seráphico padre San Francisco en el Reyno de la Nueva España,* dividida en dos tomos. Joseph González, O.F.M. Guatemala.
1937–44 *Crónica de la provincia del Santíssimo Nombre de Jesús de Guatemala de el Orden de Nuestra Seráfico padre San Francisco (1714–17).* Biblioteca Goathemala, vols. 14–17. 4 vols. Guatemala.

Vázquez de Espinosa, Antonio
1942 *Compendium and Description of the West Indies* (*ca.* 1620). Translated by Charles Upson Clark. Washington, D.C.
1968 *Description of the Indies* (*ca.* 1620). Translated by Charles Upson Clark. Washington, D.C.: Smithsonian Institution Press.

Viana, Francisco de, Lucas Gallego, and Guillermo Cadena
1955 Relación de la provincia de Verapaz hecha por los religiosos de Santo Domingo de Cobán, 7 de diciembre de 1574. *Anales de la Sociedad de Geografía e Historia de Guatemala* vol. 28:18–31. Guatemala.

Viesca Treviño, Carlos and Ignacio de la Peña Páez
1976 Las enfermedades mentales en el códice Badiano. *Estudios de Cultura Nahuatl* vol. 12:79–84. Mexico.

Villacorta Calderón, José Antonio
1926 *Monografía del departamento de Guatemala.* Guatemala: Tipografía Nacional.
1942 *Historia de la capitanía general de Guatemala.* Guatemala: Tipografía Nacional.

Villacorta Cifuentes, Dr. Jorge Luís
1976 *Historia de la medicina, cirugia y obstetricia prehispanicas.* Guatemala.

Virkki, Nilo
1962 Comentarios sobre el baño de vapor entre los indígenas de Guatemala. *Guatemala Indígena* vol. 2:no. 2, 71–85.

Vogel, Virgil J.
1973 *American Indian Medicine.* Norman: University of Oklahoma Press.

Vogt, Even Z.
1970 *The Zinacantecos of Mexico: A Modern Maya Way of Life.* New York: Holt, Rinehart and Winston.

Wagley, Charles
1949 The Social and Religious Life of a Guatemalan Village. *American Anthropological Association. Memoirs* 71.

Warren, J. Benedict
1973 An Introductory Survey of Secular Writings in the European Tradition on Colonial Middle America, 1503–1818. In *Guide to Ethnohistorical Sources,* edited by Howard F. Cline and John B. Glass. Handbook of Middle American Indians vol. 13:part 2, 42–137. Austin: University of Texas Press.

Wauchope, Robert
1948 *Excavations at Zacualpa, Guatemala.* Middle American Research Institute, Tulane University, Publication no. 14. New Orleans.

Weiner, Michael A.
1980 *Weiner's Herbal: The Guide to Herb Medicine.* New York: Stein and Day Publishers.

Winter, Evelyne
1972 *Mexico's ancient and native remedies: a handbook of testimonials and historic references for modern use.* Editorial Fournier, S.A.

Wisdom, Charles
1940 *The Chortí Indians of Guatemala.* Chicago: The University of Chicago Press.

Wood, Corinne Shear
1978 Syphilis in Anthropological Perspective. *Social Science and Medicine* vol. 12:47–55.

Woodbury, Richard B. and Aubrey S. Trik
1953 *The Ruins of Zaculeu, Guatemala.* Richmond, Va.: The William Byrd Press, Inc.

Wren, R. C.
1973 *Potter's New Cyclopaedia of Botanical Drugs and Preparations.* London: Health Science Press.

Ximénez, Francisco
1615 *Quatro libros, de la naturaleza . . .* Traducido por fray Francisco Ximénez. Mexico.

Ximénez, Francisco
1929 1929–30 *Historia de la provincia de San Vicente de Chiapa y Guatemala* (1721–22). Biblioteca Goathemala vols. 1–3. Guatemala.
1967a *Escolios a las historias de origen de los indios.* Sociedad de Geografía e Historia de Guatemala, Special Publication no. 13.
1967b *Historia natural del reino de Guatemala (1722).* Guatemala: Editorial José de Pineda Ibarra.

Index